THIAMINE

THIAMINE

EDITED BY

CLARK J. GUBLER, M.D., Ph.D.
Brigham Young University

MOTONORI FUJIWARA, M.D.
Kyoto University, Japan

PIERRE M. DREYFUS, M.D.
University of California at Davis

A WILEY-INTERSCIENCE PUBLICATION

JOHN WILEY & SONS, New York • London • Sydney • Toronto

Library of Congress Cataloging in Publication Data

United States–Japan Seminar on Thiamine, 2d, Monterey,
  Calif., 1974.
  Thiamine.

  Proceedings of the seminar held Oct. 3-5, 1974.
  "A Wiley-Interscience publication."
  Includes bibliographical references and index.
  1. Vitamin B1—Congresses. 2. Nervous system—Con-
gresses. I. Gubler, Clark J., 1913–   II. Fujiwara,
Motonori, 1915–   III. Dreyfus, Pierre M. IV. Ti-
tle. [DNLM: 1. Thiamine—Congresses. W3 UN612 1974t/
QU189 U58 1974t]

QP772.T5U54   1974   599′.01′926   75-29485
ISBN 0-471-33012-4

Printed in the United States of America

10 9 8 7 6 5 4 3 2 1

PREFACE

This volume contains the full proceedings of the papers and discussions presented at the Second Cooperative United States–Japan Seminar on Thiamine, which took place October 3–5, 1974, in Monterey, California. The seminar was jointly sponsored by the National Science Foundation, Office of International Programs, and the Japan Society for the Promotion of Science. Since the first thiamine seminar, held in Hakone, Japan, in 1969, a great deal of new information has become available and much interest generated on the functions, mechanism of action, and metabolism of thiamine. Therefore, the participants in the second seminar overwhelmingly agreed to publish these proceedings. The information contained in this book should be of interest to all who are working on thiamine research and to nutritionists and clinical people also. It not only includes reviews of the current status of various areas of thiamine research, but incorporates considerable new information as well.

The format of this volume closely follows that of the seminar. The first section deals with the thiamine diphosphate-dependent α-ketoacid dehydrogenases: their isolation, properties, and the regulation of their activity. This is of current interest because of the central role of thiamine both in the metabolism of the several biologically important α-ketoacids and in energy production. The second section includes discussions of the transport and metabolism of thiamine, the effects of thiamine deficiency, and the nutritional status of thiamine in the world. The last three sections are concerned with the roles and mechanism of action of thiamine in nerve function and transmission. Currently there is great interest in this area, since one prominent symptom of thiamine deficiency or malfunction is neuropathy, and since several hereditary disorders with mental retardation and neurological symptoms are related to the malfunction of various thiamine-dependent functions. Thiamine transport and metabolism in the brain are dealt with in the third section, the relation of malfunction of thiamine to neuropathy in the fourth, and various thiamine-related hereditary metabolic diseases in the fifth.

The successful completion of this book is largely due to the generous cooperation of the various participants, who are all active contributors to the advance of knowledge in the area of thiamine research. Thanks are also due Mrs. Anne G. Golightly and Mrs. Dorothy Dreyfus for their efforts in manuscript editing.

We hope that this volume is informative to those interested and that it will act as a catalyst for further research in this very exciting field.

CLARK J. GUBLER
MOTONORI FUJIWARA
PIERRE M. DREYFUS

Provo, Utah
Kyoto, Japan
Davis, California
November, 1975

CONTENTS

THIAMINE

OPENING REMARKS

Clark J. Gubler, Ph.D.
Department of Chemistry
Brigham Young University
Provo, Utah
United States Coordinator
Second United States-Japan Seminar on Thiamine

The first cooperative United States–Japan seminar on thiamine was held in Hakone, Japan, in August 1969. Through the talks, discussions, and social interaction a much closer bond was cemented between those working in this area in the United States and their colleagues in Japan. Since this first meeting the evidence of mutual cooperation and interest between workers in our two countries has increased. It is fitting that we should meet together since a great deal of the work done on thiamine in the past was carried out in the United States and Japan, and this trend has continued. In the 5 years between that first meeting and this second seminar in Monterey, California, a great many exciting new data have become available, particularly in the area of neurological functions. We trust that this meeting will also be very informative and stimulating.

Thanks are gratefully extended to the National Science Foundation, Office of International Programs; the United States-Japan Cooperative Science Program; and the Japan Society for the Promotion of Science for making this seminar possible. Appreciation is also due to Hoffmann-LaRoche, Inc., Nutley, New Jersey; University of California School of Medicine, Davis, California; Brigham Young University, Provo, Utah; and Mr. Jerry Hawthorne of Beckman Instruments for financial assistance in regard to

1

physical arrangements, publications, and other matter related to the seminar. We also thank the Holiday Inn, Monterey, California, for excellent physical facilities and cooperation.

Motonori Fujiwara, M.D.

Department of Hygiene
Kyoto University
Kyoto, Japan
Japan Coordinator
Second United States-Japan Seminar on Thiamine

First of all, I would like to express my hearty appreciation to Professor Gubler for the great efforts he made to realize this meeting. I am very happy that we could all come together today to hold the second United States-Japan seminar on thiamine. As you remember, we had the first such seminar in Hakone, Japan, 5 years ago. We had a very wonderful time, and through that seminar great advances in this field and mutual understanding among the investigators were achieved.

Looking back on these 5 years reminds me how time flies. But, to our satisfaction, much progress in this field has been made in this interval. During the same time many scholars have advanced our knowledge in both countries, and some of them are attending this conference.

There is no doubt that the discovery of the lipotropic derivatives of thiamine such as allithiamine and other thiamine disulfides, which have the ability to cross biological membranes with greater facility, has given a strong impetus to the study of thiamine in Japan since World War II and has been a tool for gaining a greater understanding of its functions and metabolism.

I believe that your interesting presentations, your enthusiastic discussions, and the mutual exchange of ideas will make this meeting successful.

ONE

THIAMINE-DEPENDENT ENZYMES

1. Purification and Function of α-Ketoacid Dehydrogenases in the Mammalian Multienzyme Complexes

MASAHIKO KOIKE, M.D.
MINORU HAMADA, M.D.
KICHIKO KOIKE, M.D.
TADAYASU HIRAOKA
YUTAKA NAKAULA

Department of Pathological Biochemistry
Atomic Disease Institute
Nagasaki University School of Medicine
Nagasaki, Japan

It is now well established that all thiamine-dependent enzymatic reactions, such as α-ketoacid oxidation and transketolation, require the coenzyme form of thiamine, namely, thiamine diphosphate (ThDP) (1). Recently, considerable evidence has accumulated indicating that the important intermediate metabolites in the "citric acid cycle," such as pyruvate and 2-oxoglutarate, are degraded by an oxidative decarboxylation reaction involving, sequentially, decarboxylation, acyl generation, acyl transfer, and electron transfer reactions by multienzyme complexes with high molecular weights (2, 3).

We have succeeded in isolating in soluble form two kinds of mammalian multienzyme complexes in highly purified states, namely, the pyruvate and 2-oxoglutarate dehydrogenase complexes, from Keilin-Hartree preparations of pig heart muscle by a modification of the original procedures (4, 5).

1.   Purification of the Mammalian α-Ketoacid Dehydrogenase Complexes

The amber-colored extract obtained from pig heart Keilin-Hartree preparations was fractionated with protamine sulfate into two fractions containing the 2-oxoglutarate dehydrogenase complex (OGDC) and pyruvate dehydrogenase complex (PDC), respectively (4). Thereafter, the 2-oxoglutarate dehydrogenase complex was isolated from the first fraction by Triton X-100 extraction, calcium phosphate gel-cellulose column chromatography (twice), and ammonium sulfate fractionation (6). The pyruvate dehydrogenase complex was isolated from the second fraction by ultracentrifugation, 5 to 30% sucrose density gradient centrifugation, and ammonium sulfate fractionation (7). With this procedure an approximately 105-fold purification for the 2-oxoglutarate dehydrogenase complex and a 280-fold purification for the pyruvate dehydrogenase complex were achieved.

2.   Properties of the α-Ketoacid Dehydrogenase Complexes

In addition to the overall reaction, there are ferricyanide-linked α-ketoacid dehydrogenase (decarboxylase), lipoate acyltransferase, and lipoamide dehydrogenase activities, each associated with its respective complex, as shown in Table 1.

The molecular weights are 7.4 million for the pyruvate dehydrogenase complex and 2.7 million for the 2-oxoglutarate dehydrogenase complex, as shown in Table 2. Both of the complexes are apparently giant biopolymers.

As shown in Table 3, the pyruvate dehydrogenase complex contains only two protein-bound coenzymes, lipoic acid and FAD, and lacks ThDP. Therefore, the ferricyanide-linked pyruvate dehydrogenase activity of the pyruvate dehydrogenase complex is dependent on added ThDP, and its

Table 1.   Enzymatic Activities of Pig Heart α-Ketoacid Dehydrogenase Complexes

Enzyme	Overall Reaction	Specific Activity, μmoles/(hr)(mg protein)		
		α-Ketoacid Dehydrogenase	Acyltransferase	Lipoamide Dehydrogenase
PDC	120	5.7	290	370
OGDC	375	144	76	1160

Table 2.   Hydrodynamic Parameters and Molecular Weights of Pig Heart α-Ketoacid Dehydrogenase Complexes

Enzyme	$s\,^{\circ}_{20,w}$	$D_{20,w} \times 10^{-7}$, cm^2/sec	Molecular Weight $\times$ 10^6			Electric Mobility $\times$ 10^{-5}, cm^2/V·sec
			s and D	Archibald	Sed. Equi.	
PDC	68.5S	1.35	9.7	9.0	7.4	−4.8
OGDC	36.5S	1.18	2.8	2.7	2.7	−9.9

apparent K_m is 4.2 $\times$ 10^{-6} M. In contrast, the 2-oxoglutarate dehydrogenase complex contains these three coenzymes in an enzyme-bound form.

3.   Purification of α-Ketoacid Dehydrogenases (Decarboxylases)

Each of the two α-ketoacid dehydrogenases was purified from its respective complex.

PYRUVATE DEHYDROGENASE

Pyruvate dehydrogenase (PDH) was purified by resolving the pyruvate dehydrogenase complex into its component enzymes (7). First, the pyruvate dehydrogenase complex was separated into two fractions, i.e., lipoamide dehydrogenase (PDC-Fp) and a colorless fraction, by fractionation on a gel-cellulose column in the presence of 4 M urea and 1% ammonium sulfate. The latter colorless fraction was further separated into two fractions, i.e.,

Table 3.   Contents of Protein-Bound Coenzymes of Pig Heart α-Ketoacid Dehydrogenase Complexes

Enzyme	ThDP,	Lipoic Acid,	FAD,
	moles/mole of complex		
PDC	0	24	12
	($K_m = 4.2 \times 10^{-6} M$)		
OGDC	6	8	12

pyruvate dehydrogenase and lipoate acetyltransferase (LAT), by gel filtration on Sepharose 6B in the presence of 0.7 M potassium iodide. Further purification of pyruvate dehydrogenase was achieved by ammonium sulfate fractionation.

2-OXOGLUTARATE DEHYDROGENASE

2-Oxoglutarate dehydrogenase (OGDH) was also purified by resolving the 2-oxoglutarate dehydrogenase complex into its component enzymes (6). First, the 2-oxoglutarate dehydrogenase complex was separated into two fractions, i.e., lipoamide dehydrogenase (OGDC-Fp) and a colorless fraction, by fractionation on a gel-cellulose column in the presence of 2.5 M urea and 1% ammonium sulfate. The latter fraction was then further separated into two fractions, i.e., 2-oxoglutarate dehydrogenase and lipoate succinyltransferase (LST), in the presences of 0.7 M guanidine HCl, 2 mM dithiothreitol, and 0.5% Triton X-100. Further purification of 2-oxoglutarate dehydrogenase was achieved by ultracentrifugation and ammonium sulfate fractionation.

SUBUNIT COMPOSITION OF THE TWO COMPLEXES

The molecular weights and subunit compositions of the component enzymes of both complexes are summarized in Table 4. Both complexes are

Table 4. Subunit Compositions of Pig Heart α-Ketoacid Dehydrogenase Complexes

| Enzyme | Molecular Weight | Subunit | | Per Molecule of Complex | |
		No.	Molecular Weight	Total No. of Subunit	Mole of Coenzyme
PDC	7,400,000				
PDH	153,000	2	41,000	60	ThDP = 0
		2	36,000	60	
LAT	1,800,000	24	74,000	24	LiA[a] = 24
PDC-Fp	108,000	2	54,000	12	FAD = 6
OGDC	2,700,000				
OGDH	216,000	2	97,000	12	ThDP = 6
LST	1,000,000	24	41,000	24	LiA[a] = 8
OGDC-Fp	108,000	2	55,000	12	FAD = 6

[a] Lipoic acid.

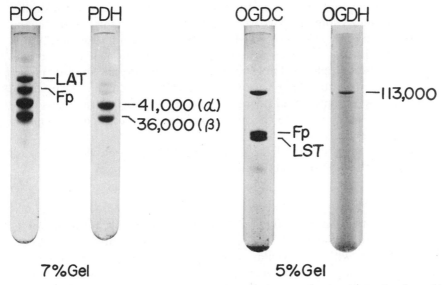

Figure 1. Polyacrylamide gel electrophoresis in sodium dodecyl sulfate of α-ketoacid dehydrogenase complexes (PDC and OGDC) and their dehydrogenase components (PDH and OGDH).

apparently constructed with a core lipoate acyltransferase (LAT or LST) to which the α-ketoacid dehydrogenase (PDH or OGDH) and lipoamide dehydrogenase (PDC-Fp or OGDC-Fp) are bound noncovalently.

4. Properties of the α-Ketoacid Dehydrogenases

HOMOGENEITY

As shown in the electropherograms (Fig. 1) of these two α-ketoacid dehydrogenases on sodium dodecyl sulfate (SDS) gels (8), both preparations are homogeneous (9, 10). Pyruvate dehydrogenase consists of two different subunits with molecular weights of 41,000 (α) and 36,000 (β), respectively. 2-Oxoglutarate dehydrogenase consists of a single subunit with a molecular weight of 113,000. Homogeneity was also confirmed by analytical ultracentrifugation.

SUBSTRATE SPECIFICITY

Thus we have obtained, in highly purified form, two kinds of mitochondrial ThDP-dependent enzymes. Pyruvate dehydrogenase shows a rather wide spectrum of substrate specificity; that is, this enzyme is capable of decarboxylating not only pyruvate but also α-ketobutyrate to a similar extent, and shows some activity with α-ketovalerate, α-ketoisocaproate, and α-ketocaproate as well (10). α-Ketobutyrate degradation activity is associated with this complex throughout the purification of the pyruvate dehydrogenase complex (11). It appears that an enzyme specific for α-ketobutyrate oxidation in pig heart tissue does not exist and that the pyruvate dehydrogenase complex itself degrades α-ketobutyrate. This finding is quite interesting in relationship to the human genetic disorder, known as maple syrup urine disease.

   In contrast to pyruvate dehydrogenase, the 2-oxoglutarate dehydrogenase is highly specific for 2-oxoglutarate (9).

OTHER PROPERTIES

The comparative data (9, 10) on characteristic properties of these two α-ketoacid dehydrogenases are summarized in Table 5. Pyruvate dehydrogenase, with a molecular weight of 153,000, apparently contains a pair of different subunits ($\alpha_2\beta_2$), as has already been shown in the electropherograms on SDS gels (cf. Fig. 1). The N-terminal group of each subunit has been determined to be alanine (α) and glycine (β). 2-Oxoglutarate dehydrogenase, with a molecular weight of 216,000, is a dimer of a single subunit with a molecular weight of 113,000 and amino-terminal alanine.

   The 2-oxoglutarate dehydrogenase contains a rather high α-helical

Table 5. Comparative Data of Properties of Pig Heart Pyruvate and 2-Oxoglutarate Dehydrogenases

Property	PDH	OGDH
Molecular weight	153,000	216,000
Subunit No.	α_2 β_2	α_2
Molecular weight	$\alpha = 41,000$ (SDS) $\beta = 36,000$ (SDS)	$\alpha = 97,000$ (sed. equi.) 113,000 (SDS)
NH$_2$-terminal, M/M of enzyme	α = Alanine (2) β = Glycine (2)	Alanine (2)
ThDP, M/M of enzyme	0 K_m app. $= 4.2 \times 10^{-6}\ M$	1
α-Helix content, %	17	34

structure, and also contains protein-bound ThDP, in contrast to pyruvate dehydrogenase, which is free of ThDP. The loose binding of ThDP to the apopyruvate dehydrogenase may permit the protein kinase to phosphorylate this enzyme (12). The results presented indicate that these enzymes are quite different structurally and functionally, although they are ThDP-dependent enzymes which catalyze analogous reactions.

Both enzymes apparently catalyze the first step of the oxidative decarboxylation of pyruvate or 2-oxoglutarate. However, Roche and Reed (13) reported that the α-subunit catalyzes the decarboxylation of pyruvate, and that the β-subunit catalyzes the successive reductive acetylation of lipoic acid in the reaction sequence. Pettit et al. (14) also reported that *Escherichia coli* 2-oxoglutarate dehydrogenase catalyzes the decarboxylation of 2-oxoglutarate and the successive reductive succinylation of lipoic acid. I regret that we cannot as yet confirm these findings.

5. Kinetic Studies of the Oxidative Decarboxylation of α-Ketoacids

INTRODUCTION

It was recently suggested by Tsai et al. (15) and Cleland (16) that the reaction of the pyruvate dehydrogenase complex from bovine kidney proceeded via a "three-site Ping-Pong mechanism." The mammalian pyruvate dehydrogenase complex has no bound ThDP, while the 2-oxoglutarate dehydrogenase complex does. Both complexes catalyze the same coordinated sequence of reactions, which involve the interaction of the lipoyl moiety (lipS$_2$) of a core enzyme, lipoate succinyltransferase or lipoate acetyltransferase, with ThDP bound to 2-oxoglutarate dehydrogenase or pyruvate dehydrogenase, with CoA bound to core enzyme, and finally with FAD bound to lipoamide dehydrogenase, as shown in Fig. 2.

THREE-SITE PING-PONG MECHANISM

The α-ketoacid dehydrogenase complexes catalyze the overall reaction of a CoA- and NAD-linked oxidative decarboxylation of α-ketoacids (Eq. 1):

$$R-CO-COOH + CoA-SH + NAD^+ \rightarrow$$
$$R-CO-S-CoA + CO_2 + NADH + H^+ \quad (1)$$

where R = CH$_3$—, HOOC—(CH$_2$)$_2$—, etc.

The reaction at each of the three sites (cf. Fig. 2) in the 2-oxoglutarate dehydrogenase complex is not random sequential and might be expected to have the same mechanism for the bovine kidney pyruvate dehydrogenase complex as reported by Tsai et al. (15). We can then diagram such

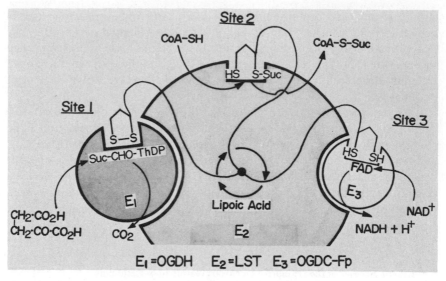

Figure 2. Schematic reaction sequence of the oxidative decarboxylation of 2-oxoglutarate. A scheme represents the possible rotation of a lipoyllysyl moiety between succinic semialdehyde (Suc-CHO)-ThDP at site 1 (E₁), the site 2 (E₂) for succinyl transfer to CoA, and the oxidized FAD at site 3 (E₃). The lipoyllysyl moiety binds to a core enzyme (E₂).

mechanisms for the 2-oxoglutarate dehydrogenase complex as shown in Fig. 3. The data obtained from initial velocity experiments fit the general equation (Eq. 2) derived by Cleland for a "three-site Ping-Pong mechanism" in the absence of products; where K_a, K_b, and K_c are Michaelis constants for 2-oxoglutarate (A), CoA (B), and NAD (C), respectively.

$$v = \frac{V}{1 + \dfrac{K_a}{[A]} + \dfrac{K_b}{[B]} + \dfrac{K_c}{[C]}} \tag{2}$$

From this equation, one can theoretically expect all lines from double reciprocal plots of B versus A, C versus B, and A versus C to be parallel.

The results obtained from the initial velocity measurement revealed that when either 2-oxoglutarate, CoA, or NAD is used as a variable substrate in the presence of various concentrations of the other substrates, the initial overall velocity of the 2-oxoglutarate dehydrogenase complex shows parallel kinetics when intramitochondrial levels of NAD are used (17), as shown in Fig. 4.

Let us consider the mechanisms of the overall reactions catalyzed by the 2-

oxoglutarate dehydrogenase complex. The reaction at site 1 can be written as in Fig. 5. The reaction at this site is mainly in one direction, so the first product P-term can be dropped. The 2-oxoglutarate and CoA are cooperatively essential for releasing the first product. This may be interpreted as indicating that the reaction at this site with bound ThDP is consistent with a random mechanism, where the combination of the second substrate at site 2 occurs before the first product is released from site 1.

At sites 2 and 3, such parallel lines are characteristic of a Ping-Pong or binary complex mechanism, where the release of the product is initiated by the binding of the next substrate.

PRODUCT INHIBITION

The rate equation of the 2-oxoglutarate dehydrogenase complex predicts that in product inhibition experiments each product will be competitive with respect to the substrate that binds at that site, and uncompetitive with respect to other substrates.

In agreement with these predictions, succinyl-CoA was competitive with respect to CoA and NADH was competitive with respect to NAD. Succinyl-CoA and NADH were both uncompetitive with respect to 2-oxoglutarate. However, noncompetitive (rather than uncompetitive) inhibition kinetics

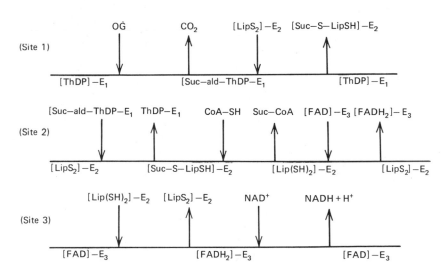

Figure 3. Diagram of the overall oxidative decarboxylation reaction mechanism catalyzed by the 2-oxoglutarate dehydrogenase complex. The abbreviations used are as follows: Suc-ald-ThDP, succinic semialdehyde-ThDP; LipS$_2$, lipoic acid; Suc-S-LipSH, S-succinyl dihydrolipoic acid; Lip(SH)$_2$, dihydrolipoic acid.

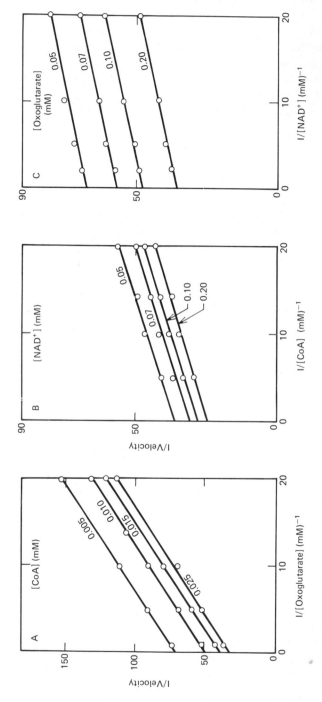

Figure 4. Initial velocity patterns for the overall reaction in the 2-oxoglutarate dehydrogenase complex. (*a*) 2-Oxoglutarate was varied with concentrations of CoA as indicated, but NAD was held constant at 0.025 mM. (*b*) CoA was varied with concentrations of NAD as indicated, but 2-oxoglutarate was held constant at 2.5 mM. (*c*) NAD was varied with concentrations of 2-oxoglutarate as indicated, but CoA was held constant at 0.02 mM.

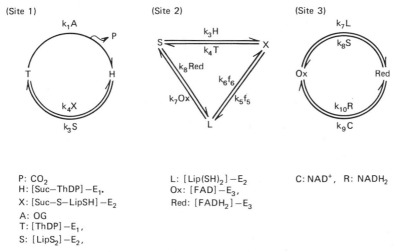

(Site 1)   (Site 2)   (Site 3)

P: CO_2
H: $[Suc-ThDP]-E_1$.
X: $[Suc-S-LipSH]-E_2$
A: OG
T: $[ThDP]-E_1$,
S: $[LipS_2]-E_2$,

L: $[Lip(SH)_2]-E_2$
Ox: $[FAD]-E_3$,
Red: $[FADH_2]-E_3$

C: NAD^+, R: $NADH_2$

Figure 5. Mechanism of the overall oxidative decarboxylation reaction of 2-oxoglutarate at each of the three sites in the 2-oxoglutarate dehydrogenase complex. k_1, k_3, k_4, k_5, k_6, k_7, k_8, k_9 and k_{10} are the rate constants and f_5 and f_6 are the fractional occupancy factors for the other sites (17).

were observed for succinyl-CoA versus NAD, and for NADH versus CoA (17). These data suggest that succinyl-CoA or NADH may be a dead-end inhibitor of the subsequent site or may in some way hinder the reaction at that site.

Such anomalous inhibition patterns could be caused by protein-protein interaction among E_1, E_2, and E_3 (cf. Fig. 2). The organization of the 2-oxoglutarate dehydrogenase complex (E_1-E_2-E_3) suggests the possibility that protein-protein interactions between (E_1 and E_2) and (E_2 and E_3) might have an effect on the reactions catalyzed by the individual enzymes. To investigate this possibility a kinetic study of the back reaction of lipoamide dehydrogenase (E_3) was undertaken in association with the lipoate succinyltransferase (E_2) as an integral part of the 2-oxoglutarate dehydrogenase complex. That no interaction occurs between E_1 and E_3 is indicated by the observation that 2-oxoglutarate had no effect on the back reaction (17). However, CoA inhibited the complexed lipoamide dehydrogenase noncompetitively with respect to NADH when the concentration of the fixed substrate was near its Michaelis constant; CoA did not inhibit the complexed lipoamide dehydrogenase with respect to lipoamide.

These observations suggest that the combination of CoA or succinyl-CoA with E_2 in some way hinders the combination of NADH or NAD with E_3.

These results are consistent with the proposed mechanisms, and such product inhibition patterns have also been observed with pyruvate dehydrogenase complex from pig heart mitochondria.

Differences in the reaction mechanism between 2-oxoglutarate dehydrogenase and pyruvate dehydrogenase were observed at greater than physiological concentration of NAD, with or without bound ThDP at each site. These differences may be due to the binding of ThDP causing the 2-oxoglutarate dehydrogenase to undergo a conformational change, or they may be caused by the swing of the lipoyl moiety from site 1 to site 2. We intend to investigate this point in more detail.

REGULATION OF THE PYRUVATE DEHYDROGENASE COMPLEX

Since the pyruvate dehydrogenase complex occupies an important branch point in glycolysis, the "citric acid cycle," and the β-oxidation system of fatty acid degradation, the complex could be a possible site for metabolic regulation. The data accumulated are summarized in Fig. 6. Previous studies (11) have revealed that the activity of the mammalian pyruvate dehydrogenase complex is inhibited by the products, such as acetyl-CoA and NADH, and that this inhibition is reversed by CoA and NAD. The sites of acetyl-CoA and NADH inhibition are the pyruvate dehydrogenase and lipoamide dehydrogenase components of the complex, respectively. The overall reaction of the pyruvate dehydrogenase complex with pyruvate was

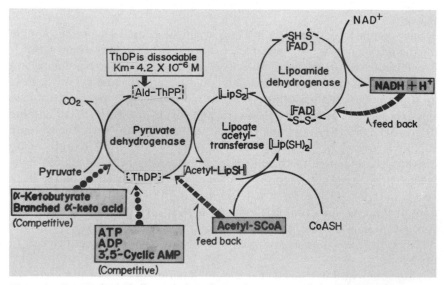

Figure 6. Proposed metabolic regulation scheme of pyruvate oxidation in mammals.

competitively inhibited by other α-ketoacids such as α-ketobutyrate, α-ketovalerate, and α-keto-β-methylvalerate.

Thiamine diphosphate in the pyruvate dehydrogenase complex is highly dissociable, and the overall activity is completely dependent on added ThDP. This activity is inhibited by nucleotides, such as ATP, ADP, AMP, cAMP, and TMP. This inhibition can be reversed by ThDP.

These studies suggest that these types of inhibition are good candidates for physiological regulation of the complex. However, the 2-oxoglutarate dehydrogenase complex which contains bound ThDP was not inhibited by these nucleotides. This supports our concept of regulation or the pyruvate dehydrogenase complex.

A new and interesting mechanism for regulation of the pyruvate dehydrogenase complex by enzymic modification of it has been reported by Reed and his associates (12).

Acknowledgments

We are indebted to Dr. K. H. Tachiki, Section of Neurobiology, Institute of Psychiatric Research, Indiana University Medical School, for his criticisms and kind help in the preparation of the manuscript. We also thank Dr. W. W. Cleland, Department of Biochemistry, University of Wisconsin, for his criticism. Finally, we wish to thank Miss M. Yoshida for her help in the preparation of the manuscript and Mrs. S. Nakao for her technical assistance.

References

1. L. O. Krampitz, *Ann. Rev. Biochem.*, **38**, 213 (1969).
2. I. C. Gunsalus, in W. D. McElroy and B. Glass, Eds., *The Mechanism of Enzyme Action*, Johns Hopkins Press, Baltimore, 1954, p. 545.
3. L. J. Reed, in M. Florkin and E. H. Stotz, Eds., *Comprehensive Biochemistry*, Vol. 14, Elsevier, Amsterdam, 1966, p. 99.
4. T. Hayakawa, M. Hirashima, S. Ide, M. Hamada, K. Okabe, and M. Koike, *J. Biol. Chem.*, **241**, 4694 (1966).
5. M. Hirashima, T. Hayakawa, and M. Koike, *J. Biol. Chem.*, *242*, 902 (1967).
6. N. Tanaka, K. Koike, M. Hamada, K. -I. Otsuka, T. Suematsu, and M. Koike, *J. Biol. Chem.*, **247**, 4043 (1972).
7. M. Hamada, K. -I. Otsuka, K. Koike, N. Tanaka, K. Ogasahara, and M. Koike, *J. Biochem.*, **78**, 187 (1975).
8. K. Weber and M. Osborn, *J. Biol. Chem.*, **244**, 4406 (1969).

9. K. Koike, M. Hamada, N. Tanaka, K. -I. Otsuka, K. Ogasahara, and M. Koike, *J. Biol. Chem.*, **249**, 3836 (1974).

10. M. Hamada, T. Hiraoka, K. Koike, K. Ogasahara, T. Kanzaki, and M. Koike, article in preparation.

11. T. Kanzaki, T. Hayakawa, M. Hamada, Y. Fukuyoshi, and M. Koike, *J. Biol. Chem.*, **244**, 1183 (1969).

12. T. C. Linn, F. H. Pettit, and L. J. Reed, *Proc. Natl. Acad. Sci. U.S.*, **62**, 234 (1969).

13. T. E. Roche and L. J. Reed, *Biochem. Biophys. Res. Commun.*, **48**, 840 (1972).

14. F. H. Pettit, L. Hamilton, P. Munk, G. Namihira, M. H. Eley, C. R. Willms, and L. J. Reed, *J. Biol. Chem.*, **248**, 5282 (1973).

15. C. S. Tsai, M. W. Burgett, and L. J. Reed, *J. Biol. Chem.*, **248**, 8348 (1973).

16. W. W. Cleland, *J. Biol. Chem.*, **248**, 8353 (1973).

17. M. Hamada, K. Koike, Y. Nakaula, T. Hiraoka, M. Koike, and T. Hashimoto, *J. Biochem.*, **77**, 1047 (1975).

2. Regulation of Mammalian Pyruvate Dehydrogenase Complex by Phosphorylation and Dephosphorylation

LESTER J. REED, Ph.D.

Clayton Foundation Biochemical Institute
and Department of Chemistry
The University of Texas at Austin
Austin, Texas

Pyruvate and α-ketoglutarate dehydrogenase systems have been isolated from microbial and eukaryotic cells as functional units with molecular weights in the millions. Two classes of complexes have been obtained, one specific for pyruvate, the other for α-ketoglutarate. In eukaryotic cells the pyruvate and α-ketoglutarate dehydrogenase complexes are located in mitochondria, apparently in the matrix space.

Much of the interest in the pyruvate and α-ketoglutarate dehydrogenase complexes derives from their key positions in metabolism (Fig. 1). Pyruvate is an intermediate in the biosynthesis of fats (lipogenesis) and carbohydrates (gluconeogenesis), and its complete oxidation via the tricarboxylic acid cycle is a major source of energy. Tricarboxylic acid cycle intermediates, including α-ketoglutarate, are also converted to precursors of protein, porphyrins, and nucleic acids.

The pyruvate and α-ketoglutarate dehydrogenase complexes possess distinctive structures (1) and catalyze a coordinated sequence of reactions (Fig. 2). Several of them have been separated into their component enzymes and have been reassembled from the isolated enzymes. They are apparently

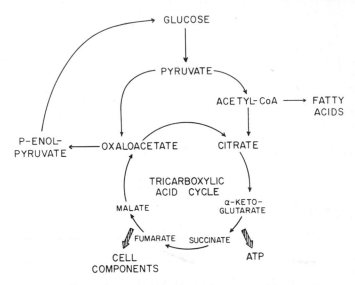

Figure 1. Diagram illustrating central positions of pyruvate and α-ketoglutarate in cellular metabolism. The abbreviations used are as follows: CoA, coenzyme A; ATP, adenosine 5′-triphosphate.

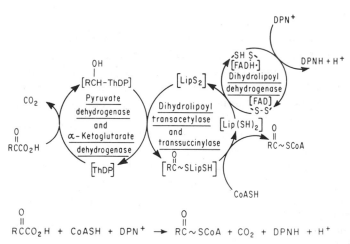

Figure 2. Reaction sequence in pyruvate and α-ketoglutarate oxidation. The abbreviations used are as follows: ThDP, thiamine diphosphate; LipS$_2$ and Lip(SH)$_2$, lipoyl moiety and its reduced form; CoASH, coenzyme A; FAD, flavin adenine dinucleotide; DPN$^+$ and DPNH, diphosphopyridine nucleotide and its reduced form.

self-assembling systems. Each of these complexes contains a core, consisting of dihydrolipoyl transacetylase or dihydrolipoyl transsuccinylase, to which pyruvate dehydrogenase or α-ketoglutarate dehydrogenase and dihydrolipoyl dehydrogenase are joined by noncovalent bonds. Thus the core enzyme plays both a catalytic and a structural role. The pyruvate dehydrogenase complex from mammalian cells, and apparently from other eukaryotic cells as well, contains, in addition to the three catalytic components, two regulatory enzymes, a kinase and a phosphatase, which are also attached to the transacetylase core (2).

1.   Subunit Composition and Structure of Mammalian Pyruvate Dehydrogenase Complex

The pyruvate dehydrogenase complexes isolated from bovine kidney and heart mitochondria have molecular weights of about 7,000,000 and 9,000,000, respectively. The subunit compositions of the two complexes are summarized in Table 1. The components of the two complexes are very similar, if not identical. The pyruvate dehydrogenase component has a molecular weight of about 154,000 and possesses the subunit composition $\alpha_2\beta_2$ (3). The molecular weights of the two subunits are about 41,000 and 36,000, respectively. The isolated dihydrolipoyl dehydrogenase has a molecular weight of about 110,000 and contains two apparently identical polypeptide chains and two molecules of FAD. The molecular weights of the kinase and phosphatase polypeptide chains are about 50,000 and 100,000,

Table 1. Subunit Composition of Pyruvate Dehydrogenase Complexes from Bovine Kidney and Heart

Enzyme	Molecular Weight	Subunit No.	Subunit Molecular Weight	Subunits per Molecule of Complex Kidney	Heart
Pyruvate	154,000	2	41,000	40	60
dehydrogenase		2	36,000	40	60
Transacetylase	3,100,000	60	52,000	60	60
Flavoprotein	110,000	2	55,000	10	12
Kinase	?	?	~50,000	~5	~5
Phosphatase	100,000	1	100,000	~5	~5

respectively. The core enzyme, the dihydrolipoyl transacetylase, consists of 60 apparently identical polypeptide chains of about 52,000 molecular weight. Each transacetylase chain apparently contains one molecule of covalently bound lipoic acid. The subunit composition of the bovine kidney and heart pyruvate dehydrogenase complexes is 60 transacetylase chains, 40 (kidney complex) or 60 (heart complex) of each of the two types of pyruvate dehydrogenase chains (i.e., 20 or 30 tetramers), and 10 to 12 flavoprotein chains (i.e., 5 to 6 dimers). The pyruvate dehydrogenase complex isolated from bovine kidney can bind about 10 additional pyruvate dehydrogenase tetramers. The apparent number of kinase and phosphatase chains per molecule of complex is small, about five chains of each enzyme. Clearly, the bovine kidney and heart pyruvate dehydrogenase complexes do not have their components present in equimolar ratios. The molecular basis of this phenomenon and its functional significance are under investigation.

The appearance of the mammalian dihydrolipoyl transacetylase in the electron microscope is that of a pentagonal dodecahedron (1, 4, 5), and its design appears to be based on icosahedral (532) symmetry. The tentative conclusion from electron microscopic studies is that the flavoprotein dimers are located at the fivefold positions (i.e., in the faces) of the transacetylase pentagonal dodecahedron and that the pyruvate dehydrogenase tetramers are located at the twofold positions (i.e., on the edges). The locations of the kinase and the phosphatase on the transacetylase are not yet known.

2.   Regulation of Mammalian Pyruvate Dehydrogenase Complex

PRODUCT INHIBITION

Mechanisms for control over the activity of the pyruvate dehydrogenase complex from mammalian cells, and apparently from other eukaryotic cells as well, include product inhibition and covalent modification (6, 7). The activity of pyruvate dehydrogenase complexes is inhibited by the products of pyruvate oxidation, acetyl-CoA and DPNH, and these inhibitions are reversed competitively by CoA and DPN, respectively. These observations have led to suggestions that the activity of these multienzyme complexes may be regulated *in vivo*, at least in part, by the [acetyl-CoA]/[CoA] ratio and by the oxidation level of the DPN-DPNH pool.

COVALENT MODIFICATION

Another regulatory mechanism, involving phosphorylation and dephosphorylation of the pyruvate dehydrogenase component of the mammalian pyruvate dehydrogenase complex (Fig. 3), was first

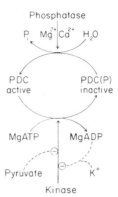

Figure 3. Interconversion of active and inactive (phosphorylated) forms of the mammalian pyruvate dehydrogenase complex (PDC). Minus sign indicates inhibition.

demonstrated in this laboratory (8, 9). We found that highly purified preparations of the bovine kidney pyruvate dehydrogenase complex were inactivated by incubation with micromolar concentrations of ATP. On the other hand, AMP, ADP, CTP, GTP, and UTP were ineffective in this regard. Using ATP labeled with ^{32}P in either the α-, $\alpha\beta$-, or γ-phosphoryl moieties, we established that the terminal phosphoryl moiety of ATP is transferred to the pyruvate dehydrogenase complex. When the phosphorylated (inactivated) complex was resolved, essentially all of the protein-bound radioactivity was found in the pyruvate dehydrogenase component. Further investigation revealed that the phosphorylated, inactivated pyruvate dehydrogenase complex was reactivated by incubation with millimolar concentrations of Mg^{2+}. Restoration of activity was accompanied by release of inorganic orthophosphate. Subsequent studies provided evidence that phosphorylation and concomitant inactivation of pyruvate dehydrogenase are catalyzed by a kinase (i.e., pyruvate dehydrogenase kinase), which is bound tightly to the transacetylase, and dephosphorylation and concomitant reactivation are catalyzed by a phosphatase (i.e., pyruvate dehydrogenase phosphatase), which is loosely associated with the complex. This control mechanism has been demonstrated with preparations of the pyruvate dehydrogenase complex from kidney, heart, liver, brain, adipose tissue, *Neurospora crassa,* and *Saccharomyces lactis* (7). However, we have found no evidence that microbial pyruvate dehydrogenase complexes or microbial or eukaryotic α-ketoglutarate dehydrogenase complexes are regulated by phosphorylation and dephosphorylation.

The site of this covalent regulation is the pyruvate dehydrogenase component of the complex. Phosphorylation occurs on seryl residues in the α-chain (mol. wt. 41,000) of bovine kidney and heart pyruvate dehydrogenase

(3). The amino acid sequence around the phosphoserine residues in bovine kidney pyruvate dehydrogenase has been determined (10):

Tyr-His-Gly-His-Ser(P)-Met-Ser-Asn-Pro-Gly-Val-Ser(P)-Tyr-Arg

Phosphorylation of the first seryl residue in this sequence results in inactivation of pyruvate dehydrogenase. The third seryl residue undergoes phosphorylation only after the first seryl residue has been phosphorylated (10, 11). The physiological significance, if any, of this latter phosphorylation site is under investigation. It appears that phosphorylation of only one α-chain in a pyruvate dehydrogenase tetramer ($\alpha_2\beta_2$) results in inactivation of that tetramer (11).

Evidence has been obtained (12) which suggests that the α-chain catalyzes the decarboxylation of pyruvate to produce α-hydroxyethylthiamine diphosphate and that the β-chain catalyzes the reductive acetylation of the lipoyl moiety of the transacetylase with α-hydroxyethylthiamine diphosphate (Fig. 1). Using ^{14}C-labeled substrates, we have shown that phosphorylation of pyruvate dehydrogenase inhibits the first, but not the second, reaction.

Thiamine diphosphate reduces the rate of inactivation (phosphorylation) of the pyruvate dehydrogenase complex by the kinase and ATP (12). This effect of thiamine diphosphate is apparently exerted on pyruvate dehydrogenase rather than on the kinase. Phosphorylation of the complex also decreases its ability to bind thiamine diphosphate (the K_D value for the pyruvate dehydrogenase-Mg-thiamine diphosphate is increased about twelvefold). It appears that the thiamine diphosphate binding site and the phosphorylation site on pyruvate dehydrogenase affect each other.

Some of the kinetic and regulatory properties of the purified pyruvate dehydrogenase kinase and pyruvate dehydrogenase phosphatase from bovine kidney and heart have been determined (13). The apparent K_m values of the kinase for its substrates, MgATP^{2-} and pyruvate dehydrogenase, are about 20 and 1 μM, respectively. Provided that K$^+$ or NH$_4$$^+$ ions are present (14), ADP inhibits the kinase competitively with respect to ATP. Pyruvate is the substrate for pyruvate dehydrogenase (apparent K_m about 40 μM), and it also inhibits the kinase. Pyruvate is noncompetitive with ATP, and its inhibitory effect appears to be more pronounced with the heart kinase than with the kidney kinase. The apparent K_i values are about 80 and 900 μM, respectively. Magnesium ion is required for pyruvate dehydrogenase phosphatase activity. The apparent K_m for Mg^{2+} is about 2 mM, i.e., about 100 times the apparent K_m of the kinase for Mg^{2+}. The apparent K_m of the phosphatase for its protein substrate, pyruvate dehydrogenase phosphate, is about 3 μM. No effect of adenosine cyclic 3′,5′-monophosphate (cyclic AMP) or guanosine cyclic 3′,5′-monophosphate (cyclic GMP) on either the kinase or the phosphatase was observed in our studies.

Recent studies indicate that Ca^{2+} is required in addition to Mg^{2+} for pyruvate dehydrogenase phosphatase activity (15–17). In the presence of Ca^{2+} the phosphatase binds to the transacetylase, thereby facilitating the Mg^{2+}-dependent dephosphorylation of pyruvate dehydrogenase phosphate (17). Half-maximal activity of the phosphatase is observed at a free Ca^{2+} concentration of about 1 μM. It appears that Ca^{2+}-facilitated binding of the phosphatase to the transacetylase increases the affinity of the phosphatase for its protein substrate (by lowering the apparent K_m about twentyfold). It is possible that Ca^{2+} serves as a bridging ligand between the phosphatase and the transacetylase. Alternatively, Ca^{2+} may bind to either the phosphatase or the transacetylase, producing a conformational change that facilitates binding of the phosphatase.

Binding of the kinase to the transacetylase also increases the affinity of the kinase for its protein substrate, pyruvate dehydrogenase, by lowering the apparent K_m about thirtyfold (13). The stimulatory effect of the transacetylase on pyruvate dehydrogenase kinase activity apparently does not involve Ca^{2+} (17).

We have obtained evidence which suggests that the activity of the mammalian pyruvate dehydrogenase complex is not regulated in a totally "on"-"off" manner by the kinase and the phosphatase (14, 18). Rather, it appears that these two antagonistic regulatory enzymes maintain steady-state levels of activity of the complex and that these levels are modulated through the actions on the kinase and the phosphatase of the factors mentioned and possibly also factors yet to be identified. Thus, when the kinase and the phosphatase are present and functional, the nearly steady-state activity of the bovine kidney pyruvate dehydrogenase complex is affected markedly by varying the concentration of Mg^{2+} or Ca^{2+} and thereby changing the activity of the phosphatase (18). On the other hand, at optimum Mg^{2+} and Ca^{2+} concentrations, the steady-state activity of the complex is affected markedly by varying the concentration of K^+ at a fixed [ADP]/[ATP] ratio or by varying the [ADP]/[ATP] ratio at a fixed concentration of K^+, and thereby changing the activity of the kinase (14). In the absence of K^+, ADP had no effect on the steady-state activity of the complex.

Although a variety of physiologically significant compounds have been tested, we have been unable to detect regulation of the bovine kidney and heart kinase and phosphatase by any substances other than those mentioned above. The results obtained with the purified pyruvate dehydrogenase system suggest that the activity of the kinase may be regulated *in vivo* by the intramitochondrial concentrations of pyruvate and K^+ (possibly NH_4^+) ions and by the [ADP]/[ATP] ratio, and that the activity of the phosphatase may be regulated by the intramitochondrial concentrations of uncomplexed Mg^{2+} and Ca^{2+} (Fig. 3). The concentrations of uncomplexed Mg^{2+} and Ca^{2+} in the mitochondrial matrix may be determined, at least in part, by the [ADP]/[ATP] ratio, since ADP forms a much weaker complex with these divalent cations than does ATP. The results obtained with the purified pyruvate dehydrogenase system have been confirmed and extended with intact mitochondria (19–21).

Regulation of the interconversion of the phosphorylated and nonphosphorylated forms of pyruvate dehydrogenase in rat adipose tissue by insulin has been reported (22–24). Insulin apparently increases the proportion of the nonphosphorylated form of pyruvate dehydrogenase. It would appear that this effect of insulin is indirect and may be mediated through changes in the intramitochondrial concentrations of pyruvate, ADP, ATP, K^+, Mg^{2+}, and Ca^{2+}.

References

1. L. J. Reed and R. M. Oliver, *Brookhaven Symp. Biol.*, **21**, 397 (1968).
2. T. C. Linn, J. W. Pelley, F. H. Pettit, F. Hucho, D. D. Randall, and L. J. Reed, *Arch. Biochem. Biophys.*, **148**, 327 (1972).
3. C. R. Barrera, G. Namihira, L. Hamilton, P. Munk, M. H. Eley, T. C. Linn, and L. J. Reed, *Arch. Biochem. Biophys.*, **148**, 343 (1972).
4. E. Ishikawa, R. M. Oliver, and L. J. Reed, *Proc. Natl. Acad. Sci. U.S.*, **56**, 534 (1966).
5. T. Hayakawa, T. Kanzaki, T. Kitamura, Y. Fukuyoshi, Y. Sakurai, K. Koike, T. Suematsu, and M. Koike, *J. Biol. Chem.*, **244**, 3660 (1969).
6. L. J. Reed, in B. L. Horecker and E. R. Stadtman, Eds., *Current Topics in Cellular Regulation*, Vol. 1, Academic Press, New York, 1969, p. 233.
7. L. J. Reed, *Acc. Chem. Res.*, **7**, 40 (1974).
8. T. C. Linn, F. H. Pettit, and L. J. Reed, *Proc. Natl. Acad. Sci. U.S.*, **62**, 234 (1969).
9. T. C. Linn, F. H. Pettit, F. Hucho, and L. J. Reed, *Proc. Natl. Acad. Sci. U.S.*, **64**, 227 (1969).
10. E. T. Hutcheson, Ph.D. Dissertation, University of Texas at Austin, 1971.
11. T. E. Roche and L. J. Reed, unpublished data, 1973–74.
12. T. E. Roche and L. J. Reed, *Biochem. Biophys. Res. Commun.*, **48**, 840 (1972).
13. F. Hucho, D. D. Randall, T. E. Roche, M. W. Burgett, J. W. Pelley, and L. J. Reed, *Arch. Biochem. Biophys.*, **151**, 328 (1972).
14. T. E. Roche and L. J. Reed, *Biochem. Biophys. Res. Commun.*, **59**, 1341 (1974).
15. R. M. Denton, P. J. Randle, and B. R. Martin, *Biochem. J.*, **128**, 161 (1972).
16. E. A. Siess and O. H. Wieland, *Eur. J. Biochem.*, **26**, 96 (1972).
17. F. H. Pettit, T. E. Roche, and L. J. Reed, *Biochem. Biophys. Res. Commun.*, **49**, 463 (1972).
18. L. J. Reed, F. H. Pettit, T. E. Roche, and P. J. Butterworth, in F. Huijing and E. Y. C. Lee, Eds., *Protein Phosphorylation in Control Mechanisms*, Miami Winter Symposia, Vol. 5, Academic Press, New York, 1973, p. 83.

19. D. L. Severson, R. M. Denton, H. T. Pask, and P. J. Randle, *Biochem. J.*, **140**, 225 (1974).
20. O. H. Wieland and R. Portenhauser, *Eur. J. Biochem.*, **45**, 577 (1974).
21. E. I. Walajtys, D. P. Gottesman, and J. R. Williamson, *J. Biol. Chem.*, **249**, 1857 (1974).
22. S. I. Taylor, C. Mukherjee, and R. L. Jungas, *J. Biol. Chem.*, **248**, 73 (1973).
23. P. J. Randle and R. M. Denton, *Symp. Soc. Exp. Biol.*, **27**, 401 (1973).
24. L. Weiss, G. Löffler, and O. H. Wieland, *Hoppe-Seylers Z. Physiol. Chem.*, **355**, 363 (1974).

DISCUSSION

Chapters 1 and 2

Dr. Cooper. Have you found any competition between sodium and potassium?

Dr. Reed. Sodium is less effective than potassium in facilitating ADP inhibition. In addition, sodium inhibits kinase activity at concentrations of 50 mM and above.

Dr. Patel. I would like to congratulate both authors and to ask a question of Dr. Reed. As you mentioned, the phosphatase and the kinase are working simultaneously to maintain pyruvate dehydrogenase complex activity. Would they constitute a futile cycle in terms of ATP-ADP conversion?

Dr. Reed. The "ATPase activity" of this enzyme system appears to be insignificant, since the molecular activities of the kinase and the phosphatase are very low, i.e., about 5 moles/(min)(mole) of enzyme. Furthermore, as pointed out by E. A. Newsholme, the wastage of energy in "futile cycles" may be compensated for by increased versatility of control.

Dr. Blass. May I ask questions of both Dr. Reed and Dr. Koike? Dr. Reed, were the concentrations of K^+ and of NH_4^+ that acted on the purified kinase *in vitro* comparable to the concentrations of NH_4^+ that might occur in intact cells *in vivo,* either in the normal state or during ammonia toxicity? Dr. Koike, is there information on the K_m for thiamine diphosphate of the purified KGDH complex?

Dr. Koike. Attempts to dissociate ThDP from the oxoglutarate dehydrogenase resulted in complete loss of its activity. We did not find direct evidence as to whether ThDP is bound covalently or noncovalently. Our results, suggest, however, that ThDP is bound noncovalently.

Dr. Connelly. You indicated in your paper that the heart enzyme has activity not only with pyruvate but also to some degree with some of the branched-chain keto acids, notably keto-isocaproic. I am wondering, first, whether or not you determined the K_m and, second, on the basis of that determination, would you consider the activity with the branched-chain keto acid a significant physiological activity? I wonder whether we need to have another enzyme to take care of the branched-chain keto acids or whether your enzyme can do it.

Dr. Koike. As previously reported (*J. Biol. Chem.,* **244,** 1183, 1969), we have measured the K_m values for branched-chain α-keto acids by using pig heart pyruvate dehydrogenase complex and its pyruvate dehydrogenase component. The data obtained suggest that the estimated activities for branched-chain α-keto acid could be considered to be significant physiologically. We have not proved yet whether the pig heart complex takes care of branched-chain α-keto acids or there are other enzymes specific for these α-keto acids.

Dr. Reed. In response to Dr. Blass's question the marked effects of potassium on the activity of the kinase in the presence of ADP are observed at concentrations of 30 to 60 mM or less.

Dr. Cooper. Dr. Koike, you mentioned before that, when you removed the ThDP from the α-ketoglutarate dehydrogenase, you lost the activity and could not reconstitute it. I wonder what would have happened if you had tried thiamine triphosphate. I am thinking of Dr. Yusa's experiment. He reported that crude oxoglutarate dehydrogenase activity was restored when incubated with ThTP and ADP, but not with ThDP. Are you aware of that experiment?

Dr. Koike. I read Dr. Yusa's experiment. After we removed ThDP from the oxoglutarate dehydrogenase, we could not reconstitute the activity with either ThDP or ThDP and ATP. We have never tried ThTP.

Dr. Cooper. Dr. Yusa found that, if he added the diphosphate, he could not restore the activity but could get the activity with ThTP and ADP (T. Yusa, and B. Marvo, *J. Biochem.* (*Tokyo*), 60: 735, 1966).

Dr. Danner. In that same vein, when adding back ThDP to the α-ketoglutarate dehydrogenase complex, is the magnesium ion required in that complex as well as in the pyruvate dehydrogenase complex, and what is the effect of other ions?

Dr. Koike. When we did the experiment in an attempt to reconstitute the activity of oxoglutarate dehydrogenase after removal of ThDP, we added ThDP and Mg^{2+}. Unfortunately we failed to reconstitute the activity. The native complex contained noncovalently bound ThDP, which did not require the addition of ThDP and Mg^{2+} or Ca^{2+}.

3. Effects of Branched-Chain and Aromatic α-Ketoacids on Pyruvate and α-Ketoglutarate Metabolism

M. S. PATEL
O. E. Owen

Departments of Medicine and Biochemistry
General Clinical Research Center
and Fels Research Institute
Temple University School of Medicine
Philadelphia, Pennsylvania

Inborn errors in the metabolism of phenylalanine (phenylketonuria) and the branched-chain amino acids (maple syrup urine disease) have been known to cause a retardation in the development and function of the brain. Although the biochemical defects in the metabolism of these amino acids are well characterized, the pathogenesis of brain malfunction in untreated patients is still not well understood. As a result of specific genetic defects in the catabolic pathways of phenylalanine and the branched-chain amino acids, the concentrations of phenylalanine and the branched-chain amino acids, namely leucine, isoleucine, and valine and their corresponding α-ketoacids, and of other metabolites are markedly elevated in the plasma of untreated patients (for reviews see refs. 1 and 2). Because of a lack of activity or very low activity of hepatic phenylalanine hydroxylase in classical phenylketonuric patients, phenylalanine is metabolized via an alternative pathway by first being converted to phenylpyruvate (1). In patients with classical maple syrup urine disease, caused by the absence of or very low activity of the branched-chain α-ketoacid dehydrogenase complex(es), the oxidative decarboxylation

31

of the branched-chain α-ketoacids is impaired (2). Several investigators have recently found toxic effects of these aromatic and branched-chain amino acids and their α-ketoacids on the transport of amino acids, the synthesis of proteins and lipids, and energy metabolism in developing brain. Because the initial reaction in the catabolic pathways of these aromatic and branched-chain α-ketoacids is similar to that of pyruvate and α-ketoglutarate, we have recently investigated the effect of aromatic and branched-chain α-ketoacids on the metabolism of pyruvate and α-ketoglutarate by developing rat and human brain.

In the mitochondria, pyruvate is metabolized to acetyl-CoA and oxaloacetate by the action of pyruvate dehydrogenase complex and pyruvate carboxylase, respectively. The latter is the major enzyme for the fixation of CO_2 in the brain (3). It has been shown that phenylpyruvate inhibits both the carboxylation of pyruvate by intact rat brain mitochondria and the activity of pyruvate carboxylase in disrupted mitochondria (Table 1) (4). Phenylalanine and phenylacetate had no effect on the fixation of CO_2 by pyruvate carboxylase. The concentration of phenylpyruvate required to inhibit pyruvate carboxylase was dependent on the concentration of pyruvate used in the assay. When the pyruvate concentration was lowered from 10 to 0.5 mM in the assay medium, phenylpyruvate exerted a greater inhibitory effect on this enzyme. It should be noted that at 0.5 mM pyruvate 50% inhibition was exerted by less than 1 mM phenylpyruvate (Fig. 1). The K_m for pyruvate and the K_i for phenylpyruvate of rat brain pyruvate carboxylase were about 0.2 mM and 2 mM, respectively (4). The carboxylation of pyruvate by human brain homogenates (Table 2) and the activity of pyruvate carboxylase (Fig. 2) were also inhibited by phenylpyruvate. Phenylalanine, the branched-chain

Table 1. Effect of Phenylalanine and Its Metabolites on Pyruvate Carboxylation and on the Activity of Pyruvate Carboxylase in Rat Brain Mitochondria[a]

Addition	Pyruvate Carboxylation by Mitochondria, nmol $H^{14}CO_3$ fixed/mg protein/15 min	Pyruvate Carboxylase, munits/mg protein
None	123 ± 7	65 ± 1.3
L-Phenylalanine (10 mM)	131 ± 6	66 ± 2.1
Phenylpyruvate (10 mM)	49 ± 6	34 ± 2.1
Phenylacetate (10 mM)	133 ± 5	62 ± 1.7

[a] The data are taken from Patel (4).

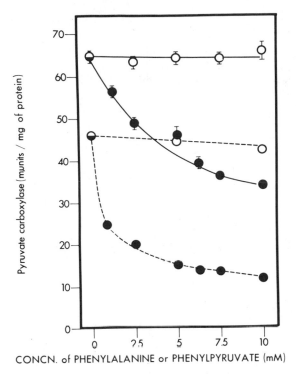

Figure 1. Effect of phenylalanine and phenylpyruvate on rat brain mitochondrial pyruvate carboxylase activity. Pyruvate was added at either 10 mM (———) or 0.5 mM (---). Phenylalanine (O) or phenylpyruvate (●) was added at the concentrations indicated. The data are taken from Patel (4).

amino acids, and their α-ketoacids had no effect on the fixation of CO_2 by cerebral pyruvate carboxylase (Table 2) (5, 6). Phenylpyruvate is also shown to inhibit pyruvate carboxylase from rat (7, 8) and human (8, 9) livers.

Pyruvate carboxylase, an anaplerotic enzyme, replenishes the C_4 compound that is required for the synthesis of dicarboxylic amino acids and for the transport of the acetyl moiety in the form of citrate across the inner mitochondrial membrane. Hyperphenylalaninemia induced in adult male and in pregnant rats lowers the concentrations of aspartate, glutamate, and glutamine in both adult and fetal brains (11, 12). Acetyl-CoA is produced in the mitochondria, whereas the *de novo* synthesis of fatty acids and acetylcholine is known to occur in the extramitochondrial compartment. Because the inner mitochondrial membrane is impermeable to acetyl-CoA, citrate is thought to be a carrier of the acetyl moiety across the mitochondrial membrane (12). In the process of the translocation of the acetyl moiety

Table 2. Effect of Phenylpyruvate and the Branched-Chain α-Keto Acids on Pyruvate Carboxylation and Pyruvate Decarboxylation by Homogenates of Human and Rat Brains[a]

Experiment	Addition	Pyruvate Carboxylation		Pyruvate Decarboxylation	
		Human Brain, μmol/g tissue/30 min	Rat Brain, μmol/g tissue/30 min	Human Brain, μmol/g tissue/15 min	Rat Brain, μmol/g tissue/15 min
1	None	1.2	5.5 ± 0.6	5.5	14.7 ± 0.7
	Phenylpyruvate (5 mM)	0.6	2.5 ± 0.5	2.8	8.6 ± 1.7
2	None	1.6	4.7 ± 0.6	5.0	13.5 ± 1.0
	α-Ketoisocaprate (5 mM)	1.7	4.7 ± 0.9	2.4	4.5 ± 0.5
	α-Keto-β-methylvalerate (5 mM)	1.6	4.7 ± 0.8	5.5	11.8 ± 2.2
	α-Ketoisovalerate (5 mM)	1.5	4.9 ± 1.1	4.2	13.4 ± 1.7

[a] The data are taken from Patel et al. (5, 6).

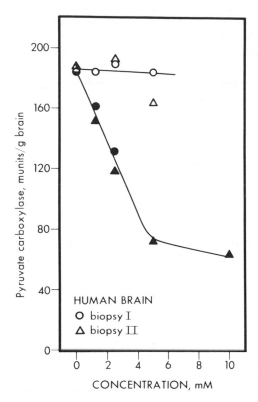

Figure 2. Effect of varying concentrations of phenylalanine (open symbols) and phenylpyruvate (solid symbols) on pyruvate carboxylase activity in homogenates of human brain. The data are taken from Patel *et al.* (5).

across the mitochondrial membrane, mitochondrial oxaloacetate is lost. It has been shown that phenylpyruvate inhibits the formation of citrate from pyruvate by rat brain mitochondria (4). This observation, together with the inhibitory effects of phenylpyruvate on citrate synthase and fatty acid synthetase (13), is consistent with a diminished cerebral lipid formation in untreated patients with phenylketonuria.

The pyruvate dehydrogenase complex plays a major role in the oxidation of pyruvate in the brain. Gallagher (14) observed a reduction in oxygen uptake by rat brain mitochondria in the presence of phenylpyruvate only when pyruvate was used as a substrate. Phenylpyruvate also inhibited the decarboxylation of $[1\text{-}^{14}C]$pyruvate to $^{14}CO_2$ by mitochondria present in whole homogenates of rat (5, 15) and human (5) brains. Although a purified pig brain pyruvate dehydrogenase complex was reported to be inhibited by phenylpyruvate (16), in recent studies phenylpyruvate had no effect on partially purified pyruvate dehydrogenase complexes from bovine (17, 18) and rat (19) brains. Furthermore, Hoffmann and Hucho (18) observed that phenylpyruvate at 10 mM concentration inhibited the interconversion of the pyruvate dehydrogenase complex from the active nonphosphorylated to the inactive phosphorylated forms, and hence protected the active form. The interconversion from the inactive to the active form of this complex was not significantly affected by phenylpyruvate (18). A discrepancy between mitochondrial studies and those involving the purified enzyme complex may be due, in part, to the effect of phenylpyruvate on the transport of pyruvate across the inner membrane, an availability of cofactors, such as CoA, and/or a possible inhibitory effect of phenylacetyl-CoA on the enzyme in intact mitochondria present in brain homogenates. Land and Clark (20) have recently observed an inhibition by phenylpyruvate and α-ketoisocaproate on the transporter system of pyruvate in rat brain mitochondria.

The branched-chain α-ketoacids have been shown to inhibit the decarboxylation of [1-^{14}C]pyruvate by rat brain (21, 22) and liver (23) preparations. We (6) have observed that, among three branched-chain α-ketoacids only α-ketoisocaproate significantly reduced the decarboxylation of [1-^{14}C]pyruvate by human and rat brain homogenates at varying concentrations of the inhibitor and the substrate (Table 2). Bowden et al. (22) and Johnson and Connelly (24) observed that α-ketoisocaproate competitively inhibited the pyruvate dehydrogenase complex from rat brain and bovine liver, respectively; however, Blass and Lewis (17) found that this enzyme complex from ox brain is not inhibited by the branched-chain α-ketoacids. Recently, Clark and Land (25) found that only α-ketoisovalerate inhibited pyruvate dehydrogenase from young rat brains. However, the other two α-ketoacids of isoleucine and valine are also found to inhibit the pyruvate dehydrogenase complex from bovine liver (24) and pig heart (26). Additional studies are needed to clarify possible variations in tissues and species.

Similar studies on the effects of aromatic and the branched-chain α-ketoacids on the α-ketoglutarate dehydrogenase complex from the brain have recently been carried out in our laboratory. As seen in Table 3, the decarboxylation of [1-^{14}C]α-ketoglutarate by rat brain mitochondria and the activity of the α-ketoglutarate dehydrogenase complex were inhibited by phenylpyruvate and the branched-chain α-ketoacids, but not by their corresponding amino acids (27). We have recently observed that phenylpyruvate competitively inhibited (K_i about 1.5 mM) the α-ketoglutarate dehydrogenase complex from rat and human brains (M. S. Patel and O. E. Owen, unpublished data). The activity of α-ketoglutarate dehydrogenase complex from brains of 2-week-old and adult rats is also

Table 3. Effect of Phenylpyruvate and the Branched-Chain α-Keto Acids on the Decarboxylation of $[1\text{-}^{14}C]\alpha$-Ketoglutarate to $^{14}CO_2$ by Mitochondria from Adult Rat Brain and on the Activity of the α-Ketoglutarate Dehydrogenase Complex from Brain Mitochondria

Experiment	Addition	α-Ketoglutarate Decarboxylation by Mitochondria, nmol/mg protein/min	Activity of α-Ketoglutarate Dehydrogenase Complex, munits/mg protein
1[a]	None	30.7 ± 0.7	56 ± 6.1
	Phenylpyruvate (1 mM)		38 ± 5.9
	Phenylpyruvate (5 mM)	13.6 ± 1.1	17 ± 1.6
2[b]	None	30.0 ± 0.7	50 ± 2.5
	α-Ketoisocaproate (5 mM)	20.8 ± 2.1	28 ± 2.1
	α-Keto-β-methylvalerate (5 mM)	16.7 ± 1.7	11 ± 1.0
	α-Ketoisovalerate (5 mM)	16.7 ± 1.0	10 ± 0.3

[a] M. S. Patel and O. E. Owen, unpublished data.
[b] The data are taken from Patel (27).

competitively inhibited by the three branched-chain α-ketoacids, with apparent K_i values of 3.8, 1.3, and 1.4 mM for α-ketoisocaproate, α-keto-β-methylvalerate, and α-ketoisovalerate, respectively (Table 4) (27). It should be noted that the last two α-ketoacids are effective inhibitors of this enzyme, and that this finding is consistent with mitochondrial studies shown in Table 3. The activity of α-ketoglutarate dehydrogenase complex from fetal and adult human brain was also competitively inhibited by α-ketoisocaproate and α-ketoisovalerate with K_i values of 4.4 and 1.4 mM, respectively (Fig. 3 and Table 4) (27). The purified α-ketoglutarate dehydrogenate complexes from pig heart (26) and bovine liver (24) have previously been shown to be inhibited by the branched-chain α-ketoacids (see also Table 4). Our findings show that a similar inhibition of this enzyme also occurs in rat and human brain preparations. The data summarized in Table 4 show that α-ketoisovalerate and α-keto-β-methylvalerate exert greater inhibitory effects on this enzyme.

The concentrations of the branched-chain α-ketoacids in the brains of patients with maple syrup urine disease are not known; however, an accumulation of these α-ketoacids in the gray matter of an infant who died of this disease has been documented by Dreyfus and Prensky (21). It should be noted that the apparent K_i values observed for the branched-chain α-ketoacids of human cerebral enzyme (Table 4) (27) are close to the levels of these α-ketoacids circulating in the plasma of untreated patients with maple

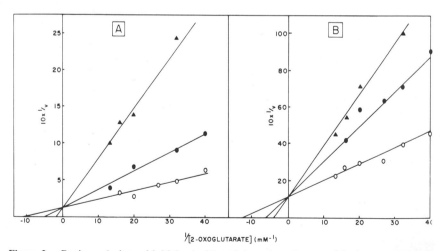

Figure 3.   Reciprocal plots of initial velocities of the α-ketoglutarate dehydrogenase complex from fetal and adult human brain against α-ketoglutarate concentrations at a fixed inhibitor concentration. The activity of the α-ketoglutarate dehydrogenase complex in fetal (A) and adult (B) human brain preparations was assayed. Other additions were as follows: O, none; ●, 6 mM α-ketoisocaproate; △, 4 mM α-ketoisovalerate. The data are taken from Patel (27).

Table 4. Comparison of K_i Values of α-Ketoglutarate Dehydrogenase Complex from Several Mammalian Tissues

Amino Acid or α-Keto Acid	Human Plasma[a,d] Normal, mM	MSUD,[b] mM	$\bar{K}_i$ Value of α-Ketoglutarate Dehydrogenase Complex — Human Brain,[c] nM	Rat Brain,[c] mM	Bovine Liver,[d] mM	Pig Heart,[e] mM
Leucine	0.1–0.4	4–6	—	—	—	—
α-Ketoisocaproate	0.1–0.4	2–4	4.5	3.6	2.4	3.4
Isoleucine	0.07–0.25	1.0–1.5	—	—	—	—
α-Keto-β-methylvalerate	0.07–0.25	1.0–1.5	N.D.[f]	1.4	1.4	1.4
Valine	0.24	1.85	—	—	—	—
α-Ketoisovalerate	0.24	1.85	1.9	1.0	0.82	2.3

[a] The data are taken from Snyderman et al. (28).
[b] MSUD: Maple syrup urine disease.
[c] The data are taken from Patel (27).
[d] The data are taken from Johnson and Connelly (24).
[e] The data are taken from Kanzaki et al. (26).
[f] N.D.: not determined.

syrup urine disease (Table 4) (28). That an inhibition *in vivo* by the branched-chain α-ketoacids of the α-ketoglutarate dehydrogenase complex occurs is supported by an increased excretion of α-ketoglutarate in the urine of untreated patients (29, 30). Although a large amount of phenylpyruvate is excreted in urine, its circulating level in the plasma of untreated phenylketonuric patients is in the range of only 0.1 mM (31).

Because of the lack of information on the levels of phenylpyruvate in the brains and other tissues of untreated patients, it is difficult to assess *in vivo* the significance of the effects of phenylpyruvate on brain metabolism. Additionally, in evaluating the effects of phenylpyruvate and the branched-chain α-ketoacids on several cerebral enzymes in patients with phenylketonuria or maple syrup urine disease, possible accumulation of high concentrations of these α-ketoacids in subcellular fractions, as well as in specific parts of the brain, should be considered.

The pyruvate dehydrogenase complex connects the glycolytic pathway and the tricarboxylic acid cycle and therefore allows further oxidation of pyruvate derived from glucose. The α-ketoglutarate dehydrogenase complex is a member of the tricarboxylic acid cycle and thus plays an important role in the oxidation of both glucose and ketone bodies. The inhibition by the branched-chain α-ketoacids and phenylpyruvate of the pyruvate dehydrogenase and the α-ketoglutarate dehydrogenase complexes would significantly reduce the oxidative metabolism of glucose and ketone bodies and, hence, energy metabolism. It has been recently observed that the developing brain effectively utilizes ketone bodies for the biosynthesis of lipids (32; also M. S. Patel and O. E. Owen, unpublished data). Succinyl-CoA is required for the formation of acetoacetyl-CoA from acetoacetate; therefore a reduction in the formation of succinyl-CoA from α-ketoglutarate in the presence of the branched-chain α-ketoacids could impair the metabolism of ketone bodies. In fact, we have recently observed that the incorporation of labeled acetoacetate and β-hydroxybutyrate into lipids by developing rat brain is inhibited by the branched-chain α-ketoacids and phenylpyruvate (M. S. Patel and O. E. Owen, unpublished data). From the data presented in Table 4 and the circulating concentrations of phenylpyruvate and the branched-chain α-ketoacids in plasma from affected patients, it is clear that the branched-chain α-ketoacids exert a greater inhibitory effect on the metabolism of ketone bodies than does phenylpyruvate.

It is appropriate to indicate here that several other cerebral enzymes, namely, hexokinase (33), 6-phosphogluconate dehydrogenase (33), citrate synthase (13, 25), fatty acid synthetase (13, 25), alanine and aspartate aminotransferases (34), and NADP-malate dehydrogenase (M. S. Patel, unpublished data), have also been found to be inhibited by phenylpyruvate

(35) and the branched-chain α-ketoacids. The diversified effects of these α-ketoacids on cerebral energy and lipid metabolism, as well as an inhibitory influence of increased levels of phenylalanine and the branched-chain amino acids on protein synthesis, may contribute greatly to the pathophysiology of mental retardation in patients with phenylketonuria or maple syrup urine disease.

Summary

The effect of aromatic and branched-chain α-ketoacids on the metabolism of pyruvate and α-ketoglutarate by rat and human brain preparations was investigated. Phenylpyruvate inhibited the carboxylation of pyruvate by intact rat brain mitochondria and also the activity of pyruvate carboxylase from rat and human brains. In contrast, phenylalanine, the branched-chain amino acids, and corresponding α-ketoacids had no effect on cerebral pyruvate carboxylase. Phenylpyruvate, as well as three branched-chain α-ketoacids, diminished the decarboxylation of pyruvate via the pyruvate dehydrogenase complex by homogenates of human and rat brain. Among three branched-chain α-ketoacids, α-ketoisocaproate appeared to exert the greatest inhibitory effect on pyruvate decarboxylation. Furthermore, aromatic and the branched-chain α-ketoacids also inhibited the decarboxylation of α-ketoglutarate by the α-ketoglutarate dehydrogenase complex from rat and human brain. α-keto-β-methylvalerate and α-ketoisovalerate had greater inhibitory effects on this enzyme. Our findings, together with those of others, show that the branched-chain α-ketoacids affect in a variety of ways, the pyruvate dehydrogenase complex and the α-ketoglutarate dehydrogenase complex from brain and other tissues. Because glucose and keton bodies are principal fuels for developing mammalian brain, an impairment in the metabolism of pyruvate and α-ketoglutarate could contribute to the pathophysiology of mental retardation in patients with maple syrup urine disease and phenylketonuria.

Acknowledgments

This work was supported in part by National Institutes of Health grants NS-10125, NS-11088, AM-16102, and RR-5624 and General Clinical Research Center grant 5-MO1-RR349.

References

1. W. E. Knox, "Phenylketonuria," in J. B. Stanbury, J. B. Wyngaarden, and D. S. Fredrickson, Eds., *The Metabolic Basis of Inherited Disease,* McGraw-Hill Book Company, New York-London, 1972, p. 266.

2. J. Dancis and M. Levitz, "Abnormalities of branched-chain amino acid metabolism," in J. B. Stanbury, J. B. Wyngaarden, and D. S. Fredrickson, Eds., *The Metabolic Basis of Inherited Disease,* McGraw-Hill Book Company, New York-London, 1972, p. 426.

3. M. S. Patel, *J. Neurochem.,* **22,** 717 (1974).

4. M. S. Patel, *Biochem. J.,* **128,** 677 (1972).

5. M. S. Patel, W. D. Grover, and V. H. Auerbach, *J. Neurochem.,* **20,** 289 (1973).

6. M. S. Patel, V. H. Auerbach, W. D. Grover, and D. O. Wilbur, *J. Neurochem.,* **20,** 1793 (1973).

7. I. J. Arinze and M. S. Patel, *Biochemistry,* **12,** 4473 (1973).

8. M. R. Sutnick, W. D. Grover, and M. S. Patel, *Pediatr. Res.,* **6,** 172 (Abs.) (1972).

9. M. C. Scrutton and M. D. White, *Biochem. Med.,* **9,** 271 (1974).

10. M. J. Carver, *J. Neurochem.,* **12,** 45 (1965).

11. M. J. Carver, J. H. Copenhaver, and R. A. Serpan, *J. Neurochem.,* **12,** 857 (1965).

12. S. Tucek, *J. Neurochem.,* **15,** 531 (1967).

13. J. M. Land and J. B. Clark, *Biochem. J.,* **134,** 545 (1973).

14. B. B. Gallagher, *J. Neurochem.,* **16,** 1071 (1969).

15. J. A. Bowden and C. L. McArthur, III, *Nature,* (London), **235,** 230 (1972).

16. M. M. Kini, Ph.D. Thesis, Yale University School of Medicine, 1965; also, references through ref. 14.

17. J. P. Blass and C. A. Lewis, *Biochem. J.,* **131,** 31 (1973).

18. B. T. Hoffmann and F. Hucho, *FEBS Lett.,* **43,** 116 (1974).

19. J. M. Land and J. B. Clark, *Biochem. J.,* **134,** 539 (1973).

20. J. M. Land and J. B. Clark, *FEBS Lett.,* **44,** 348 (1974).

21. P. M. Dreyfus and A. L. Prensky, *Nature* (London), **214,** 276 (1967).

22. J. A. Bowden, C. L. McArthur, III, and M. Fried, *Biochem. Med.,* **5,** 101 (1971).

23. J. A. Bowden, E. P. Brestel, W. T. Cope, C. L. McArthur, III, D. N. Westfall, and M. Fried, *Biochem. Med.,* **4,** 69 (1970).

24. W. A. Johnson and J. L. Connelly, Biochemistry, **11,** 2416 (1972).

25. J. B. Clark and J. M. Land, *Biochem. J.,* **140,** 25 (1974).

26. T. Kanzaki, T. Hayakawa, M. Hamada, Y. Fukuyoshi, and M. Koike, *J. Biol. Chem.,* **244,** 1183 (1969).

27. M. S. Patel, *Biochem J.,* **144,** 91 (1974).

28. S. E. Snyderman, P. M. Norton, E. Roitman, and L. E. Holt, Jr., *Pediatrics,* **34,** 454 (1964).

29. A. D. Patrick, *Arch. Dis. Child.,* **36,** 269 (1961).

30. N. C. Woody and J. A. Harris, *J. Pediatr.,* **66,** 1042 (1965).

31. G. A. Jervis, *Proc. Soc. Exp. Biol. Med.,* **81,** 715 (1952).

32. J. Edmond, *J. Biol. Chem.*, **249**, 72 (1974).
33. G. Weber, R. I. Glazer, and R. A. Ross, *Adv. Enzyme Regul.*, **8**, 13 (1969).
34. W. Lysiak, M. Pienkowska-Vogel, A. Szutowicz, and S. Angielski, *J. Neurochem.*, **22**, 77 (1974).
35. M. S. Patel and I. J. Arinze, *Am. J. Clin. Nutr.*, **28**, 183 (1975).

4. Branched-Chain α-Ketoacid Dehydrogenases

JERALD L. CONNELLY, Ph.D.
W. A. JOHNSON, Ph.D.*

Department of Biochemistry
University of North Dakota School of Medicine
Grand Fork, North Dakota

Alpha-Ketoacid dehydrogenases represent one important need for thiamine in nature. Their participation in the oxidative decarboxylation of pyruvate and α-ketoglutarate is well established. For some time it has been presumed that the catabolism of other α-keto acids very probably involves this vitamin, as well as certain other cofactors, but few efforts have been made to verify these suspicions. Among the α-keto acids in nature, particular interest is focused on the branched-chain keto derivatives of leucine, isoleucine, and valine because of the essential nature, in mammals, of these compounds and because of the relevance of this segment of amino acid metabolism to the genetic disease known, because of the associated odor, as "maple syrup urine disease" (1). This paper presents the current status of this aspect of biochemistry, as well as evidence for the direct requirement for thiamine diphosphate (ThDP) as a cofactor in the oxidative decarboxylation of branched-chain α-ketoacids.

The overall picture of branched-chain ketoacid catabolism came to light as a consequence of early metabolic studies by Meister, Coon, and others on the three essential amino acids: valine, leucine, and isoleucine (Fig. 1). Transamination converts these amino acids to ketoacids, α-ketoisovalerate (KIV), α-ketoisocaproate (KIC), and α-keto-β-methylvalerate (KMV), which are oxidatively decarboxylated to form thioesters of coenzyme A.

* Present address: Chairman, Department of Nutrition, College of Home Economics, South Dakota State University, Brookings, South Dakota.

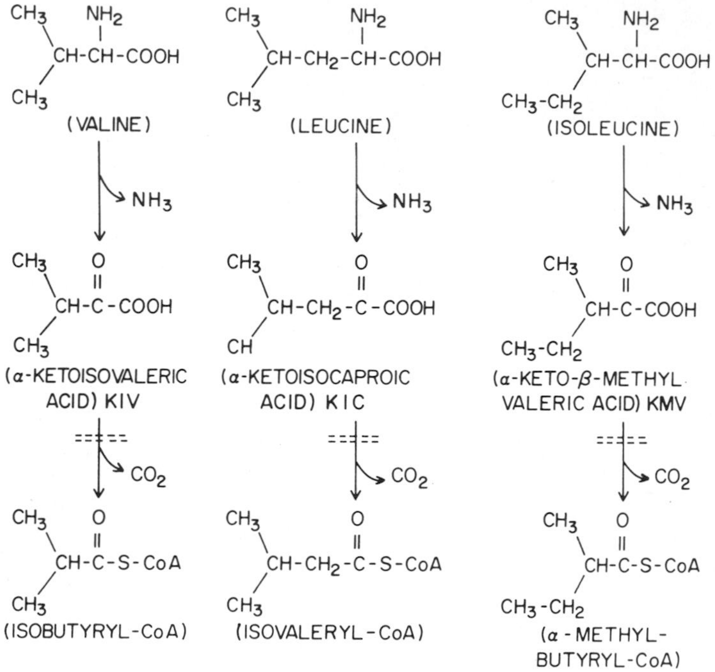

CH₃   NH₂   CH₃   NH₂   CH₃   NH₂
 \ | \ | \ |
  CH-CH-COOH   CH-CH₂-CH-COOH   CH-CH-COOH
 /   /   /
CH₃   CH₃   CH₃-CH₂
   (VALINE)   (LEUCINE)   (ISOLEUCINE)

            → NH₃   → NH₃   → NH₃

CH₃   O   CH₃   O   CH₃   O
 \   ‖   \   ‖   \   ‖
  CH-C-COOH   CH-CH₂-C-COOH   CH-C-COOH
 /   /   /
CH₃   CH   CH₃-CH₂
(α-KETOISOVALERIC   (α-KETOISOCAPROIC   (α-KETO-β-METHYL·
   ACID) KIV   ACID) KIC   VALERIC ACID) KMV

 == ‡ ==   == ‡ ==   == ‡ ==
            → CO₂   → CO₂   → CO₂

CH₃   O   CH₃   O   CH₃   O
 \   ‖   \   ‖   \   ‖
  CH-C-S-CoA   CH-CH₂-C-S-CoA   CH-C-S-CoA
 /   /   /
CH₃   CH₃   CH₃-CH₂
(ISOBUTYRYL-CoA)   (ISOVALERYL-CoA)   (α-METHYL-
                                                BUTYRYL-CoA)

Figure 1. Degradation of branched-chain amino acids. Abbreviations: KIV, α-ketoisovalerate; KIC, α-ketoisocaproate; KMV, α-keto-β-methylvalerate. = = = = indicates site of metabolic lesion in maple syrup urine disease.

Then, in a series of reactions much like those of fatty acid oxidation, these intermediates are converted to ketogenic and glycogenic compounds and steroid precursers. It was not until the early 1960s that efforts were made to isolate and characterize the branched-chain ketoacid dehydrogenases. Interest in these enzymic paths was sparked by earlier reports on "maple syrup urine disease."

This condition, first described by Menkes et al. in 1954 (1), is characterized by a marked elevation of branched-chain amino acids and their ketoacids in blood and urine. The condition is fatal very early in life unless a special diet, deficient in valine, leucine, and isoleucine, is provided. Clinical investigations disclosed that the metabolic lesion is at the point of oxidative decarboxylation, since in afflicted individuals transamination was not affected and catabolism of acyl-CoA metabolites proceeded normally (see Fig. 1).

It is currently customary to view the oxidative decarboxylation of KIV, KIC, and KMV as proceeding in a manner generally analogous to the well-defined processes of pyruvate and α-ketoglutarate catabolism (2, 3). It has thus, been presumed that the ketoacid loses CO_2 and, after an acyl transfer involving ADP and lipoic acid, combines with CoA. Reduced lipoate is then reoxidized by means of NAD-linked lipoate dehydrogenase.

Enzyme Assay

Assays used in attempts to isolate and characterize the branched-chain α-ketoacid dehydrogenase activity have been spectrophotometric (NADH production) and isotopic ($^{14}CO_2$ liberation). In addition, ferricyanide has been used as an electron acceptor in accordance with the spectrophotometric method described by Gubler (4). This technique has been useful in that it measures just the decarboxylase (dehydrogenase) component of the total activity of the complex. Both NAD^+ and $Fe(CN)_6^{4-}$ have been used as acceptors when $^{14}CO_2$ was measured, although it is generally observed that assay sensitivity is greater with NAD^+. The technique (5) employed in this assay uses a reaction flask in which a center well holds a small trapping vial containing hyamine. The reaction is stopped with acid injected through a rubber cap, and the liberated $^{14}CO_2$ is allowed to distill into the amine, which is subsequently quantitated by scintillation counting.

Tissue and Subcellular Locale

Tissue distribution studies disclosed that the highest levels of dehydrogenase activity occur in the liver, with the kidney showing considerably lower levels. Minor amounts of activity are found in brain, heart, and other tissues in various species. An interesting "division of labor" is indicated by the fact that the kidney contributes significantly to the transamination of branched-chain aminoacids, but generally provides only a small percentage of the total dehydrogenase activity. Within the cell, ketoacid dehydrogenases are localized in the mitochondrial fraction. Johnson (5), in our laboratory, and Wohlhueter and Harper (6), at Wisconsin, have observed upward to 90% of total cellular activity associated with the mitochondria. A small but significant amount of decarboxylase activity was observed in the cytosol. Both mitochondrial and cytosolic preparations gave activities linear with protein concentration. Furthermore, both laboratories have shown that the cytosolic activity is not derived from the mitochondria by solubilization processes. The physiological significance of this activity is unknown, and efforts are being made in our laboratory to purify and characterize the enzymes involved in an attempt to answer this question.

At the time of these studies techniques were available which allowed us to further investigate the question of the location of the mitochondrial activity. Removal of the outer membrane with digitonin did not remove the dehydrogenase, thus placing the activity on or within the inner membrane. In 1970 Klingenberg (7) provided a method for locating dehydrogenase activity relative to the inner membrane. He reported that some mitochondrial dehydrogenases are directly accessible to ferricyanide, itself impermeable, as electron acceptor, whereas others are accessible only through intermediates which are susceptible to inhibition by respiratory chain inhibitors. Thus antimycin A was able to distinguish between dehydrogenase activity inside and ouside the mitochondrial inner membrane. When applied to the locating of branched-chain ketoacid dehydrogenases, this technique demonstrated that the activity is on the outside of the inner membrane (5). This is in contrast to the intramitochondrial or perhaps intramembranal location of pyruvate and ketoglutaric dehydrogenases. Furthermore, this finding obviates the need for branched-chain keto acids to penetrate the inner membrane for further metabolism and thus eliminates membrane permeability as a factor in controlling the metabolism of these compounds.

Soluble Branched-Chain α Ketoacid Dehydrogenases

Before reviewing the more specific properties of these enzymic activities, it will be helpful to consider the current situation regarding nonparticulate preparations. Isolation of soluble activities has been reported by a limited number of laboratories from both bacterial and mammalian sources (Table 1). Our laboratory described a seventyfold purified enzyme from beef liver that was active with KMV and KIC but not with KIV or other ketoacids (8, 13). In 1967 Goedde and Keller (9) reported the isolation of three separate activities from beef liver. However, the complete details of the method and the enzyme kinetics have not as yet been published. A preparation of human kidney KIV dehydrogenase was reported by Ruediger and Goedde (10). The same laboratory reported a soluble bacterial (*Streptococcus faecalis*) activity having an apparent specificity for KIV (11). And, finally, in 1969 Namba et al. from Alberta, Canada, succeeded in obtaining fortyfold purified preparation from *Bacillus subtilis* (12). There is little doubt that the general instability of these activities contributes to the slow progress in this field. For example, Ruediger reports that, while preparations of pyruvate and α-ketoglutarate dehydrogenases from *S. faecalis* are stable to electrophoresis, isoelectric precipitation, and long centrifugation, the branched-chain ketoacid dehydrogenases are inactivated by these procedures. Both Wohlhueter and Harper and our laboratory lost rat liver mitochondrial

Table 1.   Soluble   Preparations   of   Branched-Chain α-Ketoacid   Dehydrogenases
Molecular weights are estimated.

	Source	Purification	Substrate Specificity	K_M	pH opt	M_W
MAMMALIAN:			KIC : KMV : KIV	Molar		Million
CONNELLY et.al.	BEEF	70x	I : I : O	KIC 3.5x10^{-3}	7.4	(2-4)
				KMV 2.5x10^{-3}	7.4	
GOEDDE et.al.	BEEF	5-20x	3 Specific Activities	KIC 2x10^{-5}	6.3	—
				KMV —	6.8	
				KIV 1.4x10^{-4}	7.4	
RUDIGER et.al.	HUMAN	30x	—	—	—	—
BACTERIAL:						
NAMBA et.al.	B. SUBTILIS	40x	I : I : 3	KMV 1.7x10^{-3}	6.5-7.0	(I)
RUDIGER et.al.	STREP. FAECALIS	90x	I : 3 : 60	—	—	—

activities during a variety of solubilization attempts, and the soluble beef liver preparation was found by us to be very sensitive to dilution, storage, temperature, and pH variations. At present, then, these contributions, although encouraging, provide a less than complete characterization of the branched-chain dehydrogenase activities in nature. Nevertheless, the collective findings of these research groups have established a basis for continued study of the problem.

Properties

Mitochondria from beef liver show all three branched-chain α-ketoacid dehydrogenase activities. Our laboratory was successful in obtaining a soluble extract that exhibited a high degree of substrate specificity for KIC-KMV. This contrasts with the activities found in whole mitochondria, where the greatest activity is shown with KIV, activities with KMV and KIC being half or less. This parallels the observations of Wohlhueter and Harper on rat liver mitochondria. It is also interesting to note that KIV was the best substrate in both soluble preparations from bacteria by Namba and Ruediger.

Particulate and soluble enzymes show varying pH optima, which generally center around pH 7.0. With beef liver mitochondria, the optimum is about 7.2 for each substrate (14). The optimum for soluble beef liver KMV-KIC dehydrogenase is about 7.4. Michaelis constants for the mitochondria activities are about 5×10^{-4} M (14) and are somewhat higher for the solubilized activity (3×10^{-3} M). Of particular interest is the substrate inhibition by KIC, reported for both beef liver (14) and rat liver (6) preparations. It is too early to speculate on the physiological significance of this phenomenon.

Mutual inhibitory effects among the branched-chain α-ketoacids have been shown to be competitive with beef liver mitochondrial dehydrogenases. Furthermore, these mutual influences and the inhibitory effects of these ketoacids on pyruvate and ketoglutaric dehydrogenases appear to be great enough to constitute a potentially significant physiological phenomenon (14). This interrelationship is probably of minimal consequence except in conditions that provide a surge of branched-chain amino acid, such as occurs after an increase in protein consumption. Such a surge could result in a condition in which the branched-chain ketoacids would promote their own catabolism, since at high levels their oxidations would be somewhat favored over those of pyruvate and α-ketoglutarate, until normal cellular levels were reattained. In the case of maple syrup urine disease, the marked build-up of branched-chain ketoacids could interrupt these central metabolic paths and lead to more serious consequences.

Cofactor Requirements

Perhaps the most obvious aspect of characterization of an enzyme activity that is suspected of being similar to the pyruvic dehydrogenase complex, with its five vitamin cofactors, is to ascertain the requirement for these and other cofactors. Although our knowledge in this respect is as yet incomplete, relatively recent findings tend to support earlier presumptions. In addition to any unsuspected cofactor requirements, the obvious targets for study are ThDP, lipoate, flavin, coenzyme A, and NAD. Since the last two compounds are reactants, it has been a relatively straightforward matter to ascertain their involvement in the oxidative decarboxylation of the branched-chain ketoacids. Thus NAD^+ has been shown to accept electrons from KIC, KMV, or KIV by our laboratory, using soluble beef liver preparations (8) or mitochondria (5); by Wohlhueter and Harper, using rat mitochondria; and by Namba et al. (12) and Ruediger et al. (11) with their bacterial preparations. Furthermore, the reduction of NAD^+ can be interrupted by ferricyanide, which presumably draws electrons from the hydroxyacyl-ThDP intermediate. Treatment of the soluble beef liver preparation at 55°C for 1 minute inactivates the NAD^+-linked but not the $Fe(CN)_6^{3-}$-linked activity (15). It has also been shown that NAD^+ is not replaceable by $NADP^+$ for either the mammalian or the bacterial enzymes.

In addition to the observation that coenzyme A is a required reactant, absolute evidence for its participation in the overall reaction derives from the isolation and identification of the acyl-CoA reaction product corresponding to the ketoacid substrate used. Thus Namba et al. (12) identified the hydroxamate of α-methylbutyrate derived from α-keto-β-methylvalerate, and Ruediger (11) also used this method as an assay.

Although there is substantial evidence for the requirements for NAD^+ and CoA in beef liver mitochondria and some evidence for the participation of NAD^+ in the cytosolic activity, the lack of CoA requirement for the latter may indicate that it is quite a different activity. It is also possible that sufficient CoA is available to obscure its need. Detailed studies were carried out in our laboratory to determine the effect of varied NAD^+ and CoA concentration on the KIC dehydrogenase activity of beef liver mitochondria. Apparent K_m's of 3.2×10^{-5} M for NAD^+ and 6.4×10^{-5} M for CoA were observed. Above 10^{-3} M, the latter exhibited an inhibitory effect. This was also observed to be the case with the soluble activity from $B.$ $subtilis$ (12). The addition of the presumptive cofactors lipoate, ThDP, and flavin to beef liver mitochondria produces no significant effect (8)—an observation expected in view of the generally tight binding of these compounds. However, some success has been reported in attempts to dissociate cofactors and subsequently reconstitute activity as a means of establishing that the cofactor is a vital component of the activity.

Ruediger reported that the enzymatic removal of lipoic acid from a soluble $S.$ $faecalis$ preparation resulted in loss of activity of the ketoacid dehydrogenase complex but that the decarboxylase and lipoate dehydrogenase remained active. The lipoic acid-dependent transacylase could be reactivated with lipoate and lipoate-activating enzyme to restore about 50% of the original activity of the complex (11). A similar finding was reported for human kidney enzyme, although the reconstitution was only 15% (10). Regular inhibition by sulfhydryl reagents such as arsenite and PCMB also supports the possible role of lipoate, although these results could as well relate to the involvement of sulfhydryl groups on protein components and are thus inconclusive for the question of lipoate.

Participation of ThDP

Although no progress has been reported regarding the possible role of flavin, definitive success has been achieved in our laboratory in establishing the participation of ThDP in branched-chain oxidative decarboxylation. This compound generally remains tightly bound to the enzymes with which it is associated. However, Morey and Juni (16) and others have shown that bound ThDP can be dissociated from enzymes by incubation of the enzyme solution at alkaline pH.

Johnson, in our laboratory, employed two methods to remove ThDP from soluble KMV dehydrogenase (Fig. 2). Method I involved the preliminary removal of Mg^{2+} by precipitation of the magnesium ammonium phosphate complex at pH 8.5. The enzyme protein was then precipitated with 55% $(NH_4)_2SO_4$, leaving the dissociated ThDP in the supernatant fraction. After repeating the last step, the protein was dissolved at pH 7.4. As shown in Fig. 3, this treatment markedly reduced the activity of the enzyme. Addition of Mg^{2+} or ThDP alone increases the activity slightly, but in concert these agents nearly triple the activity. The lower bars represent the same experiment with a more highly purified KMV dehydrogenase.

Method II (Fig. 2) also employs the pH 8.5 dissociation of ThDP, but in this procedure Mg^{2+} and ThDP are separated from the enzyme by use of a column containing Sephadex G-25, a low-molecular-weight exclusion limit gel. After precipitation of the eluted enzyme with $(NH_4)_2SO_4$, the enzyme was dissolved in phosphate buffer at pH 7.4. As shown in the second set of bars in Fig. 4, gel filtration at pH 7.4 does not alter the activity significantly.

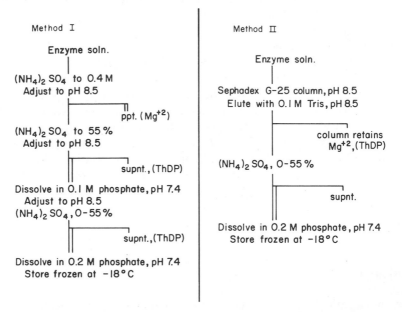

Figure 2.   Resolution of KIC:KMV dehydrogenase: Mg^{2+} and ThDP.

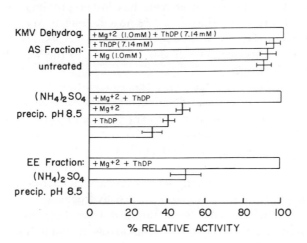

Figure 3. Effect of exogenous Mg^{2+} and ThDP on α-Ketoacid dehydrogenases: Method I. Activities of treated enzyme are relative to fully reconstituted activity, not to untreated enzyme.

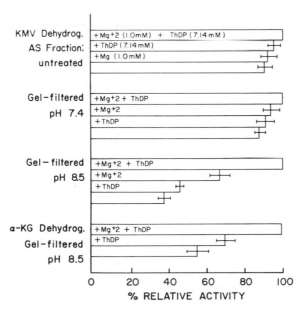

Figure 4. Effect of exogenous Mg^{2+} and ThDP on α-Ketoacid dehydrogenases: Method II. (See legend to Figure 3.)

However, at pH 8.5 the eluted enzyme has lost approximately 60% of its activity. That this technique has in fact removed requisite Mg^{2+} and ThDP is shown by the reconstitution of the activity by these factors. The bottom series of bars shows the applicability of this technique to the well-characterized ketoglutarate dehydrogenase.

It appears that Mg^{2+} most certainly acts to facilitate the binding of ThDP to the enzyme (Fig. 5). Here Mg^{2+} concentrations between 0.7 and 1.0 mM appear to provide optimum conditions for reconstitution of resolved KMV dehydrogenase with ThDP, in excess.

By way of summary we have seen the following:

1. Branched-chain ketoacid dehydrogenase activities exist and are separate from pyruvate and α-ketoglutarate dehydrogenases.
2. Soluble activities have been obtained from both mammalian and bacterial sources, an observation that emphasizes the ubiquitous character of these activities.
3. In mammals the activity appears to be predominantly in the liver and is localized in mitochondria. Some decarboxylase activity has been observed in the cytosol.
4. Thiamine has been shown to be a vital constituent of the branched-chain dehydrogenases, and, with the exception of flavin, the cofactor requirements appear to parellel those of pyruvate dehydrogenase.
5. The mutually inhibitory influences among the α-ketoacids appear to provide a potentially significant physiological regulatory mechanism.

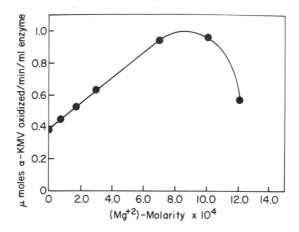

Figure 5. Effect of Mg^{2+} on beef liver KMV-KIC dehydrogenase in the presence of excess ThDP.

Acknowledgment

This work has been supported by grants from the National Science Foundation, the current grant being GB-12934.

References

1. J. Menkes, P. Hurst, and J. Craig, *Pediatrics,* **14,** 472 (1954).

2. L. J. Reed, in B. L. Horecker and E. R. Stadtman, Eds., *Current Topics in Cellular Metabolism,* Vol. 1, Academic Press, New York, 1969, p. 233.

3. T. Nayakama, T. Kanzaki, Y. Fukuyoshi, Y. Sakurai, K. Koike, T. Suematsu, and M. Koike, *J. Biol. Chem.,* **244,** 3660 (1969).

4. C. J. Gubler, *J. Biol. Chem.,* **236,** 3112 (1961).

5. W. A. Johnson and J. L. Connelly, *Biochemistry,* **11,** 1967 (1972).

6. R. M. Wohlhueter and Λ. E. Harper, *J. Biol. Chem.,* **245,** 2391 (1970).

7. M. Klingenberg, *Eur. J. Biochem.,* **13,** 247 (1970).

8. J. L. Connelly, D. J. Danner, and J. A. Bowden, *J. Biol. Chem.,* **243,** 1198 (1968).

9. H. W. Goedde and W. Keller, in W. L. Nyhan Ed., *Amino Acid Metabolism and Genetic Variation,* McGraw-Hill Book Company, New York, 1967, p. 191.

10. N. W. Ruediger, U. Langenbeck, D. Brackertz, and W. Goedde, *Biochim. Biophys. Acta,* **264,** 220 (1972).

11. N. W. Ruediger, U. Langenbeck, and H. W. Goedde, *Hoppe-Seyler's Z. Physiol. Chem.,* **353,** 875 (1972).

12. Y. Namba, K. Yoshizawa, A Ejima, T. Hayashi, and T. Kaneda, *J. Biol. Chem.,* **244,** 4437 (1969).

13. J. A. Bowden and J. L. Connelly, *J. Biol. Chem.,* **243,** 3526 (1968).

14. W. A. Johnson and J. L. Connelly, *Biochemistry,* **11,** 2416 (1972).

15. J. A. Bowden, unpublished data.

16. A. V. Morey and E. Juni, *J. Biol. Chem.,* **243,** 3009 (1968).

DISCUSSION

Chapters 3 and 4

Dr. Cooper. I have a vague recollection that four CO_2 fixation reactions exist which involve either pyruvate or phosphoenolpyruvate in a stereometric assay. Can you differentiate among them as to which is inhibited by the ketoacids?

Dr. Patel. Yes, it is possible to show that the reaction which we have measured is specific in terms of CO_2 fixation in the presence of pyruvate and that it requires acetyl-CoA, which is an obligatory cofactor for pyruvate carboxylase but not for other enzymes. There are four reactions by which CO_2 can be fixed in brain (L. Salganicoff and R. E. Koeppe; *J. Biol. Chem.*, **243**, 3416, 1968). Phosphoenolpyruvate carboxykinase is a GTP-requiring reaction, and the rate of CO_2 fixation by this enzyme is extremely low in rat brain (M. S. Patel, *J. Neurochem.*, **22**, 717, 1974). NADP-malate dehydrogenase and NADP-isocitrate dehydrogenase are reversible enzymes; however, the rate of CO_2 fixation is about one-tenth that of corresponding decarboxylation reactions. This suggests that these enzymes operate in the direction of the decarboxylation under physiological conditions. Hence a key enzyme responsible for CO_2 fixation in brain mitochondria is pyruvate carboxylase.

Dr. Dreyfus. Yesterday Dr. Cooper and I were talking about oxaloacetic acid and were wondering what the role of CO_2 fixation in the brain might be since the brain is not operating on gluconeogenesis. Is this reaction in brain of real importance? In regard to maple syrup urine disease, it is most probable that leucine is the offending amino acid; that is, the higher the leucine levels, the more mentally retarded the patient tends to be. It is of interest that isocaproic acid seems to inhibit pyruvic decarboxylation to the greatest degree (P. M. Dreyfus, and Prensky, W.).

Dr. Patel. Let me comment on the second statement first. It has been shown that α-ketoisocaproate does not inhibit the pyruvate dehydrogenase complex (J. B. Clark and J. M. Land, *Biochem. J.,* **140,** 25, 1974). The inhibitory effect of α-ketoisocaproate on the decarboxylation of [1-^{14}C] pyruvate by brain homogenate as reported here is consistent with the inhibition by α-ketoisocaproate of the transport of pyruvate across the mitochondrial membrane (J. M. Land and J. B. Clark, *FEBS Lett.,* **44,** 348, 1974). α-Ketoisocaproate inhibits the α-ketoglutarate dehydrogenase complex. In view of the high circulating concentrations of α-ketoisocaproate together with two other branched-chain keto acids, it is very likely that they would effectively inhibit the metabolism of both pyruvate and α-ketoglutarate in the brain. This might be one of the reasons why mental retardation is much more severe in cases of maple syrup urine disease than in phenylketonuric patients.

As for CO_2 fixation, it has been generally considered that pyruvate carboxylase is only a gluconeogenic enzyme. However, in adipose tissue, this enzyme also plays an important role in lipogenesis. (F. J. Ballard and R. W. Hanson, *J. Lipid Res.,* **8,** 73, 1967). In order to transport the acetyl moiety of acetyl-CoA as citrate from mitochondria, oxaloacetate is required. Any oxaloacetate lost is replenished by pyruvate carboxylase in the mitochondria. Recently we have also shown that pyruvate carboxylase plays a similar role in terms of replenishing C_4 compounds in rat brain mitochondria (M. S. Patel and S. M. Tilghman, *Biochem. J.,* **132,** 185, 1973).

Dr. Elsas. I want to make one clinical correlation in support of Dr. Patel's observations, namely, that the branched-chain ketoacids have a serious effect on the infant's brain. In maple syrup urine disease, where the branched-chain ketoacids (usually ketoisocaproic acid) are elevated in the millimolar range, there appears to be an acute effect that results in cessation of central nervous system function and development, as compared to a chronic effect seen in phenylketonuria, where an abnormality of myelin development occurs over a prolonged period of time.

I would like to ask Dr. Connelly a question relating to the relative requirements for thiamine diphosphate among the three branched-chain ketoacid decarboxylases. I noticed that in the experiments in which ThDP was not required for reconstitution it was ketoisocaproic acid that was used as substrate, but where ThDP was required after alkaline treatment KMV was used as substrate. My question is, Do you find a qualitative difference for ThDP requirement among the three branched-chain ketoacids?

Dr. Connelly. I am afraid that I have to apologize for calling the same enzyme by two different names. No, we have not investigated the ease with which ThDP can be removed from two different activities. We used a soluble enzyme that was active with both KMV and KIC, and that enzyme showed the ThDP requirement for both substrates. I would like to make another comment regarding Dr. Patel's work.

It has been shown by two or more laboratories that the effect of branched-chain ketoacids as inhibitors on all ketoacid dehydrogenases is competitive with the exception of ketoglutaric dehydrogenase, where we find a mixed type of inhibition. You mentioned, Dr. Patel, that it was recently shown that pyruvate is carried into the mitochondria by a specific transport mechanism. I do not know that this has been shown for α-ketoglutarate, but I would not be surprised if there were a mechanism for it. The fact that the results of inhibitor studies indicate that ketoglutarate is found to be inhibited by a competitive mechanism suggests that (and this has been speculated) the transport of the ketoglutarate across the membrane may constitute a significant or even a rate-limiting inhibitor site for α-ketoglutarate dehydrogenase. I am wondering whether this speculated possibility might account for the higher sensitivity of ketoglutarate dehydrogenase to branched-chain ketoacid inhibition than we see with pyruvate dehydrogenase.

Dr. Patel. It is quite possible; however, there are no available data to document this phenomenon. We have some preliminary evidence to suggest that α-ketoglutarate is transported by a specific carrier system across the inner mitochondrial membrane in rat brain (M. S. Patel, *Biochem. J.,* **144,** 91, 1974).

Dr. Blass. May I ask Dr. Connelly whether the apparent K_m for ThDP has been measured? The reason for this question is that we did not find a significant accumulation of branched amino acids or branched-chain ketoacids in the urine of thiamine-deficient rats. It is a crude approximation to go from the soluble enzyme to the intact animal, but I wondered whether the K_m's for the various thiamine-dependent enzymes might give us some clues as to which enzyme would be affected first as the animal became progressively more deficient in thiamine.

Dr. Connelly. That is a very good question. Unfortunately we have not done K_m work on that aspect.

Dr. Brin. I think that, if you want to study the appearance of or the presence of branched-chain ketoacids in thiamine deficiency, you might give them a load of the amino acid. This will stimulate the appearance of the derivative.

Dr. Itokawa. I have a minor question to ask of Dr. Connelly. Does cadmium inhibit α-ketoacid dehydrogenase? If so, at what concentrations? In Japan we have a pollution problem with cadmium.

Dr. Connelly.   Yes, effective levels of cadmium are upward to millimolar amounts.

TWO

THIAMINE-METABOLISM—GENERAL

5. Experimental Studies on the Relationships Between Thiamine and Divalent Cations, Calcium and Magnesium

MOTONORI FUJIWARA, M.D.
YOSHINORI ITOKAWA, M.D.
MIEKO KIMURA, Ph.D.

Department of Hygiene
Faculty of Medicine
Kyoto University
Kyoto, Japan

Many studies on amyotrophic lateral sclerosis (ALS) have been pursued, but a conclusive cause has not yet been identified. In 1964 Steinke and Tyler (1) suggested that an association may exist between ALS and abnormal carbohydrate metabolism. Pyruvate represents a focal point in intracellular carbohydrate metabolism, which may be deranged in ALS, as it is in some metal intoxications, notably in arsenic but also to some degree in lead and mercury poisoning. However, this opinion has not been supported by the study of Currier and Haerer (2). In 1961 Kusui (3) reported that ALS was more prevalent in the southern part of Kii peninsula. After that report Kimura began a large-scale survey in this area (4). We have collaborated with him and have examined the thiamine metabolism of ALS patients. Figure 1 shows the results of the thiamine tolerance test that we obtained.

It is clear that, despite a history of low excretion of thiamine on the day before the thiamine tolerance test, the patients excreted a very high percentage of the injected thiamine during the 24 hours after the test. These

63

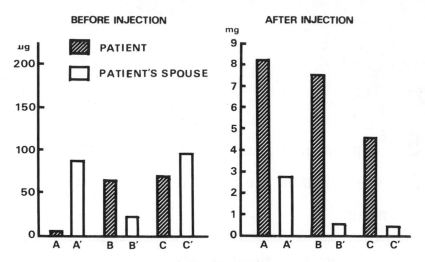

Figure 1. Urinary excretion of thiamine within 24 hours after injection of 10 mg thiamine.

observations suggest that ALS patients have lost the ability to utilize thiamine. Furthermore, Kimura discovered that the drinking water from the rivers of the Kii peninsula has, on the average, a much lower content of the metals magnesium and calcium than does river water elsewhere in Japan. As a result, the hair and nails of the ALS patients had a lower content of these metals than do the hair and nails of the average Japanese. Kimura treated the ALS patients with high doses (50 to 100 mg) of allithiamine [a lipotropic thiamine derivative discovered by Fujiwara (5)], 500 mg of

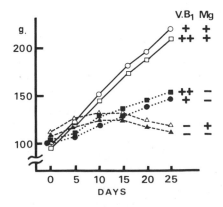

Figure 2. Growth curves (mean of five rats).

Table 1. Composition of Basal Diet

	Amount, g/100 g diet
Casein (vitamin-free)[a]	15.00
Sucrose	68.29
Olive oil	10.00
Salt mixture (calcium- and magnesium-free[b]	1.59
Cellulose	2.00
Vitamin mixture (thiamine-free)[c]	0.50
Choline chloride	0.20

	g/100 g diet
$CaHPO_4$	1.29
$CaCO_3$	0.53
$MgCl_2 \cdot 6H_2O$	0.60
	mg/100 g diet
Thiamine$\cdot$HCl	0.50

[a] Purchased from Nutritional Biochemical Corporation, Clcv(land, Ohio.

[b] The Ca- and Mg-free salt mixture contained (mg/100 g diet): NaCl, 173; $Na_2HPO_4 \cdot H_2O$, 343; K_2HPO_4, 9a5; $Fe(C_6H_5O_7) \cdot 3H_2O$, 115; $MnSO_4$, 4; KI, 0.3; $CuSO_4 \cdot 5H_2O$, 0.3; $CoCl_2 \cdot 6H_2O$, 0.3; $ZnCO_3$, 0.3; $K_2Al_2(SO_4)_4 \cdot 24H_2O$, 0.3.

[c] The thiamine-free vitamin mixture had the following contents (μg/ 100 g diet): riboflavin, 750; nicotinic acid, 5000; pyridoxine, 500; cyanocobalamin, 5; pantothenic acid, 2500; folic acid, 250; biotin, 40; ascorbic acid, 18,750; α-tocopherol, 000; menadione, 500; inositol, 9000; retinyl palmitate, 6250 I.U.; ergocalciferol, 500 I.U.

magnesium oxide, and 1 gram of calcium carbonate per day. According to his reports, this treatment had successful results: one patient was able to walk again after 2 years in bed; another became strong enough to resume his work; and all patients survived, at least for several years. Although we know that ALS must have multiple causes, our experience stimulated us to concentrate our studies on the relationships between thiamine and metals such as magnesium and calcium, aided by the atomic absorption spectrophotometer, which has only recently become available to us.

1. Relationship Between Thiamine and Magnesium

As the first experimental design we fixed calcium and thiamine or magnesium, depleted alone or together:

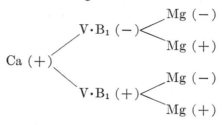

Rats of the Wistar strain, weighing from 60 to 100 grams were used. These were housed in individual stainless steel cages with raised wire bottoms. The composition of the basal diet is shown in Table 1. For the magnesium- or calcium-deficient diet, the magnesium or calcium in Table 1 was eliminated from the basal diet. The rats drank distilled deionized water *ad libitum*.

GROWTH

Figure 2 shows the growth curves. Growth was markedly inhibited by magnesium deficiency.

SEROTONIN METABOLISM

Vasodilation and erythema in ears or nose, as described by Kruse et al. (6), was observed as the first clinical symptom. It was followed by excitability or

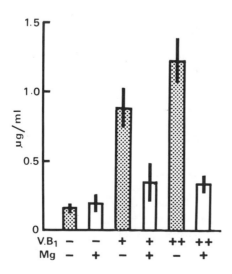

Figure 3. Blood serotonin level (mean of five rats).

convulsion. However, this symptom was not found in the rats fed a diet deficient in both magnesium and thiamine. After 4 weeks of applying these dietary regimens, blood was collected into a syringe from the descending aorta of the animals, which were anesthetized with sodium pentobarbital. Various tissues were removed, and analyses were performed.

Figure 3 shows the serotonin levels in serum of rats. There were great increases in the serotonin levels of rats fed magnesium-deficient, thiamine-supplemented diets. However, no increase of serotonin was found in the rats fed a diet deficient in both magnesium and thiamine, that is, a diet corresponding to the one which produced the symptoms of erythema or convulsion. According to Belanger et al. (7), the vasodilation of ears or nose of the magnesium-deficient rats was due to the endogenous histamine released from the mast cells destroyed as a result of magnesium deficiency. In our experiments, we also have found an elevation of histamine in liver, but the elevation of histamine in serum was not as high as was that of serotonin. In any case, which is the real cause of vasodilation, serotonin or histamine? To clarify this, we injected either histamine or serotonin (10 mg/kg body weight) into rats; vasodilation of ears or nose was observed only in the rats receiving the serotonin injection. Thus we believe now that the vasodilation in rats with magnesium deficiency is due to the increase of serotonin rather than histamine in serum.

To elucidate the mechanism of the elevation of serotonin, a study was carried out for the examination of the enzymes, one of which is the serotonin formation enzyme, namely, aromatic L-amino acid decarboxylase, and the other the serotonin-destroying enzyme, namely, monoamine

Table 2. L-Aromatic Amino Acid Decarboxylase Activity in Stomach, Liver, and Brain[a]

	Diet		Activity, $m\mu M$ 5-hydroxytryptamine/(mg protein)(min)		
Group	Thiamine	Magnesium	Stomach	Liver	Brain
1	Deficient	Deficient	4.96 ± 1.19	71.9 ± 5.4	16.9 ± 1.9
2	Deficient	Sufficient	4.73 ± 0.98	68.8 ± 2.3	16.7 ± 1.1
3	Adequate	Deficient	5.07 ± 0.68	87.6 ± 7.2	16.8 ± 0.3
4	Adequate	Sufficient	5.65 ± 0.83	91.9 ± 10.2	15.2 ± 0.9
5	Excess	Deficient	5.12 ± 0.38	89.5 ± 6.2	17.4 ± 1.1
6	Excess	Sufficient	5.04 ± 0.39	90.6 ± 5.7	17.5 ± 0.3

[a] Values represent mean $\pm$ S.E. of six rats.

Table 3.   Monoamine Oxidase Activity in Stomach, Liver, and Brain[a]

| | Diet | | Activity, mμM 5-HT-^{14}C decomposed/(mg protein)(min) | | |
Group	Thiamine	Magnesium	Stomach	Liver	Brain
1	Deficient	Deficient	0.177 ± 0.009	1.44 ± 0.07	0.72 ± 0.05
2	Deficient	Sufficient	0.175 ± 0.009	1.34 ± 0.06	0.78 ± 0.04
3	Adequate	Deficient	0.128 ± 0.011*[b]	1.15 ± 0.04*	0.74 ± 0.04
4	Adequate	Sufficient	0.160 ± 0.007	1.36 ± 0.08	0.77 ± 0.05
5	Excess	Deficient	0.121 ± 0.007*	1.10 ± 0.04*	0.78 ± 0.03
6	Excess	Sufficient	0.164 ± 0.007	1.41 ± 0.06	0.72 ± 0.09

[a] Values represent mean ± S.E. of six rats.
[b] Asterisk denotes significant difference from group 4, using Student's t test ($p < .05$), in each tissue.

oxidase. L-Amino acid decarboxylase activity was determined by the method of Lovenberg (8), and monoamine oxidase activity by the method of Wurtman and Axelrod (9).

The aromatic L-amino acid decarboxylase activity in stomach, liver, and brain is shown in Table 2. Neither magnesium supplementation nor magnesium depletion had an effect on this activity.

Table 3 shows the monoamine oxidase activity in stomach, liver, and brain. There were clear decreases of activity in both the stomach and the liver of rats fed the magnesium-deficient and thiamine-supplemented diet,

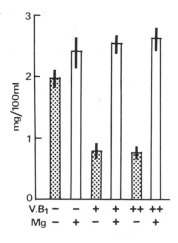

Figure 4.   Magnesium level in serum (mean of five rats).

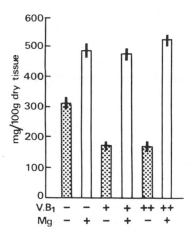

Figure 5. Magnesium level in femur (mean of five rats).

although the activity in the brain was only slightly affected. In this case also, there was no change of monoamine oxidase activities in the rats fed on both the magnesium- and the thiamine-depleted diet. From these facts it may be inferred that the elevation of serotonin was due to the decrease in activity of monoamine oxidase, though this may not be the only cause.

CHANGES IN MINERALS

For the determination of calcium and magnesium, tissues were weighed, dried in an incubator for 48 hours at 100 to 105°C, and stored for 48 hours

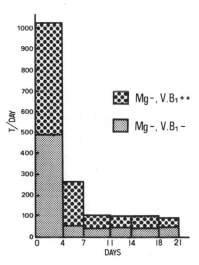

Figure 6. Urinary excretion of magnesium (paired feeding; mean of four rats).

in a desiccator containing phosphorus pentoxide. Serum and tissues thus treated were digested to a nearly colorless solution with nitric acid, and digestion was completed with perchloric acid to yield a colorless solution in the usual manner. Concentrations of magnesium and calcium were determined by atomic absorption spectrophotometry (Shimadzu, Model AA610, Japan).

The magnesium levels in the serum and femur are shown in Figs. 4 and 5. It is natural for the magnesium levels to be low in the magnesium-deficient rats, but this tendency was mitigated by thiamine deficiency in the same way as was the serotonin or monamine oxidase activity.

To solve the problem raised by the decrease in magnesium, especially in rats receiving supplementary thiamine, we examined rat feces and urine for excreted magnesium. Figure 6 shows the results of these experiments. We found a greater amount of magnesium in the urine of rats fed a magnesium-deficient and thiamine-excessive diet than in that of rats fed a diet deficient in both magnesium and thiamine. In other words, excess thiamine had accelerated magnesium excretion in the urine by forming a complex of thiamine and magnesium in the body.

Table 4 shows the calcium concentrations in various tissues. A marked elevation was found in the kidney in the magnesium-deficient rats, as many researchers have already reported (10–14). The calcium level of serum was elevated, but that of the femur was lowered.

THIAMINE METABOLISM

Thiamine levels in various tissues were determined by the fluorometric procedure of Fujiwara and Matsui (15). Figure 7 shows the thiamine levels

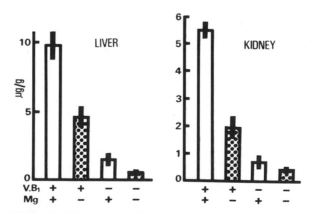

Figure 7.   Thiamine levels in liver and kidney (mean of six rats).

Table 4. Calcium Concentration in Various Tissues and Serum[a]

Diet		Concentration								
V.B₁	Mg	Brain, mg/100 g[b]	Heart, mg/100 g	Liver, mg/100 g	Spleen, mg/100 g	Kidney, mg/100 g	Testicles, mg/100 g	Muscles, mg/100 g	Femur, g/100 g	Serum, mg/100 ml
−	−	10.6 ± 0.7	15.4 ± 0.9	8.9 ± 0.3	22.1 ± 2.7	114.2 ± 22.7*[c]	22.0 ± 0.9	18.4 ± 1.2*	23.9 ± 0.8*	15.0 ± 1.3*
−	+	9.7 ± 1.3	13.4 ± 0.8	9.2 ± 0.4	24.7 ± 4.9	20.8 ± 5.4	21.6 ± 1.2	13.0 ± 1.2	28.4 ± 0.7	12.6 ± 0.5
+	−	10.2 ± 1.1	18.2 ± 0.8*	9.5 ± 0.6	19.5 ± 3.1	367.8 ± 83.3*	22.4 ± 0.9	22.4 ± 0.8*	21.1 ± 0.7*	16.7 ± 0.4*
+	+	10.6 ± 1.5	12.0 ± 0.3	8.9 ± 0.4	22.9 ± 3.6	16.3 ± 2.1	22.3 ± 1.8	10.0 ± 0.4	28.3 ± 1.2	12.7 ± 0.8
++	−	10.5 ± 0.5	17.7 ± 1.2*	9.4 ± 0.3	21.5 ± 4.2	436.7 ± 96.9*	21.7 ± 1.2	21.8 ± 1.5*	20.9 ± 0.8*	17.1 ± 1.2*
++	+	11.1 ± 1.2	10.9 ± 0.7	9.3 ± 0.7	21.0 ± 2.9	16.6 ± 5.3	21.5 ± 1.7	11.4 ± 2.6	28.6 ± 0.6	13.1 ± 1.0

[a] Values represent mean ± S.E. of five rats.
[b] Milligrams per 100 g of dry tissue weight.
[c] Asterisk denotes significant difference from group 4, using Student's t test ($p < .05$), in each tissue.

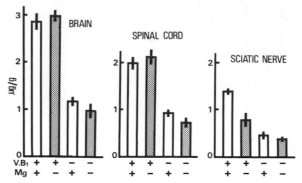

Figure 8.   Thiamine levels in various nervous tissues (mean of six rats).

in liver and kidney. It is worth noting that magnesium deficiency decreases the thiamine concentrations in these organs.

Thiamine levels in nervous tissues are shown in Fig. 8. Magnesium deficiency seems to have no effect on thiamine levels in the brain.

From previous data, it had been supposed that magnesium-deficient rats were in a state of thiamine deficiency. To confirm this, we applied the tolerance test with labeled thiamine to these rats. Radioactivity was determined by adding 0.2 ml of urine to 20 ml of counting solution, which consisted of toluene-Triton X 100-PPO-dimethyl POPOP (16), using a liquid scintillation counter (Nuclear Chicago, Mark II).

Figure 9 shows the results of urinary excretion of ^{14}C-thiamine 24 hours after 1 mg of ^{14}C-thiamine was injected. The highest excretion was found in the rats fed on the thiamine-plus-magnesium-supplemented diet; the lowest

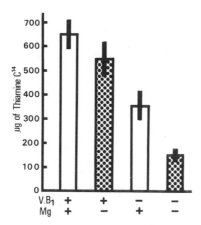

Figure 9.   Radioactive thiamine excreted in urine 24 hours after injection of 1 mg of C^{14}-thiamine (mean of three rats).

excretion occurred when both thiamine and magnesium were depleted, as expected. It may safely be concluded that the state of thiamine deficiency in ALS patients and in rats fed a thiamine- and magnesium-deficient diet is not the same. The ALS patients excreted a high percentage of thiamine in the urine, whereas in the case of the rats the excretion of thiamine was completely the reverse of that of the ALS patients. In other words, we were not able to maintain the rats in a state similar to ALS.

Transketolase activity in the tissues and blood cells of these rats was assayed by the method of Brin et al. (17), with and without *in vitro* addition of thiamine diphosphate (ThDP).

As shown in Table 5, transketolase activity in red blood cells, brain, spinal cord, and liver decreased markedly in the thiamine-deficient rats. Regardless of the organ, *in vitro* addition of ThDP to tissue homogenates from thiamine-deficient, magnesium-sufficient rats resulted in a marked recovery of the transketolase activity. However, this was not observed in rats deficient in both thiamine and magnesium. Fennelly et al. (18) reported that the addition of ThDP to red blood cell hemolysates further reduced the transketolase activity in malnourished alcoholic patients with normal livers, but frequently this effect was not seen on transketolase activity in alcoholics with cirrhotic livers. Of great interest is the fact that the latter condition is similar with respect to transketolase activity to the situation seen in rats deficient in both thiamine and magnesium.

2. Relationship Between Thiamine and Calcium

As the second experiment, dietary magnesium was fixed and either thiamine or calcium or both were depleted:

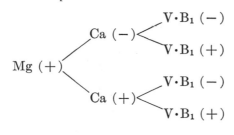

GROWTH

Figure 10 shows the growth curves. Little effect of calcium deficiency was observed.

Table 5. Transketolase Activity[a]

Group	Diet Thiamine	Diet Magnesium	In Vitro Addition	Activity, μM hexose produced/(g protein)(hr) Brain	Spinal Cord	Liver	Blood Cells
1	Deficient	Deficient	(A) None	210 ± 12*[b]	199 ± 25*	482 ± 110*	12.8 ± 2.8*
			(B) + ThDP	224 ± 17*	210 ± 28*	500 ± 100*	15.2 ± 2.6*
2	Deficient	Sufficient	(A) None	200 ± 15*	233 ± 12*	558 ± 61*	17.2 ± 3.0*
			(B) + ThDP	298 ± 20*†[c]	360 ± 15*†	998 ± 105*†	33.3 ± 1.5*†
3	Sufficient	Deficient	(A) None	480 ± 32	493 ± 40	1448 ± 166	45.6 ± 5.0
			(B) + ThDP	485 ± 33	499 ± 32	1495 ± 148	49.5 ± 4.7
4	Sufficient	Sufficient	(A) None	486 ± 32	450 ± 21	2152 ± 133	51.8 ± 6.6
			(B) + ThDP	483 ± 33	454 ± 30	2230 ± 185	60.0 ± 5.8

[a] Values represent mean ± S.E. of five rats.

[b] Asterisk denotes significant difference ($p < .05$) as compared with group 4.

[c] Dagger denotes significant difference ($p < .05$) as compared with (A) in each group.

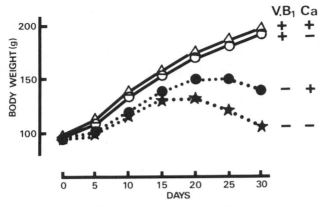

Figure 10.   Growth curves (mean of five rats).

CALCIUM LEVELS

Figure 11 shows the calcium levels in various nervous tissues. No marked change in calcium levels is evident.

THIAMINE LEVELS

Figure 12 shows the thiamine levels of liver. Little effect of calcium deficiency was found.

The concentrations of thiamine in various nervous tissues are shown in Fig. 13. Marked effects of calcium deficiency were found, especially in the

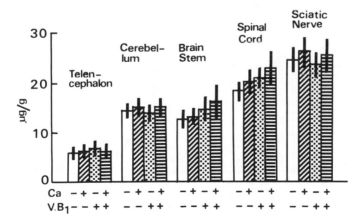

Figure 11.   Calcium level in nervous system of rats (mean of five rats).

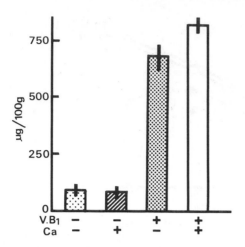

Figure 12. Thiamine level in liver (mean of five rats).

telencephalon and the brain stem. Calcium deficiency appears to have an effect on the thiamine concentration of the nervous system.

3. Relationship Between Calcium and Magnesium

To clarify the relationships among thiamine, calcium, and magnesium in greater detail, the third experiment was conducted. In this experiment,

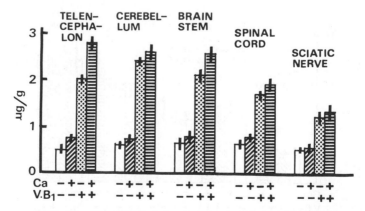

Figure 13. Thiamine levels in nervous system (mean of five rats).

thiamine was fixed, and calcium and magnesium were shifted:

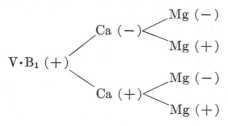

$$\text{V} \cdot \text{B}_1 \,(+) \begin{cases} \text{Ca}\,(-) \begin{cases} \text{Mg}\,(-) \\ \text{Mg}\,(+) \end{cases} \\ \text{Ca}\,(+) \begin{cases} \text{Mg}\,(-) \\ \text{Mg}\,(+) \end{cases} \end{cases}$$

SEROTONIN LEVELS

Figure 14 shows the serotonin levels in blood. Serotonin was affected by magnesium deficiency only.

THIAMINE METABOLISM

We have confirmed that there are two types of tissues, one reacting to calcium deficiency, the other to magnesium deficiency, in terms of an effect on the thiamine levels.
Figure 15 shows that the thiamine level of the blood was decreased by magnesium deficiency.

The thiamine levels of heart, liver, and kidney are shown in Fig. 16. Magnesium deficiency had a marked effect on the thiamine levels of liver and kidney, while the thiamine levels of the heart were clearly affected by calcium deficiency.

Figure 17 shows that the thiamine levels of the various nervous tissues were affected by calcium deficiency.

It seems certain that the nervous system and the heart, a series of excitable organs, so to speak, are likely to be affected by calcium deficiency, and that the other organs are likely to be affected by magnesium deficiency.

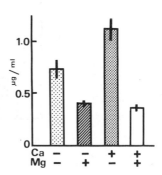

Figure 14.   Blood serotonin level (mean of six rats).

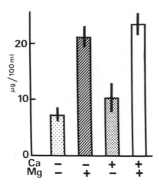

Figure 15.   Blood thiamine level (mean of six rats).

BODY TEMPERATURE

In the course of this study, we found unexpectedly that body temperature rose markedly in the rats fed the calcium-deficient and magnesium-supplemented diet, as shown in Fig. 18.

There are many references (e.g., 19–21) regarding the relationships between body temperature and calcium. These reports reveal that body temperature was lowered by calcium when it was infused into the cerebrospinal fluid or intraventricularly. However, no cases in which body temperature was elevated by low calcium status, as occurred in this experiment, have been reported.

Figure 19 shows the calcium and magnesium levels in the brain stem.

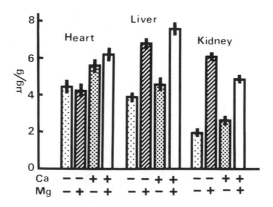

Figure 16.   Thiamine levels in various organs (mean of six rats).

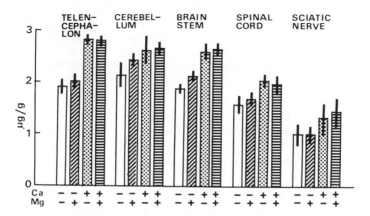

Figure 17. Thiamine levels in nervous system (mean of six rats).

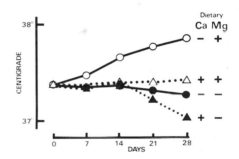

Figure 18. Body temperature (mean of six rats).

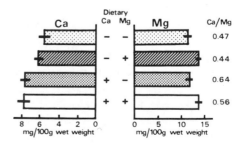

Figure 19. Calcium and magnesium levels in brain stem (mean of six rats).

From these we arrived at the following hypothesis. Body temperature is affected by the ratio of calcium and magnesium. When the Ca/Mg ratio in the brain becomes low, the body temperature rises; when the ratio becomes high, the temperature decreases (22).

4. Conclusion

There are many relationships between thiamine, magnesium, and calcium in the diet. Thiamine in the body is released by magnesium deficiency. Thiamine in the heart and nervous system is likely to be affected by calcium deficiency; in other organs, such as the liver, kidneys, and blood, thiamine is likely to be affected by magnesium deficiency. For these reasons, both calcium and magnesium are important components of a diet aimed at providing adequate thiamine nutrition.

References

1. J. Steinke and H. R. Tyler, *Metabolism,* **13,** 1376 (1964).
2. D. Currier and A. F. Haerer, *Arch. Environ. Health,* **17,** 712 (1968).
3. K. Kusui, *Nippon Seishin Shinkei Gaku Zasshi,* **64,** 85 (1961).
4. K. Kimura, *Wakayama Med. Rept.,* **64,** 177 (1965).
5. M. Fujiwara, H. Watanabe, and K. Matsui, *J. Biochem.,* **41,** 29 (1954).
6. H. D. Kruse, E. R. Orent, and E. V. McCollum, *J. Biol. Chem.,* **96,** 519 (1932).
7. L. F. Belanger, G. A. Van Erkel, and A. Jackerow, *Science,* **126,** 29 (1957).
8. W. Lovenberg, in S. P. Colowick and N. O. Kaplan, Eds., *Methods in Enzymology,* Vol. 17B, Academic Press, New York, 1971, p. 652.
9. R. J. Wurtman and J. Axelrod, *Biochem. Pharmacol.,* **12,** 1439 (1963).
10. R. Whang and L. G. Welt, *J. Clin. Invest.,* **42,** 305 (1963).
11. L. G. Welt, *Yale J. Biol. Med.,* **36,** 325 (1964).
12. E. E. Schneeberger and A. B. Morrison, *Lab. Invest.,* **14,** 674 (1965).
13. R. M. Firbes, *J. Nutr.,* **88,** 403 (1966).
14. H. Battifora, R. Eisenstein, G. H. Liang, and P. McCreary, *Am. J. Pathol.,* **48,** 421 (1966).
15. M. Fujiwara and K. Matsui, *Anal. Chem.,* **25,** 810 (1953).
16. M. S. Patterson and G. C. Greene, *Anal. Chem.,* **37,** 854 (1965).
17. M. Brin, M. Tai, A. S. Ostashever, and H. Kalinsky, *J. Nutr.,* **71,** 273 (1960).
18. J. Fennelly, O. Frank, H. Baker, and C. M. Leevy, *Am. J. Clin. Nutr.,* **20,** 946 (1967).
19. R. D. Myers, W. L. Veale, and T. L. Yaksh, *J. Physiol.,* **217,** 381 (1971).
20. W. Feldberg, R. D. Myers, and W. L. Veale, *J. Physiol.,* **207,** 403 (1970).
21. J. L. Hanegan and B. A. Williams, *Science,* **181,** 663 (1973).
22. Y. Itokawa, C. Tanaka, and M. Fujiwara, *J. Appl. Physiol.* **37,** 835 (1974).

DISCUSSION

Chapter 5

Dr. Barchi. We recognize clinically that there are a number of other causes of syndromes that present like amyotrophic lateral sclerosis with a combination of upper motor and lower motor neuron signs. This may occur in cases of arsenic, manganese, or mercury intoxication, in addition to the idiopathic variety of amyotrophic lateral sclerosis. In the cases you first referred to, do you have any idea whether there was any indication of heavy-metal or other toxicity? Did the cases appear pathologically to be instances of idiopathic ALS? If so, what is your feeling now after your studies about the relationship between thiamine and ALS?

Dr. Fujiwara. I realize that there are many causes of ALS, and I suppose that heavy-metal toxicity and ALS are different diseases. As far as the results of our experiment are concerned, it is certain that rats did not show the same thiamine metabolism as did cases of ALS. Simple magnesium or calcium deficiency in the rat could not produce the same symptoms as those of ALS patients in the Kii peninsula. We are now attempting to get rats which show changes in thiamine metabolism similar to those occurring in ALS.

Dr. Kark. Did the patients who seemed to respond to thiamine have the Guamanian form of ALS, one of the familial forms, or purely sporadic ALS?

Dr. Fujiwara. From the study of Professor Kimura, patients with ALS in the Kii peninsula showed a relatively high familial incidence, and I read that there were differences between ALS in the Kii peninsula and on Guam in terms of the content of metals in the tissues of patients. I don't know whether ALS patients on Guam show the same abnormality of thiamine metabolism as do patients on the Kii peninsula.

Dr. Barchi. There is another possible clinical correlation that you might comment on. In the last year or so, the concept that alcoholics become magnesium depleted has been raised. These patients show increased urinary magnesium excretion. Of course, we are all familiar with the concept that alcoholics can be thiamine depleted and also that they have seizures when they stop drinking. Some investigators report that the prophylactic administration of magnesium can prevent alcoholic withdrawal seizures. Do you have any opinion on that?

Dr. Fujiwara. Thiamine in tissue is fixed to divalent cations and protein. This mechanism keeps thiamine bound to tissues. Thus, increasing the supply of divalent cations results in the increased urinary excretion of thiamine and vice versa. We are presently studying the relationships between alcohol and divalent cations.

Dr. Kark. Can you speculate on possible mechanisms of interaction between divalent cations and thiamine stores, and are there any data on possible interrelations between thiamine and parathormone?

Dr. Fujiwara. There may be possibilities of interrelationships between calcium and parathormone, but we have not yet had sufficient experience to answer this question.

6. Free Thiamine Transport System in *Escherichia coli*: Evidence for the Existence of an Energy-Dependent Exit Process*

TAKASHI KAWASAKI, M.D.
KAZUO YAMADA, M.D.

Department of Biochemistry
Hiroshima University School of Medicine
Hiroshima, Japan

In the first United States-Japan cooperative seminar on thiamine, we reported on the thiamine uptake system in *Escherichia coli*. Thiamine was taken up by cells of *E. coli* K12 against a concentration gradient in a manner similar to active transport, which is an energy-, temperature-, and pH-dependent process and follows Michaelis-Menten kinetics (1). Thiamine uptake was inhibited by thiamine antagonists, pyrithiamine and oxythiamine, and transported thiamine was found in the cell mostly as thiamine diphosphate (ThDP) after a short period of incubation. The existence of a small amount of the free form was also demonstrated (1).

Thiamine is transported by the function of a carrier protein specific for thiamine. The existence of the thiamine carrier is demonstrated by isolation of a thiamine transport-negative mutant of *E. coli* K12, in which thiamine

* Abbreviations: ThMP, thiamine monophosphate; ThDP, thiamine diphosphate; HMP, 2-methyl-4-amino-5-hydroxymethylpyrimidine (thiamine pyrimidine); HMP-PP, HMP pyrophosphate; Th, 4-methyl-5-hydroxyethylthiazole (thiamine thiazole); Th-P, Th monophosphate; DNP, 2,4-dinitrophenol; CCCP, carbonylcyanide *m*-chlorophenylhydrazone; NEM, *N*-ethylmaleimide; PCMB, *p*-chloromercuribenzoate.

metabolism is not altered (2), and synthesis of the carrier is regulated by repression and derepression, depending on cellular ThDP concentration (3).

From these results, it was assumed that thiamine passes through the cell membrane in an unchanged form and then accumulates in the cytoplasm as ThDP by the coupled phosphorylation reaction (1). However, the relation between the transport across the cell membrane and the phosphorylation reaction of thiamine remains to be clarified.

In this relation, an interesting finding was recently reported by Nakayama and Hayashi (4, 5): the isolation from *E. coli* W of a mutant requiring thiamine monophosphate (ThMP) in which ThMP formation from thiamine is genetically blocked.

We have also isolated mutants of the same type from a thiamine auxotroph (KG1673) of *E. coli* K12 which is defective in thiaminephosphate pyrophosphorylase, as shown in Fig. 1. This KG1673 requires thiamine supplementation of a minimal medium (6) for growth because of the enzyme defect (7). After mutagenesis of KG1673 with nitrosoguanidine (8), five mutants lacking thiamine monophosphokinase were obtained and referred to as KG1674 to KG1678. These mutants can grow on minimal medium containing ThMP but not thiamine, and strain KG1675 or KG1676 was used in the experiments. Strains KG1675 and KG1676 showed the same characteristics with respect to the growth response as well as free thiamine transport. The other type of mutant obtained was KG1679, which grows on ThDP but not on thiamine or ThMP because of the lack of ThMP kinase.

The deficiency of the enzyme activities in these mutants as well as the parent strain was confirmed by paper chromatographic analysis of labeled thiamine transported into the cells of the mutants. In the parent strain (KG1673), labeled thiamine, ThMP, and ThDP were detected. With KG1675 or KG1676 cells, only one radioactivity peak, corresponding to free thiamine, was found, while in KG1679 labeled thiamine and ThMP, but not labeled ThDP, were demonstrated.

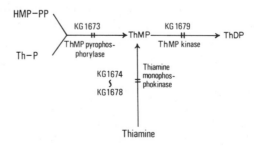

Figure 1. The pathway of thiamine diphosphate synthesis in *Escherichia coli* and the sites of genetic blocks in the mutants used.

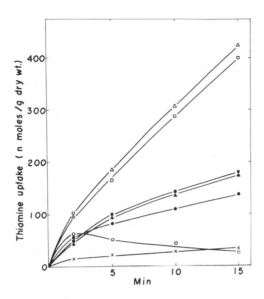

Figure 2. Time course of ^{14}C-thiamine uptake by three mutants of *E. coli* K12. Open symbols represent the uptake in the presence of 0.4% glucose; closed symbols, in the absence of glucose. △, ▲: KG1673; ○, ●: KG1675; □, ■: KG1679. x: The uptake at 0°C, which was practically identical in these strains regardless of the presence of glucose. From Kawasaki and Yamada (9).

These results indicate that the free thiamine transport system is involved in KG1675 or KG1676 and that it is possible to study thiamine transport uncoupled to the phosphorylation of thiamine in *E. coli*.

When KG1675 cells were incubated with ^{14}C-thiamine in the medium containing potassium phosphate buffer and 0.4% glucose at 37°C, a rapid transport reached a peak at 2 minutes and then decreased with time to the level found at 0°C. The parent strain, KG1673, and its ThDP auxotroph, KG1679, both of which contain the enzyme catalyzing ThMP formation from thiamine, took up labeled thiamine in the same manner, and the uptake rate was approximately 2 times faster in the presence of glucose than in its absence (9), as shown in Fig. 2.

In these experiments, it is clear that free thiamine passes first inward through the cell membrane and then outward when the phosphorylating enzyme is deficient in the cytoplasm and glucose is added as an exogenous energy source. The isolation and properties of thiamine monophosphokinase in *E. coli* K12 were described (10).

The existence of the energy-dependent exit process in KG1675, as well as in KG1676, was demonstrated by the addition of glucose to the uptake medium,

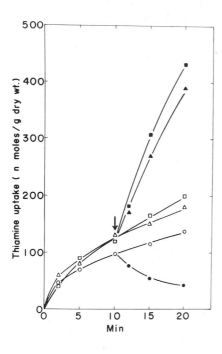

Figure 3. Effect of glucose on the uptake of thiamine by three mutants of *E. coli* K12. At the time indicated by an arrow, glucose was added at 0.4% concentration to the uptake medium without glucose and the incubation was continued for another 10 minutes. Closed symbols show the uptake after the addition of glucose. △, ▲: KG1673; □, ■: KG1679; ○, ●: KG1675. From Kawasaki and Yamada (9).

in which thiamine uptake was proceeding with no energy supply (Fig. 3). When glucose was added to the glucose-free uptake medium at 10 minutes after the incubation at 37°C, a decrease in the cellular radioactivity in KG1675 was observed, while a rapid increase in the uptake of thiamine was demonstrated in both KG1673 and KG1679 (9).

The role of glucose in bringing about thiamine exit from the cell was further confirmed by an experiment in which 2,4-dinitrophenol (2 mM) was added (Fig. 4). The uncoupler was added to the uptake medium containing glucose at 2 and 10 minutes after the incubation; this resulted in a rapid rise in the uptake of thiamine. Sodium azide at 50 mM and KCN at 1 mM showed the same effect as DNP.

The exit of thiamine was dependent on the concentrations of glucose added to the medium (Fig. 5): low concentrations, such as 20 μM, were effective in enhancing the exit for a short period, probably because of consumption of the glucose by metabolism. The increase in thiamine efflux was maximum at 0.2 mM glucose (11).

The effects of other carbon compounds as exogenous energy sources were also tested, and D-lactate and succinate at 10 mM each were found to cause the exit of thiamine from KG1676 cells, but to much lesser extents. Succinate and D-lactate added to the cell suspension of KG1673 under the same

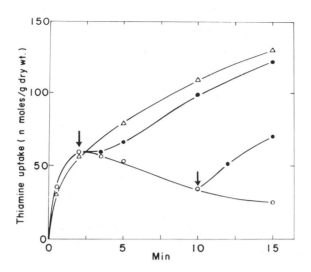

Figure 4. Effect of 2,4-dinitrophenol (DNP) on the uptake of thiamine by a ThMP auxotroph (KG1675) of *E. coli* K12. The uncoupler was added at 2 m*M* to the uptake medium containing 0.4% glucose at the times indicated by arrows, and the incubation at 37°C was continued. Closed symbols show the uptake after the addition of DNP. $\bigcirc$, $\bullet$: With glucose; $\triangle$: without glucose. From Kawasaki and Yamada (unpublished data).

Figure 5. Effect of glucose concentrations on thiamine exit from cells of a ThMP auxotroph (KG1676). To the cell suspension of KG1676 without glucose was added glucose of varying concentrations at the time shown by an arrow, and the incubation at 37°C was continued. $\bigcirc$: Without glucose; $\triangle$, $\blacktriangle$, $\square$, $\blacksquare$, and $\bullet$: glucose added at 2, 20, 50, 100, and 200 μM, respectively. From Kawasaki and Yamada (11).

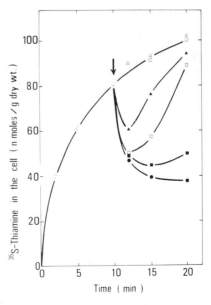

conditions as for KG1676 resulted in increases in thiamine uptake at rates approximately 66% and 31%, respectively, of the one caused by the same concentration of glucose.

The energy-dependent exit of thiamine could be demonstrated more directly with cells of KG1676 preloaded with ^{35}S-thiamine (Fig. 6). The cells were first incubated with 1 μM ^{35}S-thiamine for 30 minutes at 37°C, collected by filtration on Millipore filters, washed, and then suspended in the fresh transport medium without ^{35}S-thiamine at 37°C. The addition of glucose to the suspension of the preloaded cells resulted in an immediate rapid decrease in cellular radioactivity, indicating clearly that an energy-dependent exit process is involved in free thiamine transport. The exit of thiamine after the glucose was added proceeded linearly for at least 1 minute under the conditions employed. A slow and linear reduction in the radioactivity found in the absence of glucose was probably due to diffusion.

The exit of thiamine from the preloaded cells of KG1676 was inhibited by energy poisons and sulfhydryl reagents (Table 1). However, when the exit from the ^{35}S-thiamine-preloaded cells was measured, the inhibition of the exit by uncouplers such as CCCP was less than that caused by electron transfer inhibitors such as KCN. This may suggest that energy provided through the electron transfer system is involved in thiamine efflux in this strain.

In addition to the results indicating the involvement of the energy-dependent exit process in free thiamine transport in *E. coli*, the time course of thiamine transport by KG1675 or KG1676 (Fig. 1) shows that the entry process is also energy dependent, since the uptake of thiamine up to 2 minutes was faster in the presence of glucose than in its absence.

The existence of a carrier specific for thiamine in the cell membrane is evident functionally (1) and genetically (2). That the exit of thiamine from the

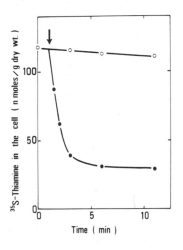

Figure 6. Exit of thiamine from ^{35}S-thiamine-preloaded cells. The cells of KG1676 preloaded with ^{35}S-thiamine were suspended at 37°C in the fresh uptake medium without glucose, and then 0.4% glucose was added at the time indicated by an arrow, followed by measurement of the radioactivity in the cells. O: No glucose added; ●: glucose added. From Kawasaki and Yamada (11).

Table 1. Effect of Metabolic Poisons and Sulfhydryl Reagents on Thiamine Exit by Glucose from ^{35}S-Thiamine-Preloaded Cells[a]

Inhibitor	Addition,[b] mM	Relative Exit, %
None	—	100
KCN	0.1	91.8
	1	22.4
Amytal	1	75.5
	5	23.8
NaN$_3$	10	75.5
	50	20.6
DNP	0.1	69.4
	1	38.8
CCCP	0.001	99.0
	0.01	95.2
Arsenate	1	102
	10	102
NEM	1	29.6
PCMB	0.5	71.2

[a] From Kawasaki and Yamada (11).
[b] All reagents of appropiate concentrations were added to the preloaded cell suspension of KG1676 just before the addition of 2 mM glucose at 37°C. Thiamine exit for 1 minute after adding glucose was measured.

cells of KG1676 is carried out by the carrier was determined from the experiment shown in Fig. 7. When nonradioactive thiamine or an antimetabolite of thiamine, either pyrithiamine or oxythiamine, was added to the suspension of the preloaded cells of KG1676 in the absence of glucose, a rapid loss of radioactivity from the cells was demonstrated. This is due to an exchange diffusion (12) which is catalyzed by the carrier protein. The addition of nonlabeled thiamine or its analogs plus glucose resulted in an additive effect of stimulation on the exit of thiamine, suggesting different mechanisms for the effect of glucose and the effects of structurally related compounds on the exit (13).

Evidence has been obtained that the same carrier protein catalyzes the passage of thiamine through the cell membrane in both directions (13).

Monovalent cations are known to affect many transport systems in microorganisms, though the mechanisms postulated vary from one system to

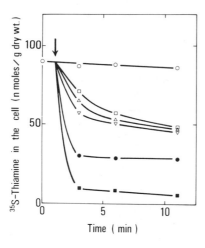

Figure 7. Effect of nonradioactive thiamine and its analogs on ^{35}S-thiamine exit from the preloaded cells. To the preloaded cell suspension of KG1676 was added nonradioactive thiamine ($\square$), pyrithiamine ($\triangledown$), or oxythiamine ($\triangle$) at 10 μM each in the absence of glucose. O: Without glucose; ●: 2 mM glucose alone; ■: 2mM glucose plus either 10 μM nonradioactive thiamine, pyrithiamine, or oxythiamine. From Yamada (13).

another. Melibiose in *Salmonella* (14), aminoisobutyrate in marine *Pseudomonad* (15), and glutamate in *E. coli* B (16) are examples of cotransport with Na^+, while proline transport by membrane vesicles of *Mycobacterium phlei* is stimulated by Na^+ without affecting the K_m value (17). Among the stimulatory effects of K^+ on microbial transports, a K^+ gradient is assumed to act at least partly as a driving force of citrate transport in *Aerobacter* (18) and of glycine transport in *Saccharomyces* (19), and in the other cases K^+ affects the accumulation process of aminoisobutyrate (15) and glutamate in *E. coli* (20). Recent studies in our laboratory have revealed that proline transport by whole cells of *E. coli* was stimulated severalfold by Li^+ without changing the K_m value (21). In any case, the effect of these cations on the exit process of a solute has not been described.

In the experiments described above (Figs. 2 to 7 and Table 1), the transport medium contained potassium phosphate as a buffer system, and, to test the effect of a given monovalent cation, harvested cells of KG1676 were washed in 50 mM $MgSO_4$ solution to deplete cellular K^+ (15) and then suspended in 50 mM Tris-HCl buffer (pH 7.3) plus 10 mM $MgSO_4$. This procedure reduced the cellular K^+ concentration to one fifth of the original level.

When glucose was added at 2 mM to the suspension of K^+-depleted cells 10 minutes after the incubation, the exit of thiamine from the cells was demonstrated (Fig. 8). However, this exit rate was greatly reduced in comparison with that in potassium phosphate buffer, as illustrated in Fig. 3. The addition of KCl with glucose enhanced the exit rate, depending on its concentrations (0.01 to 10 mM), and the effect of KCl was maximum at 1 mM (13). Although not illustrated in Fig. 8, the entry rate of thiamine in the absence of glucose was not affected by monovalent cations, including K^+, Na^+, Li^+, Cs^+, and Rb^+. This specific effect of K^+ on the exit of thiamine, but not on the entry into the cell, suggests strongly that K^+ may be required to control the functional state of thiamine carrier when it directs from inward to outward. This K^+ effect is probably the first case ever described which indicates that an exit process in the transport of a solute is affected by a monovalent cation.

Evidence has been presented that a free thiamine transport system exists in ThMP auxotrophs of *E. coli* K12. The system is composed of both energy-dependent entry and exit processes, and the latter process is controlled by K^+.

A similar exit phenomenon caused by the addition of an energy source was described in the glucose transport system of *E. coli* (22, 23). Energy coupling to active transport of a solute in microorganisms is one of the most important problems to be resolved. The energy required to support the active transport is often assumed to prevent exit of the solute (24, 25), since added uncouplers accelerate the exit.

The exit of thiamine as described is in disagreement with the explanation for the energy coupling. Therefore, the physiological significance of the energy-dependent thiamine exit found in ThMP-requiring mutants of *E. coli* remains to be clarified. One possible explanation for this exit of thiamine might be a kind of regulatory mechanism for thiamine transport, as discussed by Kepes (26) for the energy-dependent glucose exit system (22, 23).

The mechanism(s) of the stimulation by K^+ of energy-dependent thiamine exit in these mutants of *E. coli* is obscure. Preliminary data obtained by the use of K^+-specific ionophores, valinomycin and nigericin, suggest that the inflow of K^+ may be coupled to the outflow of thiamine (13).

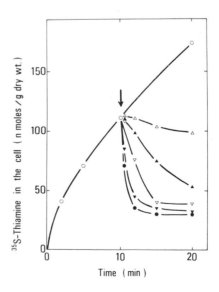

Figure 8. Effect of K^+ concentrations on thiamine exit. Glucose alone or glucose plus KCl varying in concentrations was added to the cell suspension of KG1676 without glucose at the time shown by an arrow. O: No glucose added; △: glucose (2 m*M*) alone; ▲, ▽, ▼, and ●: glucose (2 m*M*) plus 0.01, 0.1, 1, and 10 m*M* KCl, respectively. From Yamada (13).

References

1. T. Kawasaki, I. Miyata, K. Esaki, and Y. Nose, *Arch. Biochem. Biophys.*, **131**, 223 (1969).
2. T. Kawasaki, I. Miyata, and Y. Nose, *Arch. Biochem. Biophys.*, **131**, 231 (1969).
3. T. Kawasaki and K. Esaki, *Arch. Biochem. Biophys.*, **142**, 163 (1971).
4. H. Nakayama and R. Hayashi, *J. Bacteriol.*, **109**, 936 (1972).
5. H. Nakayama and R. Hayashi, *J. Bacteriol.*, **112**, 1118 (1972).
6. B. D. Davis and E. S. Mingioli, *J. Bacteriol.*, **60**, 17 (1950).
7. T. Kawasaki, T. Nakata, and Y. Nose, *J. Bacteriol.*, **95**, 1483 (1968).
8. E. A. Adelberg, M. Mandel, and G. C. C. Chen, *Biochem. Biophys. Res. Commun.*, **18**, 788 (1965).
9. T. Kawasaki and K. Yamada, *Biochem. Biophys. Res. Commun.*, **47**, 465 (1972).
10. A. Iwashima, H. Nishino, and Y. Nose, *Biochim. Biophys. Acta*, **258**, 333 (1972).
11. T. Kawasaki and K. Yamada, article in preparation.
12. J. P. Robbie and T. H. Wilson, *Biochim. Biophys. Acta*, **173**, 234 (1969).
13. K. Yamada, article in preparation.
14. J. Stock and S. Roseman, *Biochem. Biophys. Res. Commun.*, **44**, 131 (1971).
15. J. Thompson and R. A. MacLeod, *J. Biol. Chem.*, **246**, 4066 (1971).
16. L. Frank and I. Hopkins, *J. Bacteriol.*, **100**, 329 (1969).
17. A. F. Brodie, H. Hirata, A. Asano, N. S. Cohen, T. R. Hinds, H. N. Aithal, and V. K. Kalra, in C. F. Fox, Ed., *Membrane Research*, Academic Press, New York, 1972, p. 445.
18. R. G. Eagon and L. S. Wilkerson, *Biochem. Biophys. Res. Commun.*, **46**, 1944 (1972).
19. A. A. Eddy, K. J. Indge, and J. A. Nowacki, *Biochem. J.*, **120**, 845 (1970).
20. Y. S. Halpern, H. Barash, S. Dover, and K. Druck, *J. Bacteriol.*, **114**, 53 (1973).
21. T. Kawasaki and Y. Kayama, *Biochem. Biophys. Res. Commun.*, **55**, 52 (1973).
22. P. Hoffee and E. Englesberg, *Proc. Natl. Acad. Sci. U.S.*, **48**, 1759 (1962).
23. P. Hoffee, E. Englesberg, and F. Lamy, *Biochim. Biophys. Acta*, **79**, 337 (1964).
24. H. H. Winkler and T. H. Wilson, *J. Biol. Chem.*, **241**, 2200 (1966).
25. A. Kepes, *J. Membrane Biol.*, **4**, 784 (1971).
26. A. Kepes, in F. Bronner and A. Kleinzeller, Eds., *Current Topics in Membranes and Transport*, Vol. 1, Academic Press, New York, 1970, p. 101.

DISCUSSION

Chapter 6

Dr. Elsas. Dr. Kawasaki, I wonder whether the effects of glucose in stimulating the efflux of thiamine on this mutant cell line might be related to the mechanism that Kaback has proposed for other nonion substrate transports, i.e., some form of electron transfer system in which your proposed thiamine permease may have an altered configuration in the presence of an organic substrate which would effectuate electron transfer. I guess the way to approach this question would be to set up an artificial system such as PMS-ascorbate or to give other organic compounds such as lactate and study the efflux of thiamine.

Dr. Kawasaki. We have examined the effects of some carbon sources on the efflux of thiamine by glucose-grown cells. D-Lactate was effective in inducing the efflux of thiamine to a much lesser extent than was glucose. Succinate was also slightly effective. An artificial system such as PMS-ascorbate may not act in the transport by these whole cells.

Dr. Cooper. Would you say that the entrance of thiamine was independent of a monovalent cation? This is rather unusual; do you know of any other transport-facilitating system that is independent of a sodium-activated transport?

Dr. Kawasaki. Yes, I stated that the entrance of thiamine is independent of monovalent cations in *E. coli* cells. There are many microbial transport systems that are not related to monovalent cations. One of the differences between microbial and animal transport systems might be that Na^+-K^+-ATPase is not involved in the former systems. However, several transport systems in microorganisms are known to be stimulated by Na^+, K^+, or Li^+.

The mechanisms postulated for such stimulations vary from one system to another.

Dr. Barchi. Dr. Kawasaki, I am interested in the sigmoid nature of the efflux curve of thiamine as a function of internal thiamine concentration. My question is going to take you a step backward to preliminary data. In most of the curves you showed where there was an induced efflux of thiamine in a preloaded cell in response to glucose, the concentrations of thiamine dropped rapidly and subsequently reached a plateau. This seemed to be invariably the case. Do you think that this represents the existence of a pool of thiamine inside the cells in some other form, which is not accessible to efflux? And if that is the case, how do you correct your curves for efflux of thiamine in preloaded cells as a function of thiamine concentration for the possible existence of such a pool?

Dr. Kawasaki. I do not think that there exists an inaccessible pool of thiamine for efflux. Since the glucose-stimulated efflux of thiamine is catalyzed also by the thiamine carrier, an equilibrium state for efflux is existent. The initial velocity of the efflux was measured under conditions in which less than 7% of the intracellular thiamine pool was moved out into the medium after the addition of glucose.

7. Uptake of Thiamine Tetrahydrofurfuryl Disulfide and Thiamine Thiazole in *Escherichia coli* and the Relationship to Thiamine Diphosphate Biosynthesis*

TAKASHI KAWASAKI, M.D.
KAZUO YAMADA, M.D.
HIROSHI YAMASAKI, Ph.D.

Department of Biochemistry
Hiroshima University School of Medicine
Hiroshima, Japan

A disulfide derivative of thiamine, thiamine allyl disulfide, was discovered by Fujiwara and Watanabe (1), and many derivatives of thiamine disulfide have subsequently been synthesized (2).

One of the properties which explains the effectiveness of these disulfide derivatives is a fat-soluble nature that is newly given by the groups linked to the thiamine moiety through the disulfide bridge. Evidence has therefore been presented by many Japanese groups that thiamine disulfides penetrate into the red cells by passive diffusion (2–5). However, one of the derivatives, thiamine propyl disulfide (TPD), was not taken up by yeast cells in the early course of the study on metabolism of these disulfide derivatives (6).

Some properties of the thiamine transport system in *Escherichia* have been

---

* Abbreviations: TTFD, thiamine tetrahydrofurfuryl disulfide; TPD, thiamine propyl disulfide; HMP or hydroxymethylpyrimidine (thiamine pyrimidine), 2-methyl-4-amino-5-hydroxymethylpyrimidine; HMP-P, HMP monophosphate; HMP-PP, HMP pyrophosphate; Th or thiazole (thiamine thiazole), 4-methyl-5-hydroxyethylthiazole; Th-P, Th monophosphate; 2-aminothiazole, 2-amino-4-methyl-5-hydroxyethylthiazole; ThMP, thiamine monophosphate; ThDP thiamine diphosphate.

described (7), and many mutants of different types which are involved not only in thiamine transport but also in thiamine metabolism, are available.

With these various strains of *E. coli* K12, the uptake of thiamine tetrahydrofurfuryl disulfide (TTFD) and the relationship of its uptake to its metabolism have been studied (8). Since TTFD was labeled with ^{35}S at the inner side of two sulfur atoms, ^{35}S-labeled thiamine was formed when ^{35}S-labeled TTFD was reduced chemically or biologically to thiamine.

The pathway of biosynthesis of thiamine and thiamine diphosphate (ThDP) in *E. coli* is shown in Fig. 1. Thiamine monophosphate (ThMP) is synthesized in exactly the same way as occurs in yeast (9) and is then directly converted into ThDP (10, 11). On the other hand, thiamine added to the outside of the cell passes through the cell membrane via a thiamine carrier and is then converted into ThMP in the cytoplasm (7). The mutants of *E. coli* used in the experiments and the sites of their genetic block in the pathway are also shown in Fig. 1. Strain KG33 (12) was used mainly in the experiments; KG1675 is a ThMP auxotroph, which shows properties for free thiamine transport identical to those of KG1676 (7). Strains KG900 and KG905, which are derivatives of KG33 and require thiazole for growth, are lacking in thiamine transport activity; that is, they cannot take up thiamine from the medium (13).

Assay of TTFD uptake by whole cells of *E. coli* was carried out under the same conditions as those described for thiamine transport by the Millipore filtration technique (12).

The time course of TTFD uptake at three different concentrations in the

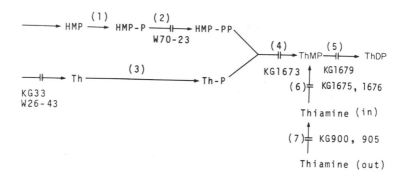

(1) HMP kinase; (2) HMP-P kinase; (3) Th kinase
(4) Thiaminephosphate pyrophosphorylase; (5) ThMP kinase
(6) Thiamine monophosphokinase; (7) Thiamine permease

Figure 1. The pathway of ThDP synthesis in *Escherichia coli* and the sites of genetic blocks in mutants.

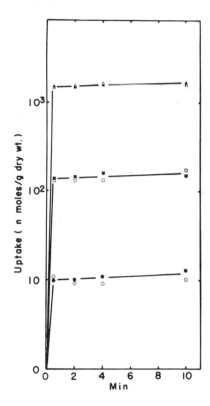

Figure 2. Time course of ^{35}S-TTFD uptake. Strains KG1673 and KG1675 were used, and both strains gave essentially identical patterns of uptake. Closed symbols show the uptake in the presence of 0.4% glucose; open symbols, in the absence of glucose. ●, ○: 0.1 μM; ■, □: 1.0 μM; ▲, △: 10 μM ^{35}S-TTFD. From Yamada and Kawasaki (8).

presence and the absence of glucose is shown in Fig. 2. The uptake rate is proportional to the concentrations of TTFD without saturation, and the uptake is rapidly equilibrated within 30 seconds. Glucose had no effect on the rate and extent of TTFD uptake. Therefore, energy poisons such as 2,4-dinitrophenol also had no effect on the uptake in the presence of glucose.

The pattern of TTFD uptake by thiamine transport-negative mutants, KG900 and KG905, is identical to that found in strains such as KG1673 and KG33, which are normal in their thiamine transport activities, as shown in Fig. 3. Moreover, the uptake of TTFD at 0°C is almost 60 to 70% of that at 37°C, indicating a temperature independence of TTFD uptake in *E. coli*.

These results indicate that TTFD uptake in *E. coli* takes place by diffusion. In the transport of a solute by diffusion, a simple diffusion mechanism is distinguishable from the mechanism of carrier-mediated facilitated diffusion. To determine which type of diffusion is involved in TTFD uptake by *E. coli* cells, the uptake of TTFD is compared with thiamine uptake, which is a typical process of carrier-mediated active transport (12, 13).

One of the SH reagents, *N*-ethylmaleimide, markedly inhibits thiamine

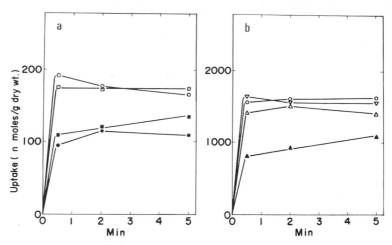

Figure 3. Uptake of ^{35}S-TTFD by various strains of *E. coli* K12. In the left side (*a*) the uptake of ^{35}S-TTFD (1 μM) by KG33 (O, ●) and W26-43 (□, ■) is seen, and in the right side (*b*) the uptake of ^{35}S-TTFD (10 μM) by KG1673 (O), KG900 (∇), and KG905 (Δ, ▲) is illustrated. Open symbols represent the uptake at 37° C; closed symbols, at 0° C. From Yamada and Kawasaki (8).

transport, depending on its concentration, while TTFD uptake by the same KG33 cells is slightly inhibited without further increase in the extent of the inhibition (Fig. 4).

Various analogs of thiamine were then added to the uptake medium of ^{35}S-TTFD or ^{35}S-thiamine at a hundredfold concentration of the labeled substrates, in order to determine the competition of the analogs with labeled TTFD or thiamine for the specific carrier in the cell membrane. As shown in Fig. 5, TTFD uptake was not affected by unlabeled thiamine and pyrithiamine, and was lowered by only 25% in the presence of nonradioactive TTFD and TPD. Thiamine uptake by cells of the same strain was inhibited about 40% by pyrithiamine and over 80% by nonlabeled thiamine.

When the amount of thiamine carrier was reduced by repression (14), i.e., by allowing KG33 cells to grow on an excess of thiamine (1 μM), thiamine transport was reduced to only 15% of the level of cells grown on a limited amount of thiamine (0.01 μM). However, TTFD uptake was only slightly influenced under these conditions (8).

It can be concluded from these results that thiamine tetrahydrofurfuryl disulfide passes through the cell membrane of *E. coli* by simple diffusion but not by facilitated diffusion.

When the TTFD in the cells of the *E. coli* was analyzed by paper chromatography and by counting the radioactivity of 1-cm strips of the paper

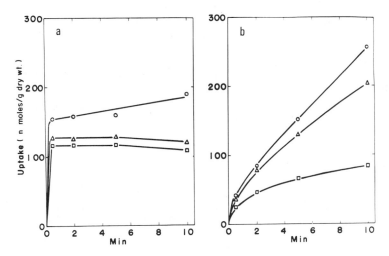

Figure 4. Effect of *N*-ethylmaleimide on ³⁵S-TTFD uptake. Parts *a* and *b* represent the uptake of ³⁵S-TTFD (1 *μM*) and of ³⁵S-thiamine (1 *μM*), respectively, by KG33. ○: No addition; △: 0.1 m*M*; □: 1.0 m*M* *N*-ethylmaleimide. From Yamada and Kawasaki (8).

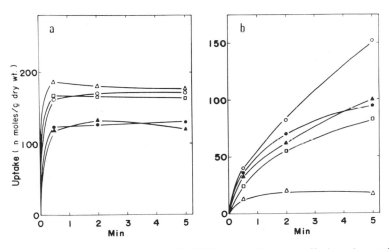

Figure 5. Effect of thiamine analogs on ³⁵S-TTFD uptake. Parts *a* and *b* show the uptake of ³⁵S-TTFD and of ³⁵S-thiamine, respectively, by KG33. Each labeled substrate was used at 1 *μM*, and the concentration of nonradioactive analogs added was 100 times that of either ³⁵S-thiamine or ³⁵S-TTFD. ○: No addition of analogs; △: thiamine; □: pyrithiamine; ●: TTFD; ▲: TPD. From Yamada and Kawasaki (8).

developed (12, 15), it was clearly demonstrated that TTFD was first converted into thiamine and then transformed into ThDP through ThMP in the cytoplasm as the incubation time increased (8).

The characteristics of the thiamine and thiamine disulfide transport systems in *E. coli* have been presented. However, little is known about the uptake of each moiety of thiamine and its regulation in relation to thiamine biosynthesis. It has been reported (16) that a mutant of *E. coli* W strain, resistant to 2-aminothiazole, an antimetabolite of thiazole, lacks the ability to take up thiazole as well as the antimetabolite from the medium. This result was obtained from experiments with nonlabeled thiazole and suggests a possible carrier-mediated uptake of the thiazole moiety of thiamine in *E. coli* cells.

We have prepared ^{35}S-labeled thiazole by bisulfite cleavage of ^{35}S-thiamine and then purified it (17). Assay of ^{35}S-thiazole uptake by *E. coli* K12, a wild strain, was carried out under exactly the same conditions as with TTFD.

The time course of thiazole uptake at three concentrations showed an almost identical pattern to that of TTFD, illustrated in Fig. 1: the uptake is proportional to the thiazole concentration gradient up to 0.1 mM with no tendency to saturate (Fig. 6).

^{35}S-Thiazole was taken up at the same rate, regardless of the presence of

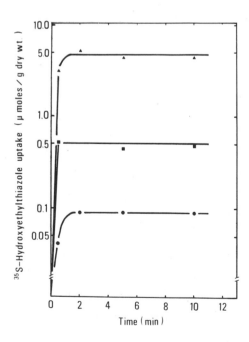

Figure 6. Effect of ^{35}S-thiazole concentrations on the rate of uptake. *E. coli* K12, a wild strain, was used. ●: 1 μM; ■: 10 μM; ▲: 100 μM ^{35}S-thiazole. From Yamasaki et al. (15).

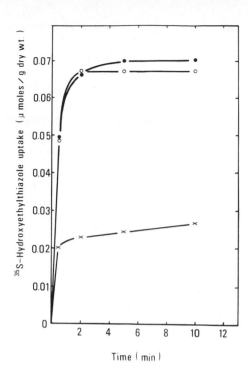

Figure 7. Effect of glucose and temperature on ^{35}S-thiazole uptake. ●: 0.4% glucose at 37°C; ○: no glucose at 37°C; ×: 0.4% glucose at 0°C. From Yamasaki et al. (15).

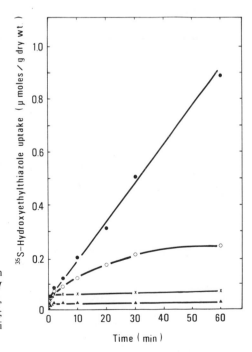

Figure 8. Effect of HMP and glucose on ^{35}S-thiazole uptake. ● and ▲: 0.1 mM HMP plus 0.4% glucose at 37 and 0°C, respectively; ○: 0.1 mM HMP at 37°C; ×: 0.4% glucose at 37°C. From Yamasaki et al. (15).

101

glucose, with a partial dependence on temperature; that is, the uptake at $0°C$ was reduced to approximately 35% of that found at $37°C$ (Fig. 7).

These results indicate that thiazole is also taken up by diffusion, as found for TTFD. However, the uptake of thiazole was inhibited about 55% when the cells were treated with 1 mM N-ethylmaleimide for 5 minutes before the initiation of the uptake, whereas 30% inhibition was observed when the uptake was initiated with the simultaneous addition of this SH reagent and ^{35}S-thiazole (15). This result suggests that facilitated diffusion, mediated by the carrier, is involved in the uptake of thiamine thiazole.

The effect of hydroxymethylpyrimidine, the other half moiety of thiamine molecule, on the thiazole uptake was then studied (Fig. 8). The rate of thiazole uptake was increased by the addition of 0.1 mM HMP and more markedly enhanced by HMP plus glucose. However, the addition of both HMP and glucose was completely ineffective at $0°C$. In the presence of glucose, about 1 μM HMP was enough to stimulate ^{35}S-thiazole uptake at the maximal rate.

Hydroxymethylpyrimidine is converted into its pyrophosphate through the formation of its monophosphate, as shown in Fig. 1. The addition of HMP-P or HMP-PP, with glucose, to the uptake medium of ^{35}S-thiazole, however, failed to increase the thiazole uptake (15). This is probably due to impermeability of the membrane for these phosphate compounds of HMP (18).

When 2-aminothiazole, a competitive inhibitor of Th kinase in *E. coli* (16), was added to the uptake medium containing HMP and glucose, complete inhibition of the ^{35}S-thiazole uptake resulted at 10 μM concentration of the antimetabolite (Fig. 9). This is due to the inhibition of Th-P formation catalyzed by Th kinase.

These results indicate that the stimulatory effect of HMP on Th uptake is brought about by the coupling of its uptake to their metabolisms via the pathway of thiamine biosynthesis shown in Fig. 1.

This assumption is supported also by the results obtained with mutants blocked in thiamine biosynthesis. Strain KG1673 is a mutant deficient in thiaminephosphate pyrophosphorylase, and in strain W70-23 HMP-P kinase is lacking. No stimulatory effect from the addition of HMP and glucose was detected with these two mutants, as compared with that obtained for a wild strain of *E. coli* K12 (15).

A disulfide derivative of thiamine, TTFD, is transported into *E. coli* cells by simple diffusion and then converted in the cell into thiamine, ThMP, and, finally, ThDP. On the other hand, thiamine thiazole moiety is taken up into the cell by carrier-mediated facilitated diffusion without the consumption of metabolic energy. The uptake of thiazole is greatly enhanced in the presence

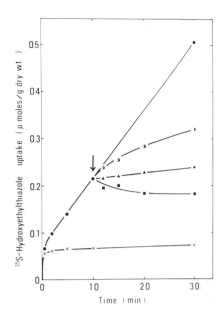

Figure 9. Effect of 2-aminothiazole on ³⁵S-thiazole uptake in the presence of HMP and glucose. At the time indicated by the arrow, 1 μM (◑), 10 μM (▲), and 100 μM (■) 2-aminothiazole were added to the uptake medium containing 10 μM HMP and 0.4% glucose (●). The control (×) contained no HMP or glucose. From Yamasaki et al. (15).

of the pyrimidine moiety of thiamine and glucose. Evidence has been presented that the enzymes involved in thiamine biosynthesis participate in this physiological regulation of thiazole uptake.

References

1. M. Fujiwara and H. Watanabe, *Proc. Jap. Acad.*, **28**, 156 (1952).

2. C. Kawasaki, in R. S. Harris, I. G. Wool, and J. A. Loraine, Eds., *Vitamins and Hormones*, Vol. 21, Academic Press, New York, 1963, p. 69.

3. Z. Suzuoki and T. Suzuoki, *J. Biochem.* (Tokyo), **40**, 11 (1953).

4. M. Morita and T. Mineshita, *Vitamins* (Japanese), **33**, 67 (1966).

5. I. Utsumi, K. Kohno, K. Noda, I. Saito, and M. Mizobe, *Vitamins* (Japanese), **37**, 243 (1968).

6. Z. Suzoki, *J. Biochem.* (Tokyo), **42**, 27 (1955).

7. T. Kawasaki and K. Yamada, article submitted for publication in this book.

8. K. Yamada and T. Kawasaki, article in preparation.

9. G. M. Brown and J. J. Reynolds, *Ann. Rev. Biochem.*, **32**, 419 (1963).

10. H. Nakayama and R. Hayashi, *J. Bacteriol.*, **109**, 936 (1972).

11. H. Nishino, A. Iwashima, and Y. Nose, *Biochem. Biophys. Res. Commun.*, **45**, 363 (1971).

12. T. Kawasaki, I. Miyata, K. Esaki, and Y. Nose, *Arch. Biochem. Biophys.*, **131**, 223 (1969).

13.   T. Kawasaki, I. Miyata, and Y. Nose, *Arch. Biochem. Biophys.*, **131**, 231 (1969).

14.   T. Kawasaki and K. Esaki, *Arch. Biochem. Biophys.*, **142**, 163 (1971).

15.   H. Yamasaki, H. Sanemori, K. Yamada, and T. Kawasaki, *J. Bacteriol.*, **116**, 1280 (1973).

16.   A. Iwashima and Y. Nose, *J. Biochem.*, **62**, 537 (1967).

17.   R. R. Williams, R. E. Waterman, J. C. Keresztesy, and E. R. Buchman, *J. Am. Chem. Soc.*, **57**, 536 (1935).

18.   H. Nakayama and R. Hayashi, *J. Vitaminol.* (Kyoto), **17**, 64 (1971).

8. Thiamine-Binding Protein of *Escherichia coli*

Y. NOSE, M.D.
A. IWASHIMA, M.D.
A. NISHINO, M.S.

Department of Biochemistry
Kyoto Prefectural University of Medicine
Kyoto, Japan

In recent years a number of binding proteins of *Escherichia coli,* released by osmotic shock, have been shown to bind small molecules such as sugar, amino acids, some vitamins, and inorganic substances, and evidence has accumulated to imply that these proteins are involved in the active transport of the molecules which they bind. With regard to a protein binding thiamine, Nishimune and Hayashi (1) first described the occurrence of a thiamine-binding protein in a thiamineless mutant of *E. coli.* We also obtained a thiamine-binding protein from a mutant of *E. coli* K12 auxotrophic for thiamine thiazole (KG33) by cold-osmotic shock treatment according to the method of Neu and Heppel (2). It has already been reported that the thiamine-binding protein is believed to participate in the thiamine transport through the cell membrane of *E. coli* according to the following findings (3). First, the activity of thiamine accumulation in the cells reduced with osmotic shock was partially restored by the addition of shock fluid as shown in Fig. 1. Second, the rate of thiamine transport, which is repressed by the addition of thiamine to the growth medium of *E. coli,* was roughly proportional to the thiamine-binding activity in shock fluids from the cells (Fig. 2). However, the exact role of the protein in the transport process in unknown.

Recently, we purified the thiamine-binding protein to homogeneity by affinity chromatography, using agarose coupled with thiamine diphosphate

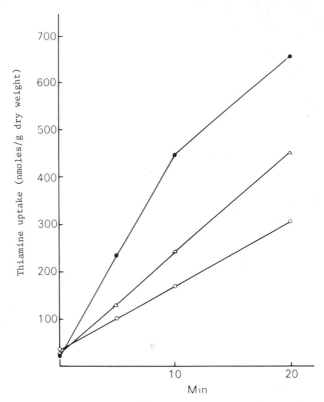

Figure 1. Partial restoration of uptake ability of shocked cells for thiamine by concentrated shock fluid. *Escherichia coli* KG33 grown at 37°C on Davis-Mingioli's medium (4) containing 0.2% glucose and 0.02 μM thiazole was harvested at early stationary phase of growth. The cells, washed once with the minimal medium, were subjected to the cold osmotic shock procedure of Neu and Heppel (2). The shock fluid was concentrated *in vacuo*. Assay of ^{14}C-thiamine uptake was carried out as previously reported (5). Symbols: ●, control cells; ○, cold-shocked cells; △, cold-shocked cells with concentrated shock fluid.

(6). We report here some properties of the purified thiamine-binding protein and discuss the relationship between the thiamine-binding protein and the thiamine transport in *E. coli* based on the inhibitory effects with thiamine analogs.

1. Properties of Thiamine-Binding Protein

Table 1 shows the result of purification of the thiamine-binding protein in the shock fluid. The specific activity, measured by the equilibrium dialysis

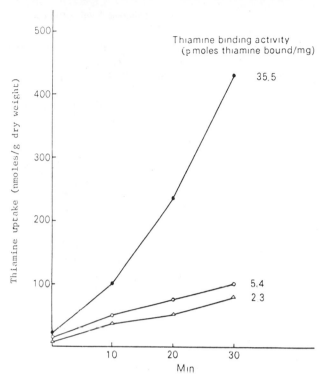

Figure 2. Effect of thiamine added to the growth medium on thiamine uptake and *in vitro* thiamine-binding activity by *E. coli* KG33, grown in the minimal medium containing various concentrations of thiamine as indicated. The rates of thiamine uptake by the cell suspensions were determined, and the thiamine-binding activity in shock fluids was assayed by the equilibrium dialysis method previously described (3). Growth medium was supplemented with 0.01 μM thiamine (●), 0.3 μM thiamine (○), or 1.0 μM thiamine (△).

Table 1. Purification of Thiamine-Binding Protein from *E. coli* KG33

Step	Total Activity, pM	Total Protein, mg	Specific Activity, pM/mg
1. Shock fluid	33,946	630	53.9
2. Ammonium sulfate fraction, 65 ~ 95%	10,506	346	30.4
3. Negative adsorption on DEAE-cellulose	7,947	43	184
4. Affinity chromatography	7,880	1.6	4925

method, represents an overall purification of approximately ninetyfold with a total recovery of 23.2%. An elution pattern of the protein adsorbed to ThDP-sepharose is shown in Fig. 3. The binding of thiamine-binding protein to the column was fairly strong, and the protein could not be eluted with 4 *M* urea. With 8 *M* urea in 0.05 *M* potassium phosphate buffer, pH 7.0, it was quantitatively eluted, resulting in a reversible inactivation. The purified protein exhibits a single band in a standard polyacrylamide gel electrophoresis performed by the method of Weber and Osborn (7).

Since the protein was eluted by 8 *M* urea with a reversible inactivation, but not by 4 *M* urea, the influence of urea on the thiamine-binding protein was examined by acrylamide gel electrophoresis in the absence and the

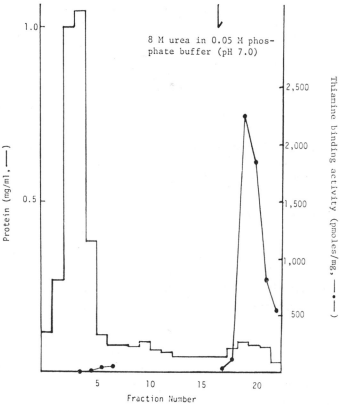

Figure 3. Affinity chromatography of partially purified thiamine-binding protein on TDP-sepharose column. The column (1.4 × 8 cm) packed with ThDP-agarose (6) was equilibrated with 0.05 *M* potassium phosphate buffer, pH 7.0, and the solution concentrated (step 3) was applied to the column. After washing, it was eluted with 0.05 *M* K-phosphate buffer, 4 *M* urea, and then 8 *M* urea in the same buffer successively.

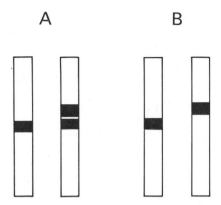

Figure 4. Polyacrylamide gel electrophoresis of the thiamine-binding protein in the absence and the presence of urea. The gels contained 7% acrylamide, 0.2% bisacrylamide, 0.1 M sodium phosphate buffer (pH 7.1), and 0.15% ammonium persulfate in the absence (left of A, B) and the presence of 4 M urea (right of A) or 8 M urea (right of B). The amount of protein applied was 0.1 mg, and the electrophoresis was run at 8 mA per tube for 2.5 hours (A) and 1.5 hours (B). The protein migrated to the anode (bottom).

presence of urea. As shown in Fig. 4, the protein, previously incubated with 4 M urea for 2 hours (right of A), gave two bands, a slower-moving and a faster-moving band, while the control without urea gave (left of A) a faster-moving band alone. The protein pretreated with 8 M urea (right of B) gave a single band, a slower-moving one.

This suggests a probable conformational change of the protein with urea. Therefore, the thiamine-binding protein pretreated with 8 M urea was subjected to electrophoresis on SDS-acrylamide gel, which can be used for determination of the subunit structure of protein. The urea-treated and untreated proteins gave the same movement as a single band on the acrylamide gel containing 1% SDS, which showed no evidence of subunit structures.

In addition, as shown in Fig. 5, the molecular weight of the protein was determined by the method of Weber and Osborn (7). It was calculated to be 38,000, in agreement with the value of 39,000 for the native protein previously obtained by gel filtration (6).

The optimum pH was between 8 and 9, when assayed in 0.1 M citrate buffer. A similar curve was obtained with 0.1 M Tris-HCl buffer, although the activity was slightly lower. The binding was sharply decreased at a higher or lower pH, but the loss of activity was almost recovered by a return to the optimum pH.

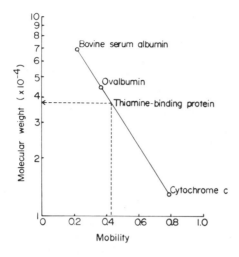

Figure 5. Determination of the apparent molecular weight of thiamine-binding protein by polyacrylamide gel electrophoresis in SDS. The protein was incubated at 37°C for 2 hours in 0.1 *M* sodium phosphate buffer (pH 7.1), 1% in SDS and 1% in β-mercaptoethanol, and then run in a polyacrylamide gel containing 1% SDS in place of urea as described in Fig. 4. The mobility of the protein was plotted against the logarithm of molecular weights of the marker proteins as indicated, which were run in the same way.

2. Inhibition of Thiamine-Binding Activity with Thiamine Analogs

It has been reported that the uptake of thiamine by *E. coli* cells was inhibited by thiamine analogs (8). As shown in Fig. 6, the rates of the uptake were inhibited about 80 to 85% at 5 minutes after incubation by the addition of thiamine analogs, except for pyrithiamine, at molar ratios to thiamine of 100:1. Thiamine sulfuric acid, oxythiamine, dimethialium, and chloroethylthiamine inhibited the thiamine uptake to almost the same extent.

Therefore the effects of the thiamine analogs on the thiamine-binding activity of the protein were examined. As can be seen in Table 2, some of the thiamine analogs, such as thiamine sulfuric acid ester and thiamine phosphoric acid esters, showed marked inhibitions at molar ratios to thiamine of 1:1. On the other hand, the inhibitions by chloroethylthiamine, oxythiamine, etc., were fairly low. The degree of inhibition by thiamine sulfuric acid or thiamine phosphates and thiamine analogs such as chloroethylthiamine and dimethialium differed greatly. This indicates that the inhibitory action of the thiamine analogs on thiamine transport and on thiamine binding to thiamine-binding protein did not coincide. The binding of thiamine to the protein is highly specific for its chemical structure, and the thiamine derivatives containing an acidic group appeared to bind more easily to the protein than did thiamine itself. This is compatible with the reason of binding of the protein to ThDP-sepharose.

Lineweaver-Burk plots of the binding as a function of thiamine concentrations gave a value for the apparent K_m for thiamine of 9.2×10^{-9}

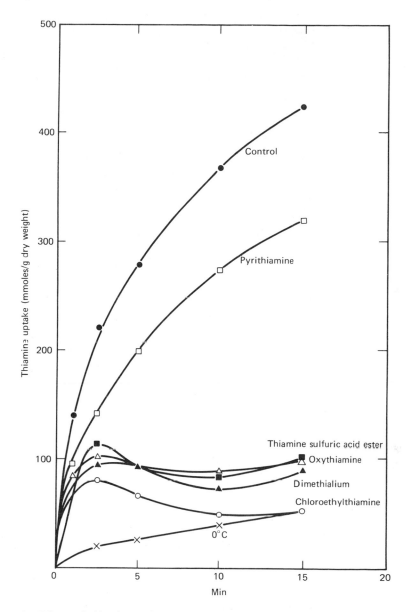

Figure 6. Effects of thiamine analogs on ^{14}C-thiamine uptake by *E. coli* KG33. The cell suspensions containing 0.4% glucose were incubated with 1 μM ^{14}C-thiamine and 100 μM thiamine analogs shown in symbols as indicated, and the rate of thiamine uptake was measured as previously reported (5).

Table 2. Inhibition by Thiamine Analogs of Thiamine-Binding Activity[a]

	Inhibition, %	
	Thiamine Analogs/Thiamine	
Addition	1	100
Thiamine sulfuric acid ester	100	
ThMP	88.6	
ThDP	69.8	
ThTP	50.8	
Chloroethylthiamine		66.0
Dimethialium		44.4
Hydroxyethylthiamine		44.7
Oxythiamine		25.3
Pyrithiamine		0
Thiamine concentration: $2 \times 10^{-8} M$		

[a] Each thiamine analog was added to the dialyzing buffer simultaneously with ^{14}C-thiamine at molar ratios as indicated; then the thiamine-binding activity was assayed by equilibrium dialysis procedure.

M (Fig. 7). This is approximately 2 orders of magnitude lower than the K_m value of $8.3 \times 10^{-7} M$ for thiamine transport by whole cells (5). The inhibitions by thiamine monophosphate and chloroethylthiamine are both competitive and showed K_i values of 3.4×10^{-9} and $6.8 \times 10^{-7} M$, respectively.

3. Chemical Modification of Thiamine-Binding Protein

Recently, studies on interactions of a tryptophan residue in the protein with thiamine diphosphate have been reported. Heinrich et al. (9) suggested an involvement of a tryptophan residue in the active site of transketolase of Baker's yeast, using a specific tryptophan modifier, water-soluble nitrobenzylsulfonium reagent.

A series of experiments using the following chemical reagents known to react with some amino acid residues in the protein was carried out, as shown in Table 3. Iodine treatment, under a fairly violent condition, caused a complete loss of the activity. N-Bromosuccinimide, known to attack tryptophan- and tyrosine-peptide bonds, brought about a 50% inactivation under the condition indicated. N-Acetylimidazole, a selective acetylating agent of tyrosine, had no effect. SH-inhibitors, such as iodoacetate, N-ethylmaleimide, and p-chloromercuribenzoate, did not affect the binding activity. Dimethyl(2-hydroxy-5-nitrobenzyl)sulfonium bromide showed a significant inhibitory effect on the thiamine-binding activity. From these results, it seems likely that a tryptophan residue is involved in the thiamine-binding site of the protein.

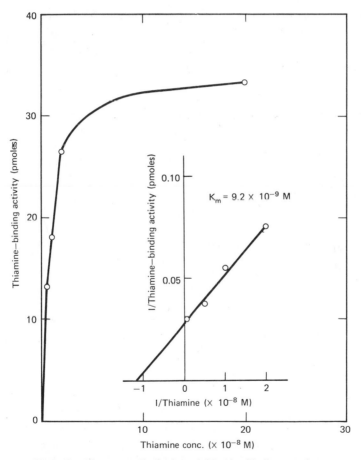

Figure 7. Lineweaver-Burk plots of thiamine-binding reaction.

Table 3. Effects of Various Chemical Treatments on Thiamine-Binding Activity[a]

Reagent	Condition of Treatment	Concentration of Reagent in Treatment M	Inactivation, %
Iodine (KI$_3$)	pH 7.0, 4°C, 4 hr	5×10^{-4}	100
N-Bromosuccinimide	pH 4.5, 25°C, 1.5 hr	2.5×10^{-6}	50
N-Acetylimidazole	pH 7.5, 25°C, 2.5 hr	1×10^{-4}	0
Iodoacetic acid	pH 5.5, 25°C, 27 hr	1×10^{-5}	2.6
N-Ethylmaleimide	pH 7.0, 4°C, 17 hr	1×10^{-3}	0
p-Chloromercuribenzoate	pH 7.0, 4°C, 17 hr	1×10^{-3}	0
Dimethyl(2-hydroxy-5-nitrobenzyl)sulfonium bromide (water soluble)	pH 3.0, 22°C, 4 hr	2×10^{-5} 2×10^{-4} 2×10^{-3}	16.9 39.4 78.7

[a] The thiamine-binding protein (10 μg) was incubated with each reagent under the indicated condition; then thiamine-binding activity was measured by the equilibrium dialysis procedure.

Table 4. Reaction of HNB-(CH$_3$)$_2$SBr with the Thiamine-Binding Protein in the Absence and Presence of Thiamine[a]

Concentration of Reagent, M	Inactivation, %	
	Thiamine Absent	Thiamine Present
2×10^{-5}	17.5	—
2×10^{-4}	47.9	16.9
2×10^{-3}	76.6	66.2

[a] Thiamine (5×10^{-7} M) was added to the thiamine-binding protein (10 μg) before the addition of the reagent; then the thiamine-binding activity was measured by the equilibrium dialysis procedure.

When cold thiamine was added to the binding protein before the addition of the sulfonium reagent, the inhibitory effect was partially reduced, as shown in Table 4. Although the concentration of the cold added thiamine was limited to 5×10^{-7} M to avoid an exchange reaction with ^{14}C-thiamine during equilibrium dialysis, it protected the protein somewhat from inactivation by the sulfonium reagent.

On the other hand, the effects of some of the chemical reagents for modification of ^{14}C-thiamine uptake by whole cells were examined. The *E. coli* cells were preincubated with the chemical modifiers at 37°C for 15 minutes and then washed and resuspended in 10 ml of the thiamine uptake system. As shown in Table 5, dimethyl(2-hydroxy-5-nitrobenzyl)sulfonium bromide inhibited thiamine binding as well as thiamine uptake. However, the thiamine uptake by the cells was markedly inhibited by the SH-inhibitors at a concentration that had no effect on the binding activity of the protein. This fact suggests the existence of a factor other than the thiamine-binding protein in the thiamine transport system of *E. coli* KG33.

4. Thiamine-Binding Protein and the Thiamine Transport System

Since ^{14}C-thiamine transported into the cells is rapidly phosphorylated, the thiamine uptake system involves a phosphorylation step of thiamine. Therefore, so far as the rate of thiamine uptake is determined by estimating thiamine transport involving phosphorylated thiamine, it is supposed to be influenced by several factors in the thiamine uptake system. Of these

Table 5. Effect of Several Reagents for Chemical Treatment of the Cells on ^{14}C-Thiamine Uptake by *E. coli* KG33[a]

Addition, M		^{14}C-Thiamine Uptake, nM/g dry weight	Inhibition, %
None		149.8	—
Iodoacetic acid	1×10^{-3}	73.4	51.0
N-Ethylmaleimide	1×10^{-3}	11.1	92.6
N-Bromosuccinimide	1×10^{-4}	5.7	96.2
Dimethyl(2-hydroxy-	1×10^{-3}	97.3	35.0
5-nitrobenzyl)-	2×10^{-3}	29.6	80.2
sulfonium bromide	5×10^{-3}	11.4	92.4

[a] Experimental conditions are described in the text.

Table 6. Activities of Main Components Involved in Thiamine Transport System of *E. coli* KG33 and KG900

Strain	^{14}C-Thiamine Uptake, nM/(g dry wt) (5 min)	Thiamine-Binding Activity, pM/mg	Thiamine-kinase, nM/(mg) (hr)	ThMP-kinase, nM/(mg) (30 min)	ThMP-PPase,[a] nM/(mg) (hr)
KG33	108.8	2.2–3.0	0.255	0.123	16.7
KG900	6.5	1.8–2.4	0.619	0.148	36.2

[a] Data described by Kawasaki et al. (1969).

factors, thiamine kinase (10) and thiamine monophosphate kinase (11) were found in *E. coli*. The former converts thiamine into thiamine monophosphate, and its reaction is significantly inhibited by chloroethylthiamine and other thiamine analogs. Furthermore, it was found that a mutant defective in thiamine uptake derived from *E. coli* KG33, reported by Kawasaki et al. (12) and designated as *E. coli* KG900, had as much thiamine-binding activity as the parent strain, and the activities of its thiamine kinase and thiamine monophosphate kinase (TMP-kinase) were equivalent to those of the parent strain. (Table 6)

This is not surprising, however, since several of the mutants isolated from *Salmonella typhimurium* were defective in transporting sulfate with high

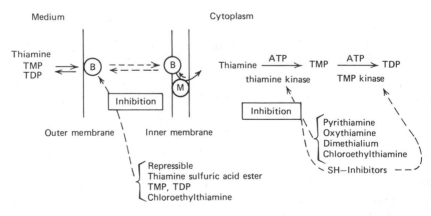

Figure 8. A model for thiamine transport system.

binding activity of sulfate (13). From these results, a model for a thiamine uptake system in *E. coli* is shown in Fig. 8.

Summary

A thiamine-binding protein that is believed to participate in thiamine transport by *E. coli* was purified to a homogeneous state from the osmotic shock fluids of *E. coli*. The molecular weight, calculated by SDS-polyacrylamide gel electrophoresis, was 38,000. There was no evidence of subunits. The apparent K_m for the binding of thiamine was 9.2×10^{-9} M, and the optimal pH was between 8 and 9. Evidence for probable involvement of a tryptophan residue at the binding site of the protein was presented.

On the basis of the difference in the inhibitory effects of thiamine analogs and some chemical modifiers on thiamine-binding activity and thiamine transport, the role of the thiamine-binding protein in the thiamine transport system of *E. coli* was discussed.

References

1. T. Nishimune and R. Hayashi, *Biochim. Biophys. Acta,* **244,** 573 (1971).
2. H. C. Neu and L. A. Heppel, *J. Biol. Chem.,* **241,** 3055 (1965).
3. A. Iwashima, A. Matsuura, and Y. Nose, *J. Bacteriol.,* **108,** 1419 (1971).
4. B. D. Davis and E. S. Mingioli, *J. Bacteriol.,* **60,** 17 (1950).
5. T. Kawasaki, I. Miyata, K. Esaki, and Y. Nose, *Arch. Biochem. Biophys.,* **131,** 223 (1969).
6. A. Matsuura, A. Iwashima, and Y. Nose, *Biochem. Biophys. Res. Commun.,* **51,** 241 (1973).
7. K. Weber and M. Osborn, *J. Biol. Chem.,* **244,** 4406 (1969).
8. A. Iwashima and Y. Nose, *J. Bacteriol.,* **112,** 1438 (1972).
9. C. P. Heinrich, K. Noack, and O. Wiss, *Biochem. Biophys. Res. Commun.,* **49,** 1427 (1972).
10. A. Iwashima and Y. Nose, *Biochim. Biophys. Acta,* **258,** 333 (1972).
11. H. Nishino, *J. Biochem.,* **72,** 1093 (1972).
12. T. Kawasaki, I. Miyata, and Y. Nose, *Arch. Biochem. Biophys.,* **131,** 231 (1969).
13. N. Ohta, P. R. Galsworthy, and A. B. Pardee, *J. Bacteriol.,* **105,** 1053 (1971).

DISCUSSION

Chapter 8

Dr. Cooper. I have a few questions for Professor Nose. First of all, you showed that, when you increased the amount of thiamine in the medium, you decreased the amount of binding or transport of thiamine; yet several illustrations later, when you did Lineweaver-Burk plots, there was no indication of any inhibition by high thiamine concentrations. I am unclear about that.

Dr. Nose. The synthesis of thiamine-binding protein is regulated and repressed by the thiamine concentrations in the growing cells associated with the rate of thiamine transport.

Dr. Cooper. Do you have any ideas concerning the physiological mechanism which releases thiamine from the thiamine-binding protein itself? And, finally, have you tried to make an antibody to the thiamine-binding protein?

Dr. Nose. Not yet, but it is most interesting to investigate the role of thiamine-binding protein on the thiamine transport of *E. coli*.

9. Biochemical Changes in Thiamine Deficiencies

CLARK J. GUBLER, M.D., Ph.D.

Department of Chemistry
Brigham Young University
Provo, Utah

Since the pioneering work of Peters and McGowan (1, 2) demonstrating a role of thiamine in pyruvate metabolism and the identification by Lohmann and Schuster (3) of thiamine diphosphate (ThDP) as the active coenzyme form, a large amount of work has been done on the functions and mechanisms of action of thiamine. It is common knowledge that ThDP serves as the coenzyme for pyruvate (PyDH) and α-ketoglutarate (αKgDH) dehydrogenases and transketolase (TK). Numerous studies have shown that the activities of these enzymes in tissues are markedly reduced when the tissues become depleted of ThDP. At the same time, the blood pyruvate level is elevated. These biochemical changes are associated with a triad of symptoms: anorexia and weight loss, cardiomegaly and bradycardia, and neuromuscular disturbances (ataxia and convulsions), along with other minor symptoms.

Two antagonists of thiamine, oxythiamine (OTh) and pyrithiamine (PTh), have been used extensively to produce experimental thiamine deficiencies. They are of particular interest because OTh produces severe anorexia and most of the other symptoms of thiamine deficiency, but never the neurological symptoms, whereas PTh produces primarily the neurological symptoms. Table 1 presents a comparison of the symptoms and related biochemical changes associated with the three types of experimental thiamine deficiency: thiamine deprivation, OTh treatment, and PTh treatment. Use has been made of these three types of deficiency to

121

Table 1. Comparison of Effects of Thiamine Deprivation and of OTh and PTh Treatment

Symptom or Effect	Thiamine Deprivation	OTh Treatment	PTh Treatment
Anorexia (loss of appetite)	+	+++	± (?) last stages
Weight loss (inanition)	+	++	+ not until terminal
Bradycardia	+	++	+ late stages
Heart enlargement	+	++	+ late stages
Adrenal hypertrophy	+	++	+ late stages
Elevation of blood corticosterone	++	++ with later exhaustion	+ late stages
Elevation of blood pyruvate	+	+++	± except in convulsions

Increased urinary thiamine excretion	0	+	+++
Depletion of tissue thiamine	decrease ++	±	+++
Inhibition of TPK	N.A.[a]	+ (very weak)	+++
Phosphorylation to –PP	N.A.	+++	± (?)
Inhibition of enzymes by inhibitor diphosphate	N.A.	+++	+
Decrease in tissue enzyme activity — PyDH Liver	+++	+++	++
PyDH Heart	+++	+++	++
PyDH Brain	+	0	+++
αKgDH Liver	+++	0	0
αKgDH Heart	+++	++	+
αKgDH Brain	0	0	++
Neurological effect (axia, convulsions)	±	0	+++

[a] N.A.: Not applicable

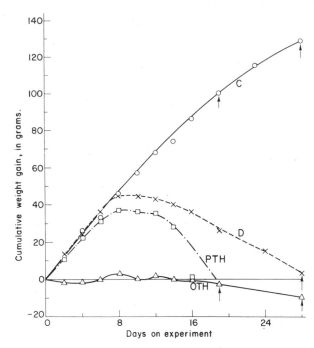

Figure 1. Typical curves for mean change in body weight of experimental rats on the standard thiamine-deficient diet: O——O, normal controls [10 μg thiamine/(100 g body weight)/(day) injected subcutaneously]; ×---×, no supplement (thiamine deprived); △——△, OTh-treated [200 μg OTh + 10 μg thiamine/(100 g) (day)]; □-·-·□, PTh-treated [50 μg PTh + 10 μg thiamine/(100 g)(day)]. Arrows indicate when rats were sacrificed.

try to determine the biochemical changes responsible for the various symptoms of thiamine deficiency. Figure 1 presents typical growth curves for rats with the three experimental thiamine deficiencies, as compared to control rats on the same standard diet. We have carried out a number of studies aimed at correlating the appearance and severity of the various symptoms with the observed biochemical changes. Since this seminar is aimed chiefly at the neurological and membrane functions of thiamine, the data presented here will relate mostly to the neurological symptoms.

Earlier work has shown that OTh enters the brain to only a slight extent or not at all, whereas PTh is actually accumulated in the brain (4, 5, and unpublished observations, C. J. Gubler). This probably explains why PTh causes rapid depletion of brain thiamine (6–8) and activity of thiamine-dependent enzymes, whereas OTh has no effect.

1. Thiamine Derivatives in the Brain after Thiamine Deprivation and Antagonist Treatment

Total thiamine, ThDP + thiamine triphosphate (ThTP), and hydroxyethylthiamine (HET) levels were determined in the brains of rats at intervals after the initiation of thiamine deprivation or treatment with OTh or PTh by methods described earlier (9). Earlier studies (10) had shown that optimum growth for the control rats could be obtained by injection of 10 μg thiamine/(100 g body wt) (day) (see Fig. 1). However, in later studies (6) it was found that, after several days on our standard thiamine-deficient diet with this thiamine supplement, tissue thiamine decreased to a new level well below those found for rats fed Purina Rat Chow. Hence, though the amount available was adequate for growth, the stores were somewhat depleted. As shown in Fig. 2, when the levels of injected thiamine were increased, total brain thiamine and ThDP increased in a proportional manner with increasing intake up to 200 μg/(100 g)(day), above which the brain levels decreased somewhat. Total HET levels remained essentially unaffected.

Figure 3 shows the changes in ThDP plus ThTP and total thiamine in rat brain with time on the treatments indicated. Pyrithiamine causes rapid depletion of total thiamine with an essentially parallel decrease in the phosphate esters. Thiamine deprivation has a much slower and more gradual effect, while OTh has no significant effect on the brain levels. Pyrithiamine accumulates rapidly in the brain in the first 4 days and then

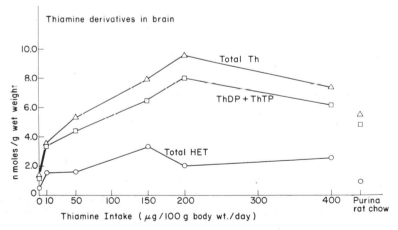

Figure 2. Levels of thiamine derivatives in rat brain after 20 days on the standard thiamine-deficient diet, supplemented with increasing daily doses of thiamine administered subcutaneously.

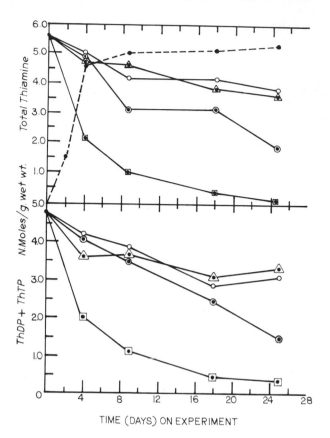

Figure 3. Brain levels of ThDP + ThTP, total thiamine, and PTh in rats on the experimental thiamine deficiencies: O——O, controls [10 μg thiamine/(100 g body weight)/(day) injected subcutaneously]; ⊙——⊙, thiamine deprived (no supplement); △——△, Oth-treated [200 μg Oth + 10 μg thiamine/(100 g)(day); ⊡——⊡, Pth-treated [50 μg PTh + 10 μg thiamine/(100 g)(day). ●----●, PTh level in PTh-treated rats. Rats were killed at various times after start of diet. From Murdock and Gubler (6).

reaches a plateau at a level comparable to the normal initial thiamine levels. Even when the total thiamine levels were markedly reduced, as in thiamine-deprived or PTh-treated rats, there was no consistent change in the total thiamine/ThDP + ThTP ratio.

As shown in Table 2, high-carbohydrate diets resulted in greater accumulation of PTh in the brain and more rapid depletion of total thiamine and ThDP in rats than occurred on a high-fat diet.

Table 2. Thiamine Compounds in Brains of Control and PTh-Treated Rats on High-Fat and High-Carbohydrate Diets

Type of Rat	Total Th		ThDP and ThTP		HET		PTh	
	High Fat	High Carbohydrate	High Fat	High Carbohydrate	High Fat	High Carbohydrate	High Fat	High Carbohydrate
Control	6.19 ±0.21	3.6 ±0.30	5.61 ±0.14	3.30 ±0.30	1.8 ±0.24	0.8 ±0.30	—	—
PTh-treated	0.62 ±0.0	0.28 ±0.0	0.49 ±1.0	0.34 ±0.10	0.32 ±0.10	0.10 ±0.10	3.8 ±0.39	5.5 ±0.39

2. Phosphorylation of Thiamine in the Brain

Since thiamine must be phosphorylated to ThDP in order to be active as the coenzyme, it is important to know more about the mechanism accomplishing this and the factors regulating this process and the ThDP levels. The reaction involved is as follows:

$$\text{Thiamine} + \text{AP}_\alpha\text{P}_\beta\text{P}_\gamma \underset{}{\overset{\text{TPK}}{\rightleftharpoons}} \text{ThP}_\beta\text{P}_\gamma + \text{AP}_\alpha$$

where TPK is thiamine pyrophosphokinase (ATP: thiamine pyrophosphotransferase). The characteristics of TPK, which has been purified 260-fold from pig brain (11), are presented in Table 3. It has an apparent pI of 4.2 and a pH opimum between 8.3 and 9.3. The K_m appears to be 5.5 to 5.9 $\times$ 10^{-2} for ATP and 4.5 to 5.6 $\times$ 10^{-6} for thiamine. Butylthiamine (BuTh), ethylthiamine (EtTH), and PTh act as potent inhibitors of TPK with K_i's even smaller than the K_m for thiamine. Oxythiamine is a relatively weak inhibitor. Optimum activity is found with a Mg^{2+}/ATP ratio of 0.6. These and other data suggest that the enzymatically active ATP species should be $Mg(ATP)_2^{6-}$. Oxythiamine has been shown to be phosphorylated by TPK (12). The question is open with PTh, although it has been reported to occur in tissues chiefly in the pyrophosphorylated form (6). Even intracerebrally injected OTh does not affect brain thiamine levels as does PTh (13).

In studies on changes in biochemical substances in the brain under conditions involving changes in brain weights, the following question has often arisen: Does brain weight bear the same relationship to body weight

Table 3. Purified Thiamine Pyrophosphokinase[a,b] of Pig Brain[c]

Property	Value	Inhibitor	K_i
K_m (ATP)	3.5–5.9 $\times$ 10^{-2}	OTh	6.8 $\times$ $10^{-4}\,M$
K_m (thiamine)	4.1–5.6 $\times$ 10^{-6}	PTh	1.4 $\times$ $10^{-6}\,M$
Optimum pH	8.3–9.3	BuTh	2.1 $\times$ $10^{-6}\,M$
Optimum Mg^{2+}/ATP ratio	0.6	EtTh	0.8 $\times$ $10^{-6}\,M$
Isoionic point (approximate)	4.2		

[a] ATP: thiamine pyrophosphotransferase.
[b] Purified 260-fold.
[c] Reaction: Thiamine $+ \text{AP}_\alpha\text{P}_\beta\text{P}_\delta \rightleftharpoons$ thiamine $\text{P}_\beta\text{P}_\delta + \text{AP}_\alpha$.

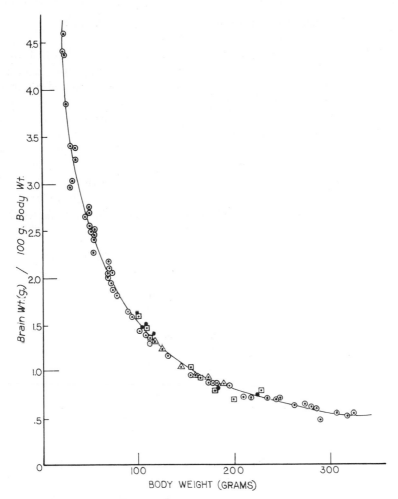

Figure 4. Relationship of brain weight to body weight in rats: ⊙ N, controls; ●, thiamine deprived; ▲, OTh-treated; ▣, PTh-treated. From Cheney et al. (14).

regardless of whether the latter was attained by steady growth, or by loss of weight after attaining a higher weight? To answer this the brain weights as percentages of body weights were plotted against body weights. The composite curve from several experiments (14) is presented in Fig. 4. This indicates that rats which attained a higher body weight and then lost weight had relative brain weights that fell on the same curve as those of rats which attained the same weight by uninterrupted growth.

3. Effect of Thiamine Deficiencies on Acetylcholine Levels in Brain

Since the biosynthesis of acetylcholine (Ach) must compete with fatty acid biosynthesis, cholesterol biosynthesis, and the TCA cycle for the common precursor component, acetyl coenzyme A (Fig. 5), we wondered whether the synthesis of Ach might not suffer if the oxidative decarboxylation of pyruvate in brain were markedly reduced as in PTh-treated rats, and whether this might bear some relation to the observed neurological involvement. As shown in Fig. 5, however, brain Ach levels were significantly lowered in all three types of experimental thiamine deficiency, whereas neurological symptoms were present only in the PTh-treated rats (14). Earlier studies by us and others have shown that brain PyDH activity is also decreased only in the PTh-treated animals. Figure 6 shows that *in*

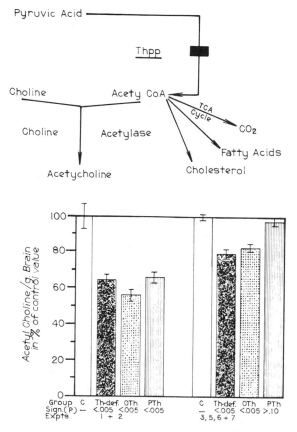

Figure 5. Effects of thiamine deficiency and thiamine antagonists on brain Ach levels.

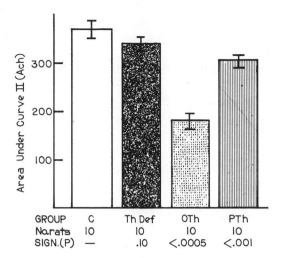

Figure 6. Conversion of [3-^{14}C]pyruvate into ^{14}C-Ach in brain homogenates *in vitro*. After removal of the brain and immediate homogenization, Ach was separated chromatographically and the ^{14}C of the Ach spot measured by a scintillation counter.

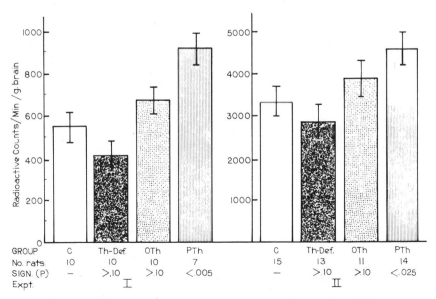

Figure 7. Conversion of injected [3-^{14}C]pyruvate to ^{14}C-Ach *in vivo* in rat brain.

vitro conversion of [3-¹⁴C]pyruvate into ¹⁴C-Ach by brain homogenates was also significantly decreased in all three deficiency types, but the effect was greatest in OTh-treated rats with no neurological involvement. On the other hand, incorporation of ¹⁴C from [3-¹⁴C]pyruvate into Ach *in vivo* was increased in PTh-treated rats but unaffected in thiamine-deprived and OTh-treated rats (Fig. 7). As the data on total radioactivity show, the total ¹⁴C recovered in the brain was markedly increased in PTh-treated rats. This finding probably indicates some breakdown in the blood-brain barrier with PTh treatment. If the cholinesterase inhibitor, eserine, was injected before PTh-induced convulsions started, a significant increase in survival time was noted, whereas no beneficial effect followed if the eserine was injected after the start of convulsions (14). Hence, though changes in Ach levels and metabolism do not correlate with the occurrence of neurological symptoms, Ach must bear some relationship to them.

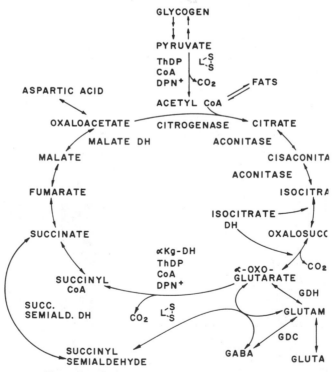

Figure 8.   The TCA cycle, showing the GABA shunt.

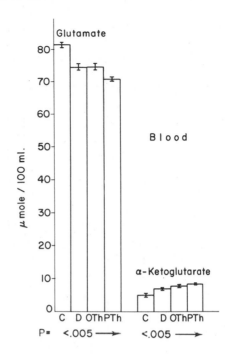

Figure 9. Blood glutamate and α-ketoglutarate levels in the three types of thiamine deficiency.

4. Thiamine Deficiencies and TCA Intermediates in the Brain

Since ThDP and ThDP-dependent enzyme activities, including PyDH and αKgDH activities, are decreased in the brains of PTh-treated rats and these changes are associated with neurological disturbances, the question arises of whether such changes, especially in αKgDH, might be associated with the development of these disturbances. When the following pathway:

$$\alpha\text{-Ketoglutanate } (\alpha\text{Kg}) \xrightarrow{\text{TDP enz.}} \text{succimyl to A} \to \text{succinate}$$

is blocked, αKg can still be converted to succinate via the γ-aminobutyric acid (GABA) shunt (Fig. 8). It has been shown that GABA is a neuroregulatory substance, and hence changes in its level or metabolism might affect brain function. A study was therefore made of the levels of some TCA intermediates in blood and brain, and the incorporation of ^{14}C from intracerebrally injected [3-^{14}C]αKg into various TCA intermediates. As shown in Fig. 9, the blood levels of glutamate were significantly reduced and those of αKg increased in all three types of thiamine deficiency. These changes corresponded to similar decreases in glutamate and increases in αKg in brain, along with significant decreases in GABA in all three

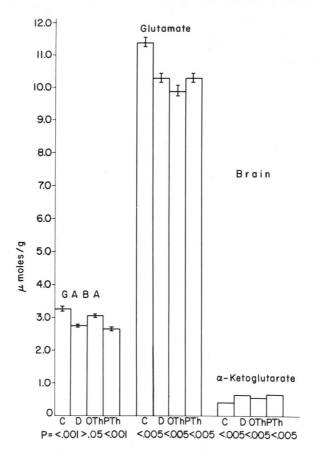

Figure 10. Brain levels of glutamate, α-ketoglutarate, and GABA in the three experimental deficiencies.

deficiencies (Fig. 10). Brain glutamate dehydrogenase activity was not affected. Thirty minutes after the intracerebral injection of $[2\text{-}^{14}C]\alpha Kg$, the ^{14}C recovered in αKg and glutamine in the brain was markedly increased, whereas that in aspartate and glutamate was markedly decreased in all three deficiencies (Fig. 11). The ^{14}C in GABA was increased in OTh-treated but not affected in Th-deprived and PTh-treated rats. The ^{14}C in succinate was decreased in deprived and PTh-treated, but unaffected in OTh-treated, rats.

From these data one would conclude that, though there are some interesting changes in TCA operation in the thiamine deficiencies, these changes do not seem to be correlated with the development of neurological symptoms.

5. Biochemical Basis for Anorexia in Thiamine Deficiencies

Anorexia and inanition are very prominent and severe symptoms in thiamine deficiency, particularly that induced by OTh treatments, and they are already evident by the second day. The anorexia associated with thiamine deprivation is less severe, except in terminal stages, and is of slower onset. There is a question as to whether anorexia is a factor after PTh treatment since inanition is really not evident until ataxia develops, when it may be due to inability to feed, caused by incoordination. The activities of PyDH and transketolase (TK) were determined in intestinal mucosa at various times after initiation of the three deficiency regimens. As shown in Figs. 12 and 13, the TK activity decreased most markedly and was most closely associated with the development of anorexic symptoms (15).

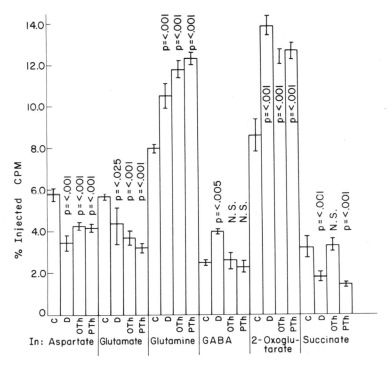

Figure 11. Distribution of ^{14}C in TCA intermediates in the brains of rats in the three experimental deficiencies.

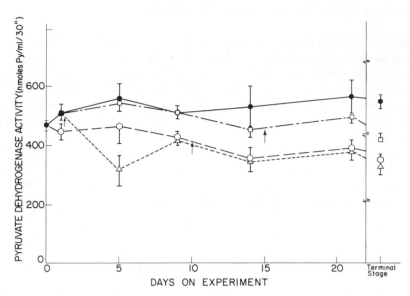

Figure 12. Pyruvate dehydrogenase activity in intestinal mucosa of rats with the three types of experimental deficiency, measured during the course of development of the deficiency. From Bai et al. (15).

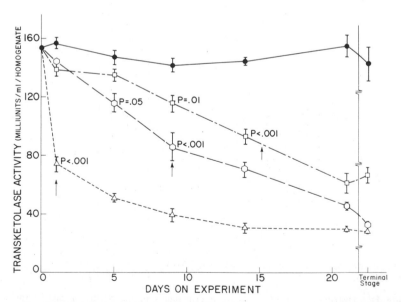

Figure 13. Transketolase activity in intestinal mucosa, measured at the same times as indicated in Fig. 12. From Bai et al. (15).

6.   Biochemical Changes in the Heart

Rats were subjected to our standard procedure for thiamine deprivation and were sacrificed at intervals after the treatment was started. Heart weight, heart rate, creatine phosphate, and ATP levels and activities of PyDH and αKgDH in the heart were then determined. The results are presented in Fig. 14 for thiamine-deprived, Fig. 15 for OTh-treated, and Fig. 16 for PTh-treated rats, where the data are expressed in percentages of the values obtained for control rats sacrificed at the same time (16). Even at the terminal stage, ATP levels were not changed in any of the deficiencies, and creatine phosphate was actually increased in OTh- and PTh-treated groups. Hence it would appear that deficiency of available energy stores is not the basis for the heart changes. As can be seen, the heart rate decreased (bradycardia) in a reciprocal fashion to the increase in relative heart weight. The changes in these heart parameters were somewhat closely correlated with the decreases in activity of PyDH and αKgDH. Since pyruvate and lactate levels are high in blood and heart tissues in the three deficiency types, hearts were removed and perfused with high levels of pyruvate and lactate in the perfusion fluid. This did not induce a slowing of the beat of the perfused hearts. The extra pyruvate and lactate did, however, produce a reduction in the force of contraction. It is interesting to note that the

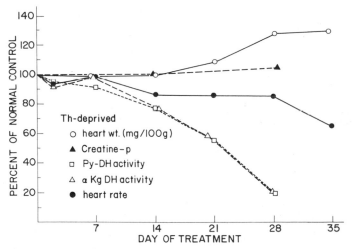

Figure 14.   Biochemical changes with time in the hearts of rats during thiamine deprivation. From Sutherland et al. (16).

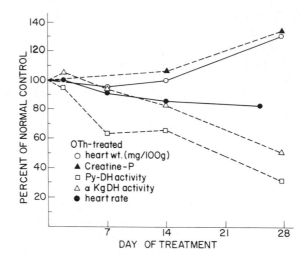

Figure 15. Changes with time in the hearts of rats on OTh treatment. From Sutherland et al. (16).

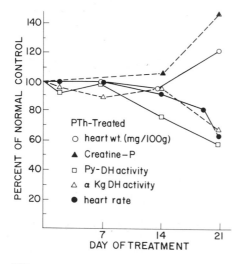

Figure 16. Changes with time in the hearts of rats on PTh treatment. From Sutherland et al. (16).

bradycardia of thiamine-deficient rat hearts persisted after they were removed and perfused with modified Krebs solution.

Acknowledgments

This work was supported by grant AM-02448 from the Institute of Arthritis, Metabolism, and Digestive Diseases, National Institutes of Health, and by the Utah Heart Association.

References

1. G. K. McGowan and R. A. Peters, *Biochem. J.*, **31**, 1637 (1937).
2. R. A. Peters, *Biochem. J.*, **31**, 2206 (1936), and **31**, 2240 (1937).
3. R. Lohmann and P. Schuster, *Naturwissenschaften*, **2**, 26 (1937).
4. G. Rindi and V. Perri, *Biochem. J.*, **80**, 214 (1961).
5. G. Rindi, L. Guiseppe, and U. Ventura, *J. Nutr.*, **81**, 147 (1963).
6. D. S. Murdock and C. J. Gubler, *J. Nutr. Sci. Vitaminol.*, **19**, 237 (1973).
7. L. DeCaro, G. Rindi, and L. DeGuiseppe, *Int. Rev. Vitam. Res.*, **31**, 333 (1961).
8. D. W. McCandless and S. Schenker, *J. Clin. Invest.*, **47**, 2268 (1968).
9. D. S. Murdock and C. J. Gubler, *J. Nutr. Sci. Vitaminol.*, **19**, 43 (1973).
10. C. J. Gubler, *J. Biol. Chem.*, **236**, 3112 (1961).
11. J. W. Peterson, C. J. Gubler, and S. A. Kuby, *Biochim. Biophys. Acta* (in press).
12. L. R. Johnson and C. J. Gubler, *Biochim. Biophys. Acta*, **1501**, 85 (1968).
13. G. Rindi, G. Sicorelli, and G. Ferrarese, *Experientia*, **25**, 706 (1969).
14. D. L. Cheney, C. J. Gubler, and A. W. Jaussi. *J. Neurochem.*, **16**, 1283 (1969).
15. P. Bai, M. Bennion, and C. J. Gubler, *J. Nutr.*, **101**, 731 (1971).
16. D. J. B. Sutherland, A. W. Jaussi, and C. J. Gubler, *J. Nutr. Sci. Vitaminol.*, **20**, 35 (1974).

DISCUSSION

Chapter 9

Dr. Itokawa. When animals were put on a thiamine-deficient diet, they lost appetite. I think that some biochemical changes in thiamine-deficient animals may be attributed to malnutrition or starvation. How are the appetites of your pyrithiamine treated rats?

Dr. Gubler. The pyrithiamine-treated rats do not seem to lose their appetites, and they do not cease eating until they get ataxia; I suppose that is the main feature there. Anorexia seems to be pretty specific for the deprived and the oxythiamine-treated rats. Changes in the gut transketolase level closely paralleled the development of the anorexia and the loss of weight related to it in the various groups.

10. Recent Information on Thiamine Nutritional Status in Selected Countries

MYRON BRIN, Ph.D.

Roche Research Center
Nutley, New Jersey

1. Introduction

Thiamine deficiency has occurred in man as a consequence of his persistence in refining grain to its white, devitaminized and demineralized, starchy eminence. Beriberi, per se, has been essentially eradicated wherever appropriate programs have been instituted to refortify the processed grain with vitamins and minerals. However, in developed countries, it still persists in alcoholics. It is unfortunate that the human species has such a compulsive predilection for pure white grain, since it is detrimental to our nutritional health. The preference persists, regardless of urban or rural dwelling, or of economic status, and is especially unfortunate for the rural village dweller who processes his own grain and has no opportunity for exposure to centrally fortified grain.

Criteria for Assessing Thiamine Status

The criteria for assessing thiamine adequacy are shown in Table 1. The dietary intake criteria are based on those of the Interdepartmental Committee on Nutrition for National Development (ICNND), *Manual for Nutrition Surveys* (1), and other sources (6). The various categories are

Table 1. Criteria for Thiamine Nutritional Adequacy

	Adequacy Grouping					
	Below Adequate		Adequate			
Criterion	Deficient	Low	Acceptable	High		Reference
Dietary						
Thiamine intake,						
mg/1000 calories	<0.2	0.2–0.29	0.30–0.4	>0.5		1
Proportion of RDA	<0.5 RDA	<0.75 RDA	0.75–1 RDA	>RDA		2–6
Biochemical						
Urine excretion,						
µg/g creatinine	<27	27–65	66–120	>120		1
Red blood cells: ThDP						
effect, % stimulation	>25	15–24	<15	—		12

established arbitrarily, being used in some similar form in Europe (2–5) and the United States. Criteria for urine excretion are those of the ICNND (23), Table 1.

After the publication in 1956 of the concept of using the red blood cells as a biopsy tissue for measuring transketolase activity to relate clinical and biochemical thiamine deficiency (7), the simple system was reported in full in 1958 (8), and in 1960 was simplified for routine use (9) and reapplied to clinical work (10). The final assay system measured the disappearance of pentose sugar and the formation of hexose sugar in the presence of hemolyzed red blood cells, both with and without added pure thiamine diphosphate (ThDP). Subsequently, another participant in this conference developed a modified assay that utilized the same buffer and substrate systems but required only microquantities of whole blood and measured the formation of sedoheptulose (11). Within 3 to 4 years, a multitude of assay choices became available (12), and additional modifications still appear (13).

The ThDP-effect criteria shown in Table 1 (14, 15) are based on studies of experimental thiamine deficiency in human beings (10), performed and assayed with the original hemolysate technique of measuring hexose formation. An illustration of the basis for these criteria is shown in Figure 1 (15). Clearly, values over 15% ThDP effect are significantly related. However, although these criteria are used almost universally by investigators, regardless of the enzyme assay system, there are no published data to show that the same criteria apply for other enzyme assays. As a matter of fact, we might have established different criteria for pentose than for hexose since, in our experience, the hexose assay was the most reliable (16).

3. Thiamine Status in Various Countries

For the last two decades, nutritional data have, for the most part, been available only from developed countries. The surveys were often performed on discrete populations or family groups; therefore reports chosen for this study may not reflect conditions prevailing throughout any country.

The dietary indices for recent reports from Switzerland, Australia, the Netherlands, Germany, and the United States are presented in Table 2. It would appear that, although large groups are consuming less than three fourths of the recommended daily allowance the (RDA) for thiamine, only scattered individuals are in the deficient category of consuming less than one half of the RDA. The exceptions are the Australian aborigines (three families reported on here), who are known to exist on bare subsistence rations in remote natural areas. The other point to be noted is the deterioration of thiamine status in the United States over a 15-year study

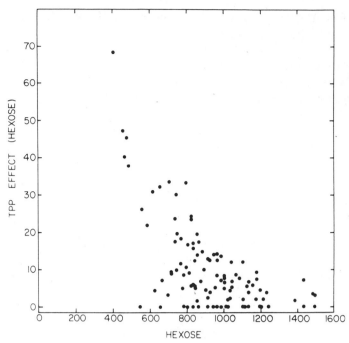

Figure 1. A scatter diagram of transketolase assay values for hexose formation and ThDP effect (hexose) for 210 subjects. A clear relationship is seen between those ThDP effect (hexose) values in excess of 15% ($p < .0001$). From Brin (15), p. 435.

period. This has been explained as being due to decreased consumption of enriched bread in favor of increased intake of refined and unenriched carbohydrate in candy, soda pop, and snack foods (6).

Certain biochemical indices have also been reported for the same group of countries. These data are shown in Table 3. In the United States, the first group of 10 institutionalized elderly men was maintained on a diet containing about 700 μg thiamine HCl/day, which is clearly inadequate (23). In the second study of 233 subjects, those institutionalized in hospitals had poorer nutrition than did those in a county home, but the self-fed (i.e., the latter) group also showed inadequate thiamine intake (24). The migrant group was at a subsistence-survival level (25) and likewise had poor thiamine status. The junior high school children had fair status for thiamine (23). *Nutrition Canada* (27) suggested that at least a quarter of the population was "at risk" on the dietary intake basis, as compared to 15 to 20% by biochemical assay. In Yugoslavia, farm families were less well nourished than were school children. Again, in the United States, 25% of the general population was below adequate biochemical levels, according to a recent compilation (20). A dietary evaluation of preschool children showed essential adequacy (22). Isolated communities in Puerto Rico also showed a high incidence of low thiamine nutrition (21).

In Table 4 are shown biochemical indices for less developed countries, as surveyed by the ICNND in cooperation with the governmental authorities of these countries over a period of years (31–37). It would appear that institutionalized groups, such as the military, have lower nutritional status for thiamine (based on urinary excretion) than do self-fed civilians, although appreciable numbers of civilians also have low values.

4. Interpretation of Findings and Recommendations

There are no universal guidelines by which one may judge how many members of a population group must be "below adequate" in the intake of a nutrient before a national public health intervention occurs. However, it is clear that major portions of the populations of many developed, as well as

Table 2. Dietary Indices for Thiamine

Country	Age Group[a]	Percent of Population below:			Reference
		RDA	0.75 RDA	0.5 RDA	
Switzerland	Aged (I)	—	72	22	2
	Students (S)	—	47	0	3
	Children (I)	—	0	0	4
Australia	Aged (I)	—	33	0	5
	Aged (S)	—	6	0	
	Aged (M)	—	67	0	
	Aborigine (S)	—	—	50	17
Netherlands	Adult (S)	—	40	3	18
	Children (S)	—	34	0	
United States	Varied (1952)	47	10	1	20
	Varied (1957)	45	9	1	
	Varied (1965)	62	13	2	

[a] I = Institution fed; S = self-fed; M = meals on wheels.

Table 3. Biochemical (Dietary) Indices for Thiamine

Country	Age Group[a]	Percent of Population below Adequate Level			Reference
		Urine	ThDP	Diet	
United States	Elderly (I)	90	43	100	24
	Elderly (I)	28	6	—	25
	Migrant (S)	38	30	—	26
	Average (S)	25	—	—	20
	Preschool (S)	—	—	2	22
	Junior high school	6	4		23
Canada	0–9 years (S)	1.0	—	17	27
	10–19 years (S)	14.0	—	27	
	20–64 years (S)	18.0	—	35	
	65+ years (S)	20.0	—	24	
	Pregnant (S)	2.0	—	21	
Yugoslavia	Farm (S)	50.0	13.0		28
	Children (S)	15.0	1.5		29
Puerto Rico	2–12 years (S)	8.3	—	—	30
	13–18 years (S)	16.0	—	—	
	19+ years (S)	4.0	—	—	

[a] I = Institution fed; S = self-fed.

Table 4 Biochemical Indices for Thiamine in Less Developed Countries

Country	Percent of Population below Adequate Level		Reference
	Military	Civilian	
Uruguay	54	27	31
Jordan	—	5	32
Colombia	51	20	33
Chile	3	1	34
Peru	34	—	35
East Pakistan	—	9	36
Thailand	13	49	37

less developed, countries have less than adequate thiamine intake. Although bread enrichment in the United States has virtually eliminated classical beriberi (38), there are still many U.S. citizens with below-adequate intake of thiamine. Perhaps this situation exists because only about 35 states have made enrichment mandatory, or it may be due to the other reasons mentioned previously (6). While enrichment of all processed grain has been recommended to eliminate hypovitaminosis (39), it has always been argued that centrally processed grain does not reach remote areas in less developed countries. What is overlooked is that enriched grain can at least reach the urban communities. Other delivery systems have been proposed for remote areas (40).

A recent bulletin of the National Academy of Science/National Research Council Food and Nutrition Board Panel on Food Standards and Fortification Policy has proposed the enrichment with six vitamins and four minerals of all grain processed in the United States, including wheat, corn, and rice. It recommends that the nutrient addition be done at the mill, to ensure uniform nutrient availability for all grain users and reprocessors (41). Carefully documented in this report are the nutritional need, the scientific justification, and the economic feasibility (42) of the proposals. Accomplishing this public health need would appear to be more complex in developing countries, but the evidence suggests that the effort is worthwhile, at least for population groups that consume centrally processed grain.

5. Summary

Thiamine status is reviewed for various developed and developing countries. About 20% of the population of developed countries have below-adequate status; in developing countries up to 50% of the population have a low thiamine intake. It has also been found that institutionalized subjects have poorer status than do free-living individuals. Delivery systems for improving thiamine status are discussed.

References

1. Interdepartmental Committee on Nutrition for National Development, *Manual for Nutrition Surveys*, 2nd ed., U.S. Government Printing Office Washington, D. C., 1963.
2. D. Schlettwein-Gsell, *Int. J. Vitam. Res.*, **39**, 457, 1969.
3. D. Schlettwein-Gsell and G. Ritzel, *Int. J. Vitam. Res.*, **40**, 95, 1970.
4. G. Ritzel and D. Schlettwien-Gsell, *Int. J. Vitam. Res.*, **40**, 548, 1970.

5. J. Woodhill et al., in M. W. Gordon, Ed., *Food and Nutrition News and Notes*, Australian Institute of Anatomy, 1970.

6. U.S. Department of Agriculture, *Household Food Consumption Survey*, Washington, D. C., 1965–66.

7. M. Brin, S. S. Shohet, and C. S. Davidson, *Fed. Proc.*, **15**, 224, 1956.

8. M. Brin, S. S. Shohet, and C. S. Davidson, *J. Biol. Chem.*, **230**, 319, 1958.

9. M. Brin, M. Tai, and A. S. Ostashever, *J. Nutr.*, **71**, 273, 1960.

10. M. Brin, *Ann. N.Y. Acad. Sci.*, **98**, 528, 1962.

11. P. Dreyfus, *New Engl. J. Med.*, **276**, 596, 1962.

12. M. Brin, in *Thiamine Deficiency-Biochemical Lesions*, Ciba Foundation Study Group, No. 28, Churchill, London, 1967, p. 82.

13. L. G. Warnock, *J. Nutr.*, **100**, 1057, 1970.

14. M. Brin, *J. Am. Med. Assoc.*, **187**, 762, 1964.

15. M. Brin, in A. A. Albanese, Ed., *Newer Methods in Nutritional Biochemistry*, Vol. 3, Academic Press, New York, 1967, p. 407.

16. M. Brin, *Methods Enzymoly*, **18**, 125, (1970).

17. M. Kamien, S. Nobile, P. Cameron, and P. Rosewear, *Aust. N. Z. J. Med.*, **4**, 126, 1974.

18. L. M. Dalderup, B. E. Van Dana, K. Schiedt, G. H. M. Keller, and F. Schouten, *Int. J. Vitam. Res.*, **40**, 633, 1970.

19. L. M. Dalderup, Netherlands Institute of Nutrition, Annual Report, 1968.

20. T. R. A. Davis, S. N. Gershoff, and D. F. Gamble, *J. Nutr. Educ.*, **1**, Suppl. I, p. 39 (Fall, 1969).

21. N. A. Fernandez, J. C. Burgos, C. F. Asenjo, and I. Rosa, *Am. J. Clin. Nutr.*, **24**, 952, 1971.

22. G. M. Owen and K. M. Kramm, *J. Am. Diet. Assoc.*, **54**, 490, 1969.

23. M. V. Dibble, M. Brin, E. McMullen, A. Peel, and N. Chen, *Am. J. Clin. Nutr.*, **17**, 218, 1965.

24. M. Brin, S. H. Schwartzberg, and D. Arthur-Davies, *J. Am. Ger. Soc.*, **12**, 493, 1914.

25. M. Brin, M. V. Dibble, A. Peel, E. McMullen, A. Bourquin, and N. Chen, *Am. J. Clin. Nutr.*, **17**, 240, 1965.

26. V. F. Thiele, M. Brin, and M. V. Dibble, *Am. J. Clin. Nutr.*, **21**, 1229, 1968.

27. *Nutrition Canada*, National Survey, Cat. #H58-36/1973, Ottawa.

28. R. Buzina, M. Jusic, A. Brodarec, N. Milanovic, G. Brubacher, S. Christeller, and J. P. Veuilleumier, *Int. J. Vitam. Res.*, **41**, 289, 1971.

29. R. Buzina, M. Jusic, J. Sapunar, N. Milanovic, A. Zinolo, A. Rajaic, G. Brubacher, and S. Christeller, *Int. J. Vitam. Res.*, **42**, 170, 1972.

30. N. A. Fernandez, J. C. Burgos, I. C. Plough, L. J. Roberto, and C. F. Asenjo, *Am. J. Clin. Nutr.*, **17**, 305, 1965.

31. Interdepartmental Committee on Nutrition for National Development, Report: *Nutrition Survey of Republic of Uruguay*, U.S. Government Printing Office, Washington, D.C., May 1963.

32. Interdepartmental Committee on Nutrition for National Development, Report: *Nutrition Survey of Hashemite Kingdom of Jordon*, U.S. Government Printing Office, Washington, D.C., May 1963.

33. Interdepartmental Committee on Nutrition for National Development, Report: *Nutrition Survey of Columbia,* U.S. Government Printing Office, Washington, D.C., December 1961.

34. Interdepartmental Committee on Nutrition for National Development, Report: *Nutrition Survey of Chile,* U.S. Government Printing Office, Washington, D.C., August 1961.

35. Interdepartmental Committee on Nutrition for National Development, Report: *Nutrition Survey of Peru Armed Forces,* U.S. Government Printing Office, Washington, D.C., December 1959.

36. Interdepartmental Committee on Nutrition for National Development, Report: *Nutrition Survey of East Pakistan,* U.S. Government Printing Office, Washington, D.C., May 1966.

37. Interdepartmental Committee on Nutrition for National Development, Report: *Nutrition Survey of the Kingdom of Thailand,* U.S. Government Printing Office, Washington, D. C., February, 1962.

38. *United States Federal Register,* p. 10788, U.S. Government Printing Office, Washington, D.C., August 3, 1943.

39. M. Brin, in A. Berg et al., Eds., *Nutrition, National Development and Planning,* W. H. Freeman, San Francisco, 1973, p. 309.

40. M. Brin, in A. A. Altschul, Ed., *New Protein Foods,* Vol. II, (in press).

41. National Academy of Science-National Research Council, *Proposed Fortification Policy for Cereal-Grain Products,* Washington, D.C., 1974.

42. S. H. Rubin and W. M. Cort, in M. Milner, Ed., *Protein-Enriched Cereal Foods for World Needs,* American Association of Cereal Chemists, St. Paul, Minn., 1969.

DISCUSSION

Chapter 10

Dr. Fujiwara. How many states enrich bread with thiamine?

Dr. Brin. About 35. As a matter of fact, I attended a meeting in Washington about 2 years ago, where I met the chief nutritionist of Florida and asked her whether bread is enriched in Florida. She said, "No, how do you go about it?" We suggested that she talk to people at the University of Florida at Gainesville. They and some other professionals in the area of nutrition sat down with some legislators in the state, and finally, last year, an enrichment bill for bread was passed in Florida. The legislators really provided a great service, which was not previously available.

Dr.Warnock. I would like to mention that I was on the Lebanese survey; the Lebanese government had a law against the enrichment of bread at the time, and our survey changed that.

Dr. Brin. This is the fallout or spinoff of good work and good collaboration. I had, of course, read many papers about nutrition in Japan, where there is an extensive program of bread enrichment not only with vitamins but in some cases also with amino acids.

Dr. Fujiwara. Do you have any speculation on the relationship between thiamine and alcohol ingestion?

Dr. Brin. Some people have asked why beriberi appears in alcoholics before other vitamin deficiencies. This is the classical syndrome which is observed when an alcoholic comes to the hospital. Our studies on the effects of fasting on erythrocyte transketolase activity have shown that the body is depleted of thiamine in 4 days. The alcoholic often consumes a poor diet, although it is inferior in many nutrients. The probability is that thiamine is depleted the most rapidly, and thus symptoms of thiamine deficiency are the first to become clinically manifest.

Dr. Kark. Along these lines, were there, in any of the studies that you mentioned, correlations with the risk level of either measurements or estimates of peripheral nerve function or of cardiac output such as arm-to-tongue circulation time?

Dr. Brin. Well, Dr. Warnock can probably speak more clearly on the evaluation of neurological status because his surveys probably involved some neurological examinations.

Dr. Warnock. We did not do any neurological work at all in the Lebanese survey. You have to bear in mind that most of these surveys are done out in the field in the back of a truck, and very little neurological work can be done under these conditions.

Dr. Brin. I once attended a Gordon conference in which Colonel Plough presented data on the loss of knee jerk and its relationship to thiamine status. The loss of knee jerk was more highly correlated with the age of the subject than with thiamine status, but that material has never been published. In some of the surveys, the medical team did a superficial neurological examination such as eliciting an ankle or a knee jerk, but that is about all. This kind of study is often done by dieticians and biochemists who do not have supporting medical teams. The medical students whom we had on controlled thiamine intake and from whom these data are derived (there were probably 15 in each group in the series of two studies) experienced only one incident of loss of knee jerk, in a control subject.

Dr. Blass. To add to that list of negative findings in regard to thiamine deficiency, a recent paper in the *Journal of Neurochemistry* claimed that acetylcholine and acetyl coenzyme A levels dropped in the brains of thiamine-deficient animals (C. P. Heinrich, H. Stadler, and H. Weiser, *J. Neurochem.*, **21**, 1273–1281, 1973). We had looked at that aspect previously and found no drop; our note is now in press. The authors of that report pointed out that there are about six or eight papers on the levels of acetyl-CoA in thiamine-deficient brain. Half report a drop, and the other half do not. One theory is that there is a change in the small pool of acetylcholine which turns over in the brain with a half-life of the order of a second or less. Now that ways are being found to inactivate brain enzymes in that time, it may become possible to make better measurements.

Dr. Gubler. I think one difference involves how soon and how the brain is removed. There has been a lot of variation in that respect. We pretreated our rats with the cholinesterase inhibitor, eserine, so there should have been little destruction of acetylcholine before the extraction was accomplished.

THREE

THIAMINE METABOLISM IN BRAIN

11. Thiamine Uptake by Rat Brain Slices

Y. NOSE, M.D.
A. IWASHIMA, M.D.
H. NISHINO, M.D.

Department of Biochemistry
Kyoto Prefectural University of Medicine
Kyoto, Japan

It has been accepted that thiamine is taken up by animal cells via an active transport process through the cell membrane and that this process is closely associated with the phosphorylation of thiamine during or after its transport (1, 2). However, in the experiment by Sharma and Quastel, using rat brain cortex slices, the concentration of ^{14}C-thiamine which was transported was calculated only from the thiamine concentration in the tissue cell water (2). Therefore this was investigated by using rat brain slices regardless of whether or not the thiamine accumulation against a concentration gradient is dependent on the phosphorylation process, and exactly calculating the intracellular to extracellular concentration ratio of ^{14}C-thiamine in the slices, especially with regard to free thiamine.

1. Experimental

CHEMICALS

Thiamine ([2-^{14}C]thiazole) hydrochloride (14 mCi/mM) and ^{3}H-inulin were purchased from the Radiochemical Centre, Amersham, England. Thiamine monophosphate (ThMP) was kindly supplied by Dr. S. Yurugi, Takeda Chemical Industries, Osaka. Thiamine triphosphate (ThTP) and chloroethylthiamine were the gifts of Dr. T. Yusa, Sankyo Company, Tokyo. Thiamine diphosphate (ThDP), pyrithiamine, and oxythiamine were the products of Sigma Chemical Company. Ouabain was purchased from Merck Company, and Dowex 1 × 4 resin from Dow Chemical Company. Other chemicals were obtained from commercial sources and were of reagent grade.

PREPARATION OF BRAIN SLICES AND INCUBATION

Rats weighing 150 to 250 grams were decapitated, and the brains were removed and placed in Krebs-Ringer bicarbonate buffer solution (pH 7.4) (3). Brain slices, about 0.3 mm in thickness, were quickly prepared by cutting both hemispheres. The slices (80 to 130 mg wet weight) were transferred to vessels containing Krebs-Ringer bicarbonate buffer with 10 mM glucose. After preincubation for 10 minutes at 37°C under gassing with a mixture of O_2 and CO_2 (95:5, v/v), ^{14}C-thiamine was added and the incubation was continued under the same conditions for an appropriate time, usually 60 minutes.

ESTIMATION OF ^{14}C-THIAMINE UPTAKE

After the incubation, the slices were rinsed with Krebs-Ringer bicarbonate buffer, gently blotted on filter paper, weighed, and homogenized with a Potter-Elvehjem homogenizer. The homogenate was heated at 90°C for 5 minutes and then centrifuged at 10,000 × g for 30 minutes. The radioactivity in the extracts and in the incubation medium was determined using a liquid scintillation counter (Packard Tri-Carb 3375).

The total tissue water was determined to be 82.4% of the wet weight after 60 minutes of incubation, from the difference between the wet tissue weight and the weight after drying at 80°C for 24 hours. The extracellular space (ECS) was determined as follows. ^{3}H-Inulin was incubated with the brain slices in the same way as that used for ^{14}C-thiamine uptake, and the radioactivity was determined in the extracts and the medium. The ECS was calculated according to the following equation:

ECS (% wet weight)

$$= \frac{\text{cpm in total tissue water/cpm in ml of medium}}{\text{wet tissue weight}} \times 100$$

The ECS value obtained was 17.5% of the wet weight. The concentration of ^{14}C-thiamine in the intracellular fluid (C_{ICF}) was calculated according to the following equation:

$$C_{ICF} = \frac{C_{tissue} - C_{medium} \times ECS \times 1/100}{(\text{total tissue water} - ECS) \times 1/100}$$

where

C_{ICF} = thiamine content/ml ICF,

C_{tissue} = thiamine content/g wet tissue,

C_{medium} = thiamine content/ml medium ($= C_{ECF}$).

The tissue accumulation of ^{14}C-thiamine was expressed as a ratio, C_{ICF}/C_{ECF}.

DETERMINATION OF FREE ^{14}C-THIAMINE AND ITS PHOSPHATE

Extracts of the slices obtained by heating were lyophilized and dissolved in a small amount of water, and then subjected to paper chromatography using an ascending method with the following solvent system: isopropanol-0.5 M acetate buffer (pH 4.5)-H_2O = 65:15:20, v/v. The developed paper chromatogram was cut into small strips and counted differentially in 10 ml of Bray's solution. The R_F values for authentic thiamine, its monophosphate, and its diphosphate were 0.70, 0.41, and 0.22, respectively.

ASSAY OF THIAMINE PYROPHOSPHOKINASE ACTIVITY

Thiamine pyrophosphokinase activity was measured as follows. The reaction mixture contained 100 μM of Tris-HCl (pH 7.5), 10 μM of ATP, 10 μM of $MgCl_2$, 6 nM of thiamine, and the enzyme solution [a fraction precipitated by 0.5 to 0.6 $(NH_4)_2SO_4$ saturation from the crude extracts of rat brains], in a total volume of 3 ml. The reaction mixture was incubated for 1 hour at 37°C. After adding 1 ml of sodium citrate buffer (pH 6.0), the reaction was stopped by heating at 90°C for 5 minutes, followed by centrifugation to remove denatured protein. Thiamine diphosphate in an aliquot (2 ml) of the deproteinized solution was determined manometrically by carbon dioxide liberation from pyruvate after recombination of yeast apocarboxylase with ThDP (4).

SEPARATION OF THIAMINE TRIPHOSPHATE BY THE ION-EXCHANGE METHOD

The procedure was based on the method of Koike and Yusa (5) with a slight modification. Three pieces of the brain slice were incubated with ^{14}C-thiamine for 1.5 hours under the same conditions as those in the uptake experiment. After the incubation the slices were homogenized with 5% trichloroacetic acid, using a Potter-Elvehjem homogenizer. The supernatant from the centrifuged homogenate was adjusted to pH 6.8 with NaOH and treated batchwise with Norit A, previously activated, instead of the "charcoal column" described in the original method. The charcoal was washed successively with water, 0.5 N HCl, and water, after which the thiamine compounds, which were adsorbed on Norit, were eluted with 20% pyridine solution. The pyridine in the eluate was removed by mixing four times with an equal volume of chloroform. The aqueous layer was applied to a column of Dowex 1 × 4 resin (1 × 40 cm, 200~400 mesh, acetate form) by adding nonlabeled ThTP as the carrier. After the thiamine and ThMP which were adsorbed on the column, were removed by washing, elution of ThTP was performed by a linear gradient of acetate buffer, pH 4.5, from 0 to 1 M. Measurement of OD_{245} and radioactivity in each 3-ml fraction was carried out.

2. Results and Discussion

UPTAKE AND ACCUMULATION OF ^{14}C-THIAMINE BY RAT BRAIN SLICES

Figure 1 shows the time course of ^{14}C-thiamine uptake at 37°C by the brain slices, which were incubated with an initial thiamine concentration of 1 × 10^{-7} M. The uptake of thiamine showed a linear increase during the first hour of incubation, after which it continued to rise more slowly for at least 3 hours.

The ratio of intracellular to extracellular concentration of ^{14}C-thiamine compounds (C_{ICF}/C_{ECF}) exceeded unity after 30 minutes of incubation. This is shown in Fig. 2. The effect of thiamine concentration on the thiamine uptake for 1 hour was examined by varying the initial concentration of ^{14}C-thiamine in the medium. As shown in Fig. 2, an accumulation of the radioactivity against the concentration gradient was observed up to 2 μM for the external thiamine concentration. At 0.2 μM for the external concentration of thiamine, the C_{ICF}/C_{ECF} value was 3.8. This ratio decreased concurrently with external thiamine concentration, and the shape of the uptake curve showed a saturable hyperbola at low external thiamine concentrations. Figure 2 also shows a temperature dependence of the thiamine uptake. When the incubation temperature was lowered to 0°C, the ^{14}C-thiamine uptake was reduced to an almost negligible amount. An apparent K_m of the uptake for thiamine gave 3.6 × 10^{-7} M.

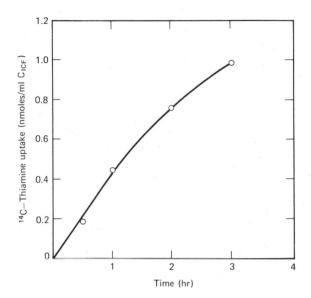

Figure 1. Time course of ¹⁴C-thiamine uptake. Rat brain slices were incubated at 37°C for the times indicated with the initial thiamine concentration of 1×10^{-7} M. Assay conditions are described in the text.

ENERGY REQUIREMENT FOR UPTAKE OF ¹⁴C-THIAMINE

The energy requirement for ¹⁴C-thiamine uptake by the brain slices is shown in Table 1. Anaerobiosis or omission of glucose from the incubation medium markedly inhibited thiamine uptake. To support this result, the effect of metabolic inhibitors on the uptake was determined. The brain slices were preincubated for 10 minutes with 2,4-dinitrophenol (DNP) or potassium cyanide (KCN), followed by the addition of ¹⁴C-thiamine and subsequent incubation for 1 hour. The uptake of ¹⁴C-thiamine was markedly inhibited by both DNP and KCN.

These effects resulted from an apparent active transport mechanism of thiamine at low external concentrations, as already reported by other investigators.

ACCUMULATION OF PHOSPHORYLATED FORMS OF ¹⁴C-THIAMINE

It has already been reported that ¹⁴C-thiamine compounds transported into brain slices appear to a considerable extent in phosphorylated form. The effects of variation of the external thiamine concentration on the accumulation of free and phosphorylated ¹⁴C-thiamine were examined. After 1 hour of incubation with various low concentrations of ¹⁴C-thiamine,

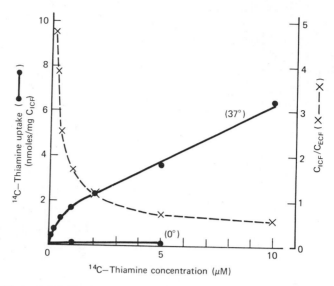

Figure 2. Effect of ¹⁴C-thiamine concentration on ¹⁴C-thiamine uptake. Incubation was carried out for 1 hour with different initial ¹⁴C-thiamine concentrations at 37 and 0°C (solid curve as indicated). Dotted curve shows the ratio of intracellular to extracellular thiamine concentration at 37°C.

Table 1.   Effect of Anaerobiosis, Omission of Glucose, and Addition of Some Metabolic Inhibitors on ¹⁴C-Thiamine uptake[a]

Incubation Conditions	¹⁴C-Thiamine Uptake, nM/ml C_{ICF}	(% inhibition)
Control	0.660	
$- O_2 + N_2$	0.194	(70.6)
$-$ Glucose	0.312	(52.7)
$+$ 2,4-Dinitrophenol (1 mM)	0.141	(78.6)
$+$ KCN (10 mM)	0.179	(72.9)

[a] The brain slices were incubated aerobically or anaerobically for 1 hour at 37°C at the initial ¹⁴C-thiamine concentration of $2 \times 10^{-7} M$. Metabolic inhibitors were added to the medium at the concentration as indicated before the preincubation.

the brain slices were homogenized and the ^{14}C-thiamine compounds extracted were measured by paper chromatographic analysis. As shown in Table 2, the ^{14}C-thiamine compounds that were accumulated were found to be mostly in phosphorylated form, and the ratio of intracellular to extracellular concentration of total (free and phosphorylated) thiamine exceeded unity and increased with a decrease in the external concentration of thiamine. However, with respect to free thiamine, the $C_{\text{ICF}}/C_{\text{ECF}}$ ratio did not exceed unity in all cases.

Since the ratio ($C_{\text{ICF}}/C_{\text{ECF}}$) of total ^{14}C-thiamine concentration exceeded unity after 30 minutes of incubation (as shown in Fig. 1), a similar experiment was carried out with brain slices incubated for 30 minutes. It was found that the ratio ($C_{\text{ICF}}/C_{\text{ECF}}$) of free thiamine for a short-time incubation was slightly smaller than that following a 1-hour incubation.

These results suggest that the accumulation of ^{14}C-thiamine compounds against the concentration gradient in the brain slices is probably due to the phosphorylation activity for thiamine in the slices.

EFFECT OF THIAMINE ANALOGS ON ^{14}C-THIAMINE UPTAKE

The effects on thiamine uptake by brain slices of thiamine analogs which had inhibitory effects on the thiamine transport system of *Escherichia coli* were examined. As shown in Table 3, ThMP and ThDP inhibited thiamine uptake to almost the same extent. The inhibition by pyrithiamine and chloroethylthiamine was strongest at molar ratios of 10:1 to ^{14}C-thiamine. In contrast, oxythiamine, which is a typical thiamine antagonist and a strong inhibitor of the bacterial thiamine transport system, showed a much weaker inhibitory action. Therefore the effects of pyrithiamine,

Table 2. Determination of Free and Phosphorylated ^{14}C-Thiamine in Brain Slices^a

Concentration of Initial External ^{14}C-Thiamine	^{14}C-Thiamine Uptake, nM/ml C_{ICF}		
	Total	Free	Phosphorylated
$2 \times 10^{-8}\ M$	0.117 (5.38)	0.017 (0.84)	0.100
$2 \times 10^{-7}\ M$	0.771 (3.86)	0.129 (0.65)	0.642
$2 \times 10^{-6}\ M$	2.34 (1.17)	0.922 (0.46)	1.418

^{a} The brain slices were incubated at 37°C for 1 hour with different concentrations of ^{14}C-thiamine. ^{14}C-Thiamine compounds were paper chromatographically analyzed as described in the text. The data in parentheses are the values of the intracellular to extracellular concentration ratio ($C_{\text{ICF}}/C_{\text{ECF}}$) for total and free thiamine.

Table 3. Effect of Thiamine Analogs on ^{14}C-Thiamine Uptake by Brain Slices[a]

Addition (2 μM)	^{14}C-Thiamine Uptake, nM/ml C_{ICF}	(% inhibition)
None	0.660	
ThMP	0.330	(50.0)
ThDP	0.342	(48.2)
Pyrithiamine	0.175	(73.5)
Oxythiamine	0.556	(15.7)
Chloroethylthiamine	0.150	(77.2)
Dimethialium	0.310	(53.1)

[a] The brain slices were incubated for 1 hour at 37°C at the initial ^{14}C-thiamine concentration of 2×10^{-7} M. Thiamine analogs (2×10^{-6} M) were added to the preincubated medium just before the addition of ^{14}C-thiamine. The rate of thiamine uptake was measured as described in the text.

chloroethylthiamine, and oxythiamine on the activity of thiamine pyrophosphokinase were examined in order to determine a role of pyrophosphorylation activity of the brain in the thiamine uptake system. As shown in Table 4, oxythiamine had almost no effect on the enzyme activity. However, some difference between pyrithiamine and chloroethylthiamine was found in the degree of inhibition. This suggests that ^{14}C-thiamine accumulation in the brain cannot be accounted for by the phosphorylation

Table 4. Effect of Thiamine Analogs on Thiamine Pyrophosphokinase Activity[a]

Addition (2 μM)	ThDP Formed, pM/mg protein	(% inhibition)
None	29.9	
Pyrithiamine	9.3	(69.0)
Oxythiamine	31.3	—
Chloroethylthiamine	22.3	(25.3)

[a] Enzyme reaction and determination of enzyme activity were carried out as described in the text. The thiamine concentration of the reaction mixture was 2×10^{-7} M.

process of thiamine alone, since other specific mechanisms in which chloroethylthiamine showed a strong inhibitory action are involved. This fact cannot exclude the existence of a specific thiamine carrier in the brain slices.

EFFECT OF OUABAIN AND VARIOUS CATIONS ON ^{14}C-THIAMINE UPTAKE

Ouabain is a specific inhibitor of the active transport of sodium ion and has been thought to be an agent reducing the ATP level in brain slices (6). The effect of ouabain on thiamine uptake at a concentration of 0.1 mM was compared with that of pyrithiamine. As shown in Table 5, ouabain caused 52.1% inhibition of the total thiamine uptake, but it did not affect the free thiamine content transported into the cells. The inhibitory effect of ouabain differs from that of pyrithiamine, and it may act on the phosphorylation step of thiamine due to a reduced level of ATP in the brain slices. Furthermore, replacement of Na$^+$, Ca^{2+} or Mg^{2+} in the incubation buffer solution by sucrose to preserve iso-osmolarity did not have a significant effect on thiamine uptake (Table 6). The inhibitory effect of high K$^+$ concentrations on thiamine uptake was also observed.

Finally, it is of interest to know whether the synthesis of thiamine triphosphate from ^{14}C-thiamine transported into brain slices occurs during such a short incubation. The experiment was performed by isolation of the ^{14}C-thiamine compounds in the tissue, using column chromatography on Dowex 1 × 4. The extraction and isolation of ^{14}C-thiamine compounds from the incubated brain slices was carried out as described in the experimental section. Figure 3 shows an elution pattern of ^{14}C-thiamine compounds after chromatography on a Dowex 1 × column. Authentic ThTP, added to the

Table 5. Effects of Ouabain and Pyrithiamine on ^{14}C-Thiamine Uptake[a]

	^{14}C-Thiamine Uptake, nM/ml C_{ICF}		
Addition	Total	Free	Phosphorylated
None	0.660	0.110	0.550
Pyrithiamine (2 μM)	0.175 (73.5%)	0.075	0.110
Ouabain (0.1 mM)	0.316 (52.1%)	0.103	0.213

[a] The brain slices were incubated for 1 hour at 37°C at the initial ^{14}C-thiamine concentration of 2 × 10^{-7} M. Ouabin and pyrithiamine were added as described in the legend for Table 3. The data in parentheses represent percentages of inhibition.

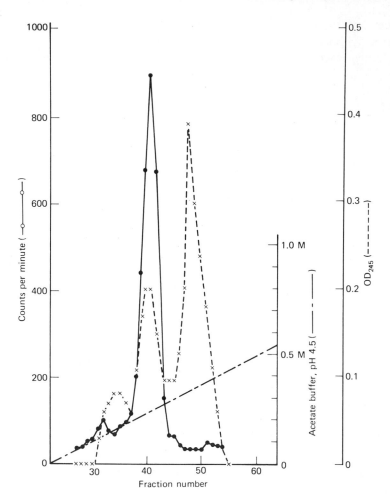

Figure 3. Analysis of ^{14}C-thiamine compounds in brain slices by Dowex 1 column chromatography. The procedure for chromatography is described in the text. Solid line: the radioactivity; dotted line: OD_{245}.

sample before adsorption on the column, was detected as a peak of OD_{245} around fraction No. 50. However, the radioactivity of synthesized ^{14}C-thiamine triphosphate was negligible around fraction No. 50, and a large peak of the radioactivity was found around fraction No. 40 (ThDP). This indicates that hardly any synthesis of ThTP occurred under the conditions employed.

Table 6.   Effect of Cations on ^{14}C-Thiamine Uptake[a]

Incubation Medium	^{14}C-Thiamine Uptake, nM/ml C_{ICF}	(% inhibition)
Complete	0.746	
− NaCl	0.558	(25.2)
− KCl, −K$_2$HPO$_4$, and + Na$_2$HPO$_4$ (1.3 mM)	0.575	(22.9)
− CaCl$_2$	0.750	—
− MgCl$_2$	0.637	(14.6)
+ KCl (50 mM)	0.579	(22.4)

[a] The brain slices were incubated with 2×10^{-7} M ^{14}C-thiamine at 37°C for 1 hour. Cations in the incubation medium were replaced by sucrose by the sodium chloride equivalent method in *The Merck Index*, 8th ed., 1968, p. 1281.

3.   Conclusions and Summary

Rat brain slices, when incubated aerobically with ^{14}C-thiamine at 37°C in Krebs-Ringer bicarbonate solution containing glucose, accumulated ^{14}C-thiamine compounds against a concentration gradient at low thiamine concentrations in the medium. This thiamine uptake showed an apparent active transport nature and also temperature dependence, apparent saturation kinetics, and an energy requirement. However, the ^{14}C-thiamine compounds transported into the brain slices were mostly the phosphorylated forms, and, with respect to free thiamine, the ratio of intracellular to extracellular concentration did not exceed unity at various low external concentrations of thiamine. This indicates that the accumulation of ^{14}C-thiamine compounds is based on the phosphorylation of thiamine in brain slices. This result differs from the data obtained by Sharma and Quastel. The discrepancy may depend on a difference in the preparation of rat brain slices, in our experiment slices were obtained from the whole brain. Or it may depend on our method of calculating thiamine concentrations in the tissue cells; these were determined by estimating the ^{14}C-thiamine concentration in the intracellular fluid (C_{ICF}).

On the other hand, the studies on inhibition of thiamine uptake with thiamine analogs and other compounds suggest a transport process mediated with a membrane carrier specific for thiamine. The thiamine compound transported into the brain slices was mostly thiamine diphosphate, probably indicating little or no synthesis of thiamine triphosphate.

References

1. G. Rindi and U. Ventura, *Experientia,* **23,** 175 (1967).
2. S. K. Sharma and J. H. Quastel, *Biochem. J.,* **94,** 790 (1965).
3. A. H. Krebs and K. Henseleit, *Z. Phys. Chem.,* **210,** 33 (1932).
4. Y. Aoshima, *Seikagaku,* **29,** 861 (1965).
5. H. Koike and T. Yusa, in D. B. McCormick and L. D. Wright, Eds., *Methods Enzymol.,* **18,** 105 (1970).
6. P. D. Swanson and H. McIlwain, *J. Neurochem.,* **12,** 877 (1965).

12. The Blood-Brain Barrier in Thiamine Deficiency

LAREN G. WARNOCK

Research Division
Veterans Administration Hospital
Nashville, Tennessee

1. Introduction

Dissolved elements in the blood do not pass into the tissue spaces of the brain as easily as they pass into tissue spaces elsewhere in the body. Therefore a special hematoencephalic barrier ("blood-brain barrier") is said to exist in the central nervous system. In summary, it appears that the capillaries of the brain, of the choroid plexus, and of the arachnoidal trabeculae all have far less permeability than do capillaries elsewhere in the body.

Labeling patterns in brain glutamic acid *in vivo* after administration of radioactive pyruvate or its precursors have been used to show the routes of pyruvic acid metabolism (1). Pyruvate can be metabolized in mammalian tissue via acetyl coenzyme A, the precursor of carbons 4 and 5 of α-ketoglutarate, or via a dicarboxylic acid, the precursor of carbons 1, 2, and 3 of α-ketoglutarate. This α-ketoglutarate can then be converted to glutamate with no mixing of the labeled carbons. With the use of sodium [2-^{14}C]pyruvate the resulting acetyl-CoA will be carboxyl-labeled, which will label glutamate in carbon 5 only on the first turn of the Krebs cycle. Subsequent turning of the cycle labels carbons 5 and 1. Conversion of pyruvate to oxaloacetate and thence to glutamate will label carbons 2 and 3 of glutamate, with carbons 1, 2, and 3 being labeled on further cycling. Labeling in carbon 4 can come only from conversion of the original pyruvate to oxaloacetate or malate and thence to a precursor of pyruvate, as in gluconeogenesis. On conversion of such an intermediate to pyruvate, carbons 2 and 3 will be labeled, resulting in [1,2-^{14}C]acetyl-CoA. Conversion of this doubly labeled acetyl-CoA will label carbons 4 and 5 of the glutamate. In the present study these labeling patterns were used to examine the pyruvate metabolism of normal and thiamine-deficient rats. The results suggest that the blood-brain barrier may be malfunctioning or degenerating in thiamine deficiency, and that this could be responsible, directly or indirectly, for the neuropathy usually present.

2. Materials and Methods

Male rats of the Sprague-Dawley strain, with initial weights of 50 to 65 grams, were fed a thiamine-deficient diet as described by Pearson et al. (2). As controls, animals pair-fed a thiamine-adequate diet were used. Characteristic deficiency signs were seen in the thiamine-deficient animals: loss of appetite, loss of weight, weakness, development of curvature of the spine, and dragging of the hind quarters. Neuropathy was not observed in the pair-fed control animals. When used, the thiamine antimetabolite, oxythiamine, was incorporated in the diet in a 50:1 ratio to the thiamine. Animals on this diet did not develop the polyneuritis observed in the thiamine-deficient animals; however, they did exhibit the other deficiency characteristics.

When the first signs of neuropathy occurred, the deficient animals, along with their pair-fed controls, were injected via the femoral vein with 0.2 ml of a solution containing 0.2 mg (10 μCi) of sodium [2-^{14}C]pyruvate. Ten minutes after receiving the isotope, the animals were decapitated. The brains were rapidly removed, usually within 1 minute, blotted on filter paper, weighed, and frozen in liquid nitrogen.

The brain tissue from each animal was homogenized with 1.3 ml 0.6 N HClO$_4$/g tissue (3). The precipitate was removed by centrifugation and rehomogenized with a volume of 0.33 N HClO$_4$ equal to that of the first supernatant solution. The supernatant solutions were combined, neutralized with 2 N KOH, refrigerated overnight, and centrifuged to remove KClO$_4$. The neutral perchlorate-free filtrates were passed over a Dowex 1-acetate column, washed with water, and eluted with 0.5 N acetic acid (4). This method readily separates aspartic and glutamic acids from the other acid components of brain. The glutamic acid fraction was removed, diluted to 50 ml with water, and quantitatively determined by the ninhydrin method of Rosen (5). Forty milliliters of this glutamic acid solution was added to

2 mmoles (294 mg) of unlabeled glutamic acid and evaporated to dryness at 60° under an air jet.

The glutamic acid was degraded by the Schmidt reaction, as described by Mosbach et al. (6) and modified by Hill et al. (7). Chloramine T was used to oxidize the glutamic acid to succinic semialdehyde, which was then reduced with hydrazine to butyric acid. The butyric acid was isolated and purified by steam distillation and Celite chromatography. Decarboxylation of the butyric acid was carried out using hydrozoic acid, resulting in carbon dioxide, representing carbon 5 of the glutamic acid, and propylamine. The amine was oxidized with alkaline permanganate to propionic acid, which was steam-distilled and purified by Celite chromatography. Alternate application of the Schmidt reaction produced carbon dioxide and the next lower amine, which was oxidized to the corresponding acid, until methylamine was finally obtained. The methylamine was distilled into hydrochloric acid. The hydrochloride was obtained by evaporation to dryness and then combusted to yield carbon 2 of glutamic acid as carbon dioxide. In each step the liberated carbon dioxide was collected and measured manometrically, and the radioactivity was determined with a vibrating reed electrometer.

Perfusion studies were carried out using the apparatus and procedures described by Exton and Park (8). The perfusate contained 30 grams of bovine serum albumin per liter of Krebs-Henseleit bicarbonate buffer and sufficient washed red blood cells from normal rats to give a hematocrit of 22%. Sodium [2-^{14}C]pyruvate was infused into the perfusate at a rate necessary to maintain a pyruvate concentration of 10 mM at constant specific activity. The rate of incorporation of radioactivity into glucose was considered a reflection of the rate of gluconeogenesis.

3. Results and Discussion

The radioactive labeling in carbon 4 of the free glutamic acid in brain tissue can be useful in determining whether a given compound entered the tissue directly or by way of liver gluconeogenesis. If sodium [2-^{14}C]pyruvate was converted to glucose via the liver, the glucose would be labeled in the 1, 2, 5, and 6 positions. This heavily randomized glucose would result in abundant label in carbon 4 of the brain glutamic acid. If the [2-^{14}C]pyruvate entered the brain directly across the blood-brain barrier, the glutamic acid would be labeled mainly in carbon 5. This technique was used by Koeppe and Hahn (9) to show that pyruvate does not enter the brain of adult animals. These results were confirmed by McMillan and Mortensen (10) in their labeling pattern studies on intracisternal injections of [2-¹⁴C]pyruvate. The results in Table 1 show that [2-¹⁴C]pyruvate entered the brain directly in adult thiamine-deficient animals. The percentage randomization from [2-¹⁴C]pyruvate in thiamine-deficient rats is comparable to that obtained when [2-¹⁴C]glucose, a precursor of [2-¹⁴C]pyruvate, is used in normal rats. Thus it is apparent that the selective transport system was not functioning in a normal fashion.

Since animals treated with oxythiamine do not develop polyneuritis, it was of interest to investigate whether pyruvic acid entered the brains directly. It can be seen in Table 1 that the percentage randomization is comparable to that for the pair-fed controls. Oxythiamine apparently does not penetrate the blood-brain barrier, whereas thiamine does (11). When oxythiamine is fed in combination with thiamine, there is a natural separation of the two compounds. The thiamine entering the brain is then sufficient to maintain brain metabolism and brain function.

It might be argued that the radioactivity in carbon 4 of brain glutamic acid could also be affected if the rates of gluconeogenesis were different in deficient and normal animals. If the rate of gluconeogenesis was slower in the deficient animal, the circulating [2-¹⁴C]pyruvic acid might have greater opportunity to penetrate directly by exchange or diffusion. To investigate this possibility, liver perfusion studies were carried out. No difference in the rates of gluconeogenesis between normal and thiamine-deficient liver is apparent. Radioactive isotope exchange and diffusion thus are not of consequence in the present interpretation. The data suggest that some sort

Table 1. Distribution of ¹⁴C in Carbons 4 and 5 of Brain Glutamic Acid after Administration of [2-¹⁴C] Pyruvate

Nutritional State	Percentage of Total in Carbon Atoms		Randomization in Carbon 4, %
	No. 4	No. 5	
Normal diet *ad libitum* (10)	21	56	55
Thiamine-deficient diet *ad libitum* (15)	2.4	56	8.2
Normal diet pair-fed (15)	8.7	46	32
Oxythiamine (50–1)-treated (7)	7.6	48	27

Numbers in parentheses indicate number of animals in each experiment.

of malfunction, affecting the selectivity for compounds entering the brain, exists in thiamine deficiency.

Histological examination of brain tissue from thiamine-deficient rats treated with trypan blue 24 hours before killing failed to show any trace of the dye. Since sensitivity of detection for radioisotopes far exceeds that of visual dye detection, we believe that the metabolic studies show the change in transport at a much earlier stage than can be demonstrated with vital stains.

The blood-brain barrier is undoubtedly important in maintaining cerebral homeostasis and in the regulation of available metabolites. By responding to changes and needs, it may also have an important role in the regulation of metabolic pathways and metabolic needs in the brain. In thiamine deficiency, where the barrier is not functioning normally, pyruvic acid and perhaps other extracranial metabolites enter the brain. These metabolites may alter the metabolic pathways in this specialized tissue, producing undesirable effects.

Whether the selectivity is a direct effect of thiamine cannot be answered here. It has been suggested (12) that glial cells have a very active hexose monophosphate pathway. It is tempting, therefore, to postulate that this alteration in selectivity reflects a change in the glial metabolism due to inadequate thiamine.

Such a postulate is supported by Robertson et al. (13) in their electron microscopic studies on thiamine deficiency. Using thiamine-deficient rats, they found no anatomical differences to explain the regional susceptibility of the brain to thiamine deficiency. The earliest observed lesion was extracellular edema, which occurred at a time when glial, vascular, and other formed elements were essentially intact. Later a ballooning and disintegration of the myelin sheaths and a swelling of the astrocytes occurred. These authors thus postulated that the earliest lesions represent an alteration in the blood-brain barrier.

It was with great interest that we reviewed the work of Lonergan et al. (14) on erythrocyte transketolase in uremia. They reported an inhibitor to transketolase and therefore postulated that the decreased activity of transketolase in uremic patients receiving thiamine-adequate diets caused the neuropathy so prevalent in these cases. Isolation of such an inhibitor would certainly be of great interest to those studying thiamine deficiency and transketolase. All our efforts to isolate such an inhibitor, however, were unsuccessful. In fact, we have not even been able to find any transketolase inhibition and thus cannot confirm the data of Lonergan et al.

References

1. R. E. Koeppe and R. J. Hill, *J. Biol. Chem.*, **216,** 813 (1955).
2. W. N. Pearson, E. Hung, W. J. Darby, Jr., M. Balaghi, and R. A. Neal, *J. Nutr.*, **89,** 133 (1966).
3. H. Busch, R. B. Hurlbert, and V. R. Potter, *J. Biol. Chem.*, **196,** 717 (1952).
4. C. H. Hirs, S. Moore, and W. H. Stein, *J. Am. Chem. Soc.*, **76,** 6063 (1954).
5. H. Rosen, *Arch. Biochem. Biophys.*, **67,** 10 (1957).
6. E. H. Mosbach, E. F. Phares, and S. F. Carson, *Arch. Biochem. Biophys.*, **33,** 179 (1951).
7. R. J. Hill, D. C. Hobbs, and R. E. Koeppe, *J. Biol. Chem.*, **230,** 169 (1958).
8. J. H. Exton and C. R. Park, *J. Biol. Chem.*, **242,** 2622 (1967).
9. R. E. Koeppe and C. H. Hahn, *J. Biol. Chem.*, **237,** 1026 (1962).
10. P. J. McMillan and R. A. Mortensen, *J. Biol. Chem.*, **238,** 91 (1963).
11. I. Ostrovskii, *Vopr. Med. Khim.*, **11,** 95 (1965).
12. P. M. Dreyfus and R. Moniz, *Biochim. Biophys. Acta,* **65,** 181 (1962).
13. D. M. Robertson, S. Wasan, and D. B. Skinner, *Lab. Invest.*, **16,** 665 (1967).
14. E. T. Lonergan, M. Semar, and K. Lange, *Arch. Intern. Med.*, **126,** 851 (1970).

DISCUSSION

Chapters 11 and 12

Dr. Blass. Is there a thiamine-binding protein in brain?

Dr. Nose. In the case of *E. coli*, we obtained a thiamine-binding protein by osmotic shock. We could not obtain positive data for brain slices, which have more protein than the shock fluid of *E. coli*. Osmotic shock is a favorite technique to isolate a binding protein from cells. It is difficult to isolate a specific protein (thiamine-binding protein) from brain slice extracts.

Dr. Cooper. I would like to confirm Dr. Nose's findings, or lack of findings. We tried the same experiments, and we also could not show any synthesis of thiamine triphosphate in either brain or liver slices. This is very disturbing to us, since we know that the compound is there but we cannot synthesize it.

Dr. Barchi. Dr. Warnock, I am wondering whether there is a possibility that the techniques you are using can be reduced to a microscale for looking at regional differences and susceptibility of the brood-brain barrier to thiamine deficiency.

Dr. Warnock. I am not an authority on the various brain structures, but I believe that it would be very difficult to do that. As you know, there are many different kinds of cells in the brain (about 15 different kinds of mitochondria), and each one may have a specialized metabolism of its own.

Dr. Dreyfus. I would like to make two comments. In many meetings dealing with thiamine, the neurological symptoms of thiamine deficiency have been referred to as "polyneuritis." I believe that this terminology is

175

erroneous. The neurological symptoms, which consist of ataxia, abnormal postures, and peculiar movements that the animals display at the end stages of deficiency, should be referred to as "an encephalopathy," since they are manifestations of disturbed central nervous system function. The major histologic and ultrastructural changes have been shown to affect the central nervous system, while the peripheral nerve changes are minimal at best and may well aggravate the CNS symptoms.

I am not surprised to hear that you were unable to observe an abnormality of transketolase activity in patients afflicted with uremic polyneuropathy. This parallels our own experience. Some years ago, we had the opportunity to measure transketolase activity in the white cells of normal and uremic patients which had been cross-incubated in the serum of normal and uremic patients, hoping to demonstrate the presence of an inhibitory factor in uremic serum or white cells that might account in part for the polyneuropathy. These experiments were entirely negative.

You talked about high hexose monophosphate shunt activity in glial cells as though this were an established fact. I am afraid that I am partially responsible for this notion, which I postulated and incorporated in one of my earlier publications; I have been quoted ever since. The idea stems from experiments in which we estimated transketolase activity in tissue rich in astrocytes and oligodendrocytes, i.e., glial tumors that we had obtained during neurosurgical procedures. Indeed, the transketolase activity was higher in astrocytomas, oligodendrogliomas, and human white matter. We thought that perhaps increased transketolase activity in glial cells reflected high hexose monophosphate shunt activity in these cells. Unfortunately the crucial experiment has not as yet been done. At this point I am not entirely certain that transketolase activity in the central nervous system is essential for its function, and there still remains considerable controversy regarding the importance of this particular metabolic step and of the hexose monophosphate shunt in general in the function of the adult nervous system. In the young, developing animal, the hexose monophosphate shunt may play an important role in the function of the nervous system by virtue of active nucleic acid synthesis.

Dr. Warnock. Sometimes our postulates catch up with us.

Dr. Cooper. My question goes back to the original design of your experiment, i.e., your comparing pair-fed control to thiamine-deficient animals. I wonder what happens, in terms of distribution of carbon, if you use starved animals.

Dr. Warnock. When we did this experiment, we had not carried out studies to see whether the pair-fed controls are true, good control models. Since then we have found that a thiamine-deficient animal reacts more as a fed animal. His metabolic pathways for the metabolism of pyruvate mimic those of a fed rather than a starved animal. Now this makes it a little hard to look at the gluconeogenesis rates. Why they are the same I am not sure. Pyruvate can go in starved conditions to oxalolacetate, and under fed conditions to acetyl-CoA. As I said, the thiamine-deficient animal seems to be more in a fed state than in a starved state. Yet these animals are losing weight. You see, whether they are starved or not, they are actually eating *ad libitum* even though they are thiamine deficient. Now whether they are really starved or not I cannot say. You have to put quotation marks around what you want to call "starved" and define this term before you can answer that type of question.

Dr. Dreyfus. I think that any pair-fed control in thiamine deficiency is a grossly undernourished animal. There is no question about the fact that these animals are grossly starved, yet they may be thiamine adequate. Have you done the experiment using just pyrithiamine?

Dr. Warnock. No, we did not use pyrithiamine at all.

Dr. Dreyfus. Pyrithiamine would circumvent the central issue of undernutrition.

Dr. Warnock. We measured pyruvic dehydrogenase using pair-fed, thiamine-deficient, and *ad libitum* fed animals on a high-carbohydrate diet. The CO_2 count in the thiamine-deficient animal was 800 and in the pair-fed animal about 1700, indicating a 50 to 60% drop in pyruvic dehydrogenase activity; however, when we examined the animal fed *ad libitum* on a high carbohydrate diet, we got a CO_2 count of 1100. That would indicate that the inhibition is approximately 30%. A pair-fed animal may not be a good laboratory control animal.

Dr. Patel. I would like to comment on a similar problem. About 5 years ago we observed that pair-feeding, which equalizes the food intake of the animals, induces many metabolic alterations (M. S. Patel and S. P. Mistry, *J. Nutr.,* **98,** 235, 1969). When you pair-feed a normal animal, it consumes the allotted food in a much shorter time and starves for the rest of the day. I think that in some nutritional experiments this can be a critical problem because pair-fed controls (meal-eaters) are being compared with deficient animals nibbling *ad libitum*. Additional controls are needed in such cases.

I have a question for Dr. Warnock in terms of gluconeogenesis. Thiamine is not directly involved in gluconeogenesis from pyruvate. However, pyruvate carboxylase requires acetyl-CoA for its activation. Acetyl-CoA is, in part, formed from pyruvate by pyruvate dehydrogenase complex. As you mentioned, you used medium containing albumin, and I wonder whether the albumin was totally free of fatty acids.

Dr. Warnock.   Yes, I believe that it was fairly close to being free of fatty acids, since we obtained the albumin from Dr. Philip Felts, who has been doing a lot of work on fatty acid stimulation of gluconeogenesis. He worked with me on this problem, and he has albumin containing very small amounts of fatty acids.

Dr. Itokawa.   When thiamine was injected intravenously, the thiamine concentration in the brain was not increased very much even if blood thiamine levels rose. From this fact I believe that some blood-brain barrier for thiamine exists. Have you done any experiments concerning this problem?

Dr. Warnock.   I am at the present time trying to develop a method for measuring ThTP in serum. If any of you know the normal levels of ThTP in serum, I would like to talk to you about it. We have got the assay to the point where we are in the ball park—in the neighborhood of 5 to 15 ng/ml serum, which is a very small amount, but we have to work on this a little more.

Dr. Gubler.   Using pair-fed controls leaves a lot to be desired. I just want to comment that we have studied pyrithiamine-treated animals in experiments involving ^{14}C distribution after the injection of ^{14}C-pyruvate subcutaneously. We found much higher labeling of the brain components in the pyrithiamine-treated animals than in others. The only way we can explain this is that the pyrithiamine must have broken down the blood-brain barrier.

13. Ultrastructural Cytochemistry of Phosphatases Related to Thiamine Metabolism

KAZUO OGAWA, M.D.
YASUHIRO AGO, M.D.
TERUO TANAKA, D.D.S.

Department of Anatomy
Kansai Medical University
Moriguchi, Osaka, Japan

Attempts were made in our laboratory to investigate the fine structural localization of the activity of phosphatases related to thiamine metabolism, such as thiamine monophosphatase (ThMPase), thiamine diphosphatase (ThDPase), and thiamine triphosphatase (ThTPase), in the brain (cerebrum and cerebellum) of normal adult rats, weighing 130 to 150 grams, and of adult male rats fed a thiamine-deficient diet for 1 to 3 weeks. The localization of the activities was compared with that of choline acetylase (ChA) in the nervous tissue, including the nerve endings at the neuromuscular junction.

The lead citrate method (1, 2) was used for the ultracytochemical demonstration of ThMPase, ThDPase, and ThTPase, and the cobalt-ferrocyanide method (3, 4) for the ChA activity. For phosphatases the enzyme reaction was carried out mainly at pH 9.2 and in some cases at pH 6.5. The reaction for the demonstration of the ChA activity was performed at pH 6.8.

For the ultracytochemical demonstration of phosphatases, nonfrozen Vibratome sections, 20 to 40 μ in thickness (5), of unfixed or fixed specimens were incubated in the incubation medium (Tris-HCl buffer, pH 8.5, 28 mM, magnesium sulfate or chloride 3.9 mM, alkaline lead citrate

2.0 mM, ThMP, ThDP, or ThTP 2 mM, sucrose 240 mM, final pH adjusted to 9.2 to 9.4; when the reaction was carried out at pH 6.5 0.1 N HCl was added to the medium to lower the pH) for 30 minutes at 37°C, postosmificated in buffered osmium tetroxide, and embedded in epon. Thin sections made by an LKB ultrotome were poststained with uranyl and/or lead acetate and examined under a JEM 7 or Hitachi 12A microscope. When specimens were fixed, this was done by perfusion fixation with 2 to 4% buffered formaldehyde, pH 7.2, for 30 to 60 minutes at 0 to 4°C, followed by immersion of the dissected specimens in the same fixative for 10 minutes or by perfusion fixation with 1% buffered glutaraldehyde, pH 7.2, for 10 minutes. Occasionally the immersion fixation was omitted. The effects of substrate protection (SP) on the enzymatic activity were also tested; that is, 1 mM ThMP, ThDP, or ThTP was incorporated in the fixative or in the buffer used before the incubation for the enzymatic reaction. In some other cases, calcium (chloride) was used instead of magnesium. The substrate-free incubation medium served as a control.

For the ultracytochemical demonstration of the ChA activity, nonfrozen Vibratome sections of tissues, fixed by perfusion fixation (4% buffered formaldehyde, pH 7.2, for 30 minutes or 1% buffered glutaraldehyde, pH 7.2, for 10 minutes at 0 to 4°C; 0.06 mM acetyl CoA and/or 5 mM choline chloride added to the fixative for the substrate protection of the enzymatic activity), were incubated in an incubation medium containing 6.0 ml of 0.1M phosphate buffer, pH 7.0 (final concentration 60 mM), 5 mg of acetyl-CoA (0.6 mM), 1.0 ml of 0.1 M choline chloride (10 mM), 0.3 ml of 0.1 M sodium citrate (3 mM), 1.0 ml of 30 mM cobalt chloride (3 mM), 1.0 ml of 5 mM potassium ferricyanide (0.5 mM), 3.4 mg of tetraisopropylpyrophosphoramide (1 mM, cholinesterase inhibitor), 1.5 g of sucrose (440 mM), and 0.7 ml of double-distilled water (total volume 10 ml, final pH adjusted to 6.8 to 7.0) for 40 to 60 minutes at 37°C. After incubation, sections were fixed in 1% buffered osmium tetroxide and processed for electron microscopy. In some cases, osmium fixation was omitted. Thin sections were observed with or without poststaining. In the case of the ChA activity the effects of SH inhibitors (3 mM N-ethylmaleimide or sodium iodoacetate), ChA inhibitor [40 mM tetramethyl ammonium chloride, or 1 to 10 mM N-hydroxyethyl-4-(1-naphthylvinyl)pyridinium bromide], and activators (100 to 300 mM KCl and 40 mM NaCN) have been examined.

The results of ultracytochemical localization of the activities of phosphatases (ThMPase, ThDPase, and ThTPase) are summarized in Table 1 and shown in Figs. 1 to 15. The fine structural localization of the activity of ThMPase and ThDPase near neutral pH has previously been reported (6, 7). The activities of phosphatases related to thiamine are localized in the

Table 1. Subcellular Localization of Phosphatases Related to Thiamine in the Nervous Tissue

Type of Tissue	ThMPase pH 9.2			ThDPase pH 9.2			ThTPase pH 9.2 (and 6.5)		
	Fixed	Unfixed		Fixed	Unfixed		Fixed	Unfixed	
	SP		SP in buffer	SP		SP in buffer	SP		SP in buffer
Neuronal plasmalemma (perikaryon and processes)	+	+	+	+	+	+	+	+	+
Synapse									
Membranes (pre- and post-)	+	+	+	+	+	+	+	+	+
Vesicles	±	+	+	±	±	±	?	?	+
Cleft	–	–	–	–	–	–	±	–	–
Mitochondria	–	+	+	–	?	?	–	+	+
Golgi apparatus	–	–	–	+	+ +	+ +	+	+	+
Endoplasmic reticulum	–	–	–	+ + +	?	?	–	–	–
Nucleus	–	–	–	–	–	–	pH 9.2: – / pH 6.5: +	pH 9.2: – / pH 6.5: +	pH 9.2: – / pH 6.5: +
Capillary endothelium									
Apical and basal membrane	+	+ +	+	+	+ +	+ +	+	+ +	+
Pinocytotic vesicles	+	+ +	+ +	+	+ +	+ +	+ +	+ +	+ +
Membrane of end-feet	±	±	±	±	=	±	±	±	±
Calcium inhibition				Inhibited			Inhibited		

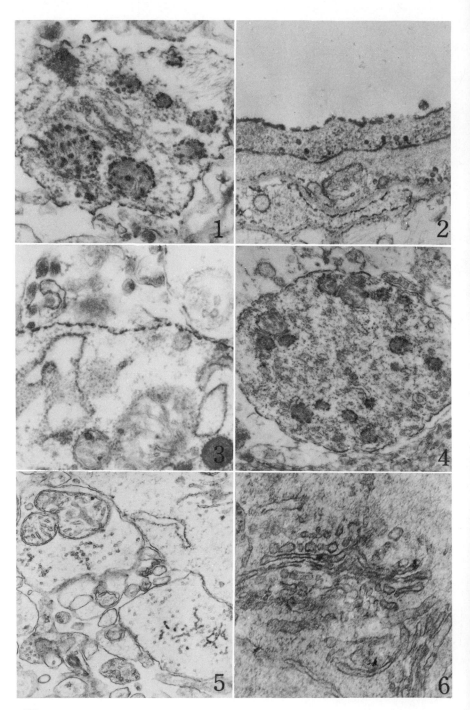

neuronal plasma membrane (perikaryon and processes) (Figs. 1, 3, 4, 9, and 11); the synapse (membranes, synaptic vesicles, some of which may be coated, and occasionally the cleft) (Figs. 5, 10, 11, and 12); occasionally the mitochondria in neurons (particularly in unfixed specimens) (Figs. 1 and 4); the Golgi apparatus (particularly in fixed specimens) in neurons except for the ThMPase activity (Figs. 7, 13, and 14, as compared to Fig. 6); and the apical as well as basal membrane and pinocytotic vesicles of the capillary endothelium (Figs. 2 and 8). By and large, there were no apparent differences in the localization of the enzymatic activities between pH 9.2 and pH 6.5. Occasionally reaction products of an obscure nature were observed in the nucleus at pH 6.5. It should be noted here that not all of the synapses are positive for the enzymatic activity (Fig. 12). Incorporation of calcium in lieu of magnesium in the incubation medium for the ThTPase activity produced some inhibitory effects on the activity at pH 6.5 and even at pH 9.2. Longer fixation in glutaraldehyde completely inhibited the enzymatic activity (Fig. 15).

The phosphatase activity in the brains of rats fed a thiamine-deficient diet for 1 to 3 weeks did not show any marked changes (Figs. 22 to 24), although the brains from rats on a thiamine-deficient diet for 3 weeks seemed to exhibit slightly lower enzymatic activity in the neuronal Golgi apparatus.

The fine structural localization of the ChA activity is shown in Figs. 16 to 21. Reaction products indicating ChA activity were observed in the plasma membrane (Fig. 16), occasionally in the mitochondria, and rarely in the Golgi apparatus in the nerve cells (Figs. 17 and 19). In some nerve cells, reaction products were observed in the endoplasmic reticulum, particularly at the ribosomal side of membrane (Fig. 18), and in the coated vesicles (Fig. 19). In synapses and the nerve endings at the neuromuscular junction, they were observed in the synaptic vesicles and the presynaptic membrane (Fig. 20 and 21). Occasionally, the synaptic cleft showed reaction products. Since KCl did not affect the activity markedly and NaCN made the medium turbid, neither KCl nor NaCN was added to the incubation medium. An

---

Figure 1. All electron micrographs are from the adult rat. Cerebrum: unfixed (substrate protection, SP). ThMPase in the plasma membrane and mitochondria of the neuronal process. ×38,000.

Figure 2. Cerebellum: 4% formaldehyde (FA) perfusion (SP) for 30 minutes, followed by immersion in 4% FA (SP). ThMPase in the capillary endothelium. ×32,000.

Figure 3. Cerebrum: unfixed (SP). ThDPase in the neuronal plasma membrane. ×32,000.

Figure 4. Cerebellum: unfixed (SP). ThDPase in the plasma membrane and mitochondria of the neuronal process. ×20,000.

Figure 5. Cerebrum: unfixed (SP). ThDPase in the synaptic vesicles. ×24,000.

Figure 6. Cerebellum: unfixed. Almost no ThDPase activity in the Golgi apparatus of a Purkinje cell. ×48,000.

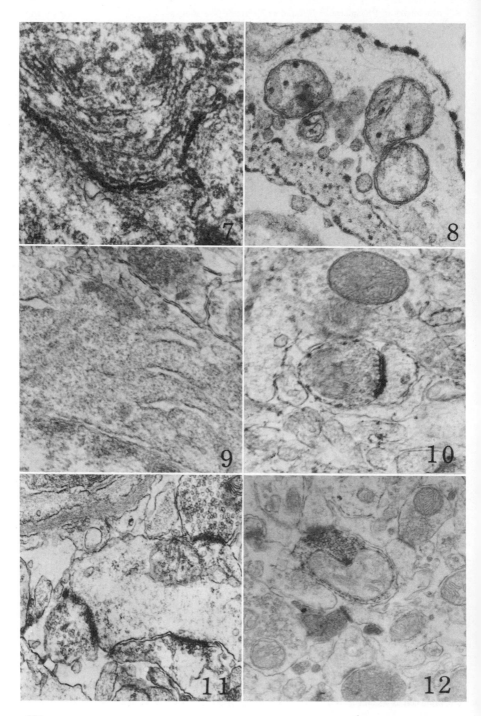

excess amount of ions might cause diffusibility of the enzyme. SH inhibitors and *N*-hydroxyethyl-4-(1-naphthylvinyl)pyridinium bromide inhibited, and tetramethyl ammonium chloride markedly affected, the enzymatic activity. The localization of the ChA activity obtained by our method is in general agreement with previous results using the lead method (8–10), although some discrepancies exist, which await further clarification.

In the present report, we specifically emphasize the striking spatial proximity or similarity of the localization of the ChA activity to that of phosphatases related to thiamine at the subcellular level, although there are minor differences. The spatial proximity alone may not mean anything; on the other hand, it may offer certain clues as to the role of thiamine in nervous tissue per se.

In this connection, it would be of great interest to pursue the enzymatic activity at the synapse, particularly in vesicular components, such as synaptic vesicles and coated vesicles. Kadota and Kadota (11) performed biochemical experiments indicating that the coated vesicle fraction from guinea pig brain possesses high nucleoside diphosphatase (NDPase) and rather low ThDPase activity, further suggesting that the coated vesicle may have some control over energy metabolism and subsequent acetylcholine synthesis in brain nerve endings through the coated vesicle NDPase. However, their experiment was performed at neutral pH. If it had been carried out at alkaline pH, a higher ThDPase activity might also have been observed in the coated vesicle fraction. Griffith and Bondareff (12) have shown the presence of ThDPase activity in the synaptic vesicles in rat brain. The relationship of the coated vesicle to the synaptic vesicle needs to be clearly identified.

In conclusion, it can be said that the correlation of thiamine metabolism with the mechanism concerning neurotransmission in the nerve endings at the subcellular level should be studied in more detail in order to clarify the role of thiamine in nervous tissue.

Figure 7. All electron micrographs are from the aduct rat. Cerebrum: 2% FA perfusion for 30 minutes. ThDPase in the Golgi apparatus of a nerve cell. ×35,000.

Figure 8. Cerebrum: unfixed. ThDPase in the capillary endothelium. ×47,000.

Figure 9. Cerebrum: 4% FA perfusion for 60 minutes. ThTPase in the neuronal plasma membrane. ×32,000.

Figure 10. Cerebrum: 4% FA perfusion for 60 minutes. ThTPase in the synaptic membrane and the plasma membrane of the neuronal process. ×38,000.

Figure 11. Cerebrum: 2% FA perfusion for 30 minutes. ThTPase in the synaptic membrane and the neuronal plasma membrane. ×27,000.

Figure 12. Cerebrum: 4% FA perfusion for 60 minutes. ThTPase in the synaptic vesicles. Not all of the synapses are positive for the ThTPase activity. ×25,000.

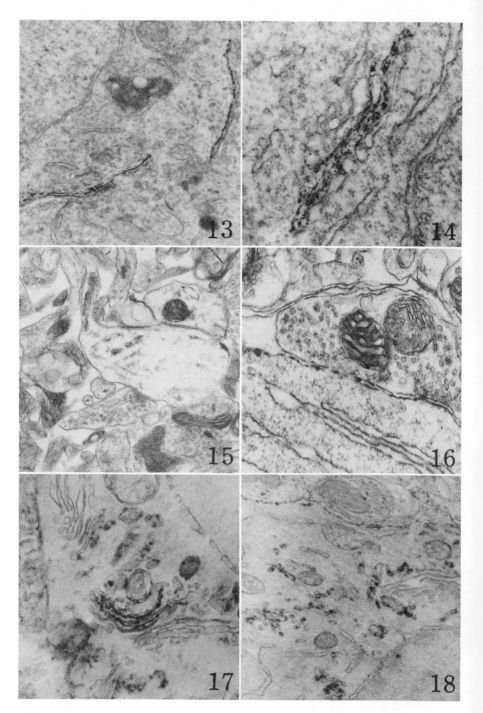

186

Figure 13. All electron micrographs are from the adult rat. Cerebrum: 2% FA perfusion (SP) for 60 minutes. ThTPase in the neuronal Golgi apparatus. ×17,000.

Figure 14. Cerebrum: 2% FA perfusion (SP) for 60 minutes. ThTPase in the neuronal Golgi apparatus. ×44,000.

Figure 15. Cerebrum: immersion fixation in 1% glutaraldehyde for 60 minutes. The ThTPase activity is completely inhibited. ×24,000.

Figure 16. Cerebrum: 4% FA perfusion (SP) for 30 minutes. ChA in the neuronal plasma membrane. ×48,000.

Figure 17. Cerebrum: 4% FA perfusion (SP) for 30 minutes. ChA in some of the neuronal Golgi apparatus. The thin section is not poststained. ×32,000.

Figure 18. Cerebrum: 4% FA perfusion (SP) for 30 minutes. ChA in the ribosomes of the rough endoplasmic reticulum and the plasma membrane of a nerve cell. ×22,000.

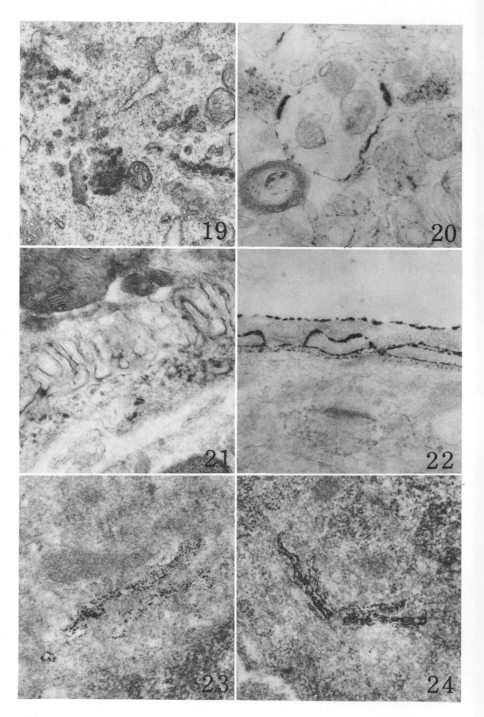

Figure 19. All electron micrographs are from the adult rat. Cerebrum: 4% FA perfusion (SP) for 30 minutes. ChA in the coated vesicles and the Golgi apparatus of a nerve cell. ×36,000.

Figure 20. Cerebrum: 4% FA perfusion (SP) for 30 minutes. ChA primarily in the synaptic vesicles and cleft. ×26,000.

Figure 21. Diaphragm: 4% FA perfusion (SP) for 30 minutes. ChA in the vesicles in the nerve endings at the neuromuscular junction. ×28,000.

Figure 22. Cerebrum of a rat fed a thiamine-deficient diet for 1 week: 4% FA perfusion for 60 minutes. ThDPase in the capillary endothelium and the synaptic membrane. ×26,000.

Figure 23. Cerebrum of a rat fed a thiamine-deficient diet for 3 weeks: 4% FA perfusion for 60 minutes. ThDPase in the neuronal Golgi apparatus. ×48,000.

Figure 24. Cerebrum of a rat fed a thiamine-deficient diet for 3 weeks: 4% FA perfusion for 60 minutes. ThDPase in the neuronal Golgi apparatus. ×48,000.

References

1. H. Mayahara, H. Hirano, T. Saito, and K. Ogawa, *Histochem,* **11,** 88 (1967).

2. H. Mayahara, H. Hirano, and K. Ogawa, *Shinryo,* **22,** 1461 (1969) (in Japanese).

3. Y. Ago and K. Ogawa, *8th International Congress on Electron Microscopy, Canberra,* Vol. II, 1974, p. 148.

4. Y. Ago and K. Ogawa, *Acta Histochem. Cytochem.,* **1,** 69 (1974).

5. Y. Ago and K. Ogawa, *Acta Histochem. Cytochem.,* **6,** 1 (1973).

6. T. Saito and K. Ogawa, *Arch. Histol. Jap.,* **27,** 473 (1966).

7. Y. Ishikawa, T. Saito, and Ogawa, K., *J. Electron Microsc.,* **16,** 344 (1967).

8. P. Kása, S. P. Mann, and C. Heff, *Nature,* **226,** 814 (1970).

9. P. Kása, *Progr. Brain Res.,* **34,** 337 (1971).

10. A. M. Burt, *Progr. Brain Res.,* **34,** 327 (1971).

11. K. Kadota and T. Kadota, *Brain Res.,* **56,** 371 (1972); S. Goldfischer, E. Essner, and B. Schiller, *J. Histochem, Cytochem.,* **19,** 349 (1971).

12. D. L. Griffith and W. Bondareff, *Am. J. Anat.,* **136,** 549 (1973).

DISCUSSION

Chapter 13

Dr. Barchi. Dr. Ogawa, did I understand correctly that in your reaction mixture for thiamine triphosphatase specifically you have 2 mM lead and that it is present during the entire reaction time?

Dr. Ogawa. In the icubation medium?

Dr. Barchi. Yes, in the incubation mixture. Have you ever studied the effects of lead citrate itself on the membrane-associated enzymes?

Dr. Ogawa. Yes, for ATPase.

Dr. Barchi. Specifically for ThTPase? We have looked at the membrane-associated ThTPase, at a pH optimum of 6.5 to 7.0, and the enzyme is extremely unhappy around heavy metals.

Dr. Ogawa. But this was added to the biochemical medium, right?

Dr. Barchi. Essentially, it is in a medium that contains substrate, a divalent cation, the membrane fractions, and heavy metals, yes.

Dr. Ogawa. That is the main point. It has been our experience that biochemical data obtained for ATPase and phosphatases biochemically cannot be compared directly with histochemical data obtained when we use a slightly different composition.

Dr. Barchi. The composition of the medium is not too different from the one that you have shown, but I do worry about it a little. I think that somehow we have to devise controls that will show definitively that the presence of heavy metals during the reaction does not inhibit the activity of the membrane-associated enzymes and possibly lead to erroneous localizations.

Dr. Ogawa. Well, of course this factor might affect the activity partly, but I do not think it makes a big difference; the situation for the histochemical demonstration of phosphatase is entirely different from the one for quantitative estimation. For instance, we use lead citrate instead of lead nitrate, and citrate in the medium chelates lead, so that 2 mM lead may not act as 2 mM lead.

Dr. Barchi. I would say that a concentration of lead in the order of 1×10^{-4} can inhibit membrane-associated ThTPase.

Dr. Ogawa. For purposes of histochemical demonstration, some investigators believe that lead should be higher than 2 mM—perhaps as high as 4 mM—because if you have lower concentrations of lead than someone else uses, you have much less concentration of the capture reagent than is needed, causing diffusion of the products. I continue to use 2 mM lead because I try to use the same concentration of the capture reagent as that of the substrate. ThMP, ThDP, or ThTP. I should also mention that there is a difference between nitrate and citrate. Nitrate is not a chelator, whereas citrate is. I do not know what form of lead you used. Therefore the situation may be a little different from the one you are talking about.

Dr. Cooper. I am halfway between you two. I think that there are situations where *in vitro* lead can be a very potent inhibitor of enzyme activity, yet in a histochemical investigation it can be used to demonstrate activity. You may be losing some of the activity but still have enough for visualization. I was going to ask you about the choline acetylase localization. You are aware that two or three different groups have developed an enzyme-metal method for ChA.

Dr. Ogawa. Yes.

Dr. Cooper. The method I was thinking of particularly is that of Feigenson and Barrnett. They have shown the ChA to be on the outside border of the vesicle, not in the vesicle membrane itself.

Dr. Ogawa. Actually, I have not seen their pictures.

Dr. Cooper. I do not think anybody else has found ChA in the endoplasmic reticulum. Have other people shown that? I was curious about your demonstration.

Dr. Ogawa. Some who used lead to trap SH groups have shown ChA in some of the neurons.

Dr. Cooper.   That is a curious place for the enzyme to be located.

Dr. Ogawa.   But it may be the site of the ChA synthesis. It is conceivable that ChA molecules are formed in the rough endoplasmic reticulum and transported to the periphery in vesicles via the Golgi apparatus, although this is mere speculation.

14. Thiamine Triphosphatases in the Brain

ROBERT L. BARCHI, M.D., Ph.D.

Departments of Neurology and Biochemistry
University of Pennsylvania School of Medicine
Philadelphia, Pennsylvania

The role of thiamine diphosphate (ThDP) as a coenzyme in decarboxylation and two-carbon transfer reactions has been recognized for decades; an extensive literature exists on the mechanism by which this unique molecule catalyzes the cleavage reactions involved and on the molecular organization of the multienzyme systems that require ThDP as a coenzyme for their function. The presence in mammalian cells of free thiamine and thiamine monophosphate (ThMP), respectively the precursor and the dephosphorylation product of the active coenzyme, can easily be understood in light of the importance of ThDP. It is well documented, however, that 5 to 9% of the total thiamine in most animal tissues exists in the form of thiamine triphosphate (ThTP) (1). This triphosphate is not able to substitute for ThDP in enzyme reactions requiring that cofactor, and its niche in the cellular economy has remained an elusive mystery.

Considerable experimental support exists for the involvement of thiamine compounds in nerve conduction and is reviewed elsewhere in this book. A number of recent observations have suggested that ThTP is the specific compound associated in some unique manner with the function of the excitable membrane. Cooper and his coworkers have demonstrated a preferential enrichment of ThTP as a percentage of total thiamine compounds in membrane fragments as they are progressively purified from nervous tissue, suggesting a specific association of ThTP with these membranes (2). A dose-related release of thiamine compounds from these membranes in response to physiologic concentrations of neuroactive agents such as tetrodotoxin and acetylcholine has been observed, although the relationship of this release to normal membrane function remains undefined. This release correlates with that observed in intact tissue preparations under physiologic conditions and appears to result in a preferential depletion of the triphosphate in both systems (3). Clearer support for the specific involvement of ThTP in the function of neural tissue is given by recent observations on the pathobiochemistry of subacute necrotizing encephalomyelopathy (SNE), a fatal hereditary illness of children that pathologically resembles closely the well-characterized encephalopathy of thiamine deficiency. In this disease the young brains reveal an absolute deficiency of ThTP, while levels of other thiamine compounds, including the coenzyme form (ThDP), remain normal, and enzyme activities requiring the presence of ThDP are found to have normal specific activities (4). An inhibitor of ThTP synthesis has been implicated as the cause of this syndrome (see Chapter 24).

As a result of widespread interest in the coenzyme form of thiamine, enzymes catalyzing the synthesis of ThDP from free thiamine and enzymes catalyzing the hydrolysis of ThDP to ThMP and inorganic phosphate have been extensively studied. Again, however, little is known about the enzymes involved in the synthesis and degradation of ThTP. Synthesis of small quantities of ThTP *in vivo* was reported by Gurtner in a study using S^{35}-thiamine as a precursor (5). More recently an activity catalyzing the synthesis of ThTP from ThDP and ATP has been partially characterized by Itokawa and Cooper (6). A detailed discussion of this enzyme appears in Chapter 25 of this publication.

If an analogy to ATP and the various ATPases may be drawn, a clue to the functional role of ThTP should be found in the enzymes that specifically catalyze the hydrolysis of the high-energy phosphate bond in this compound. An understanding of the distribution of these enzymes, the physiologic conditions required for their maximal activation, and the conditions that result in their inhibition may constitute the first step toward delineation of this role. This section will be restricted to a consideration of such enzymes and will deal mostly with recent progress in the characterization of a membrane-associated thiamine triphosphatase first observed in neural tissue.

1. Thiamine Triphosphatases in Mammalian Tissue

Thiamine triphosphatase (ThTPase) catalyzes the hydrolysis of the γ-phosphate from ThTP to yield inorganic phosphate and ThDP:

$$\text{ThTP} \xrightarrow{\text{ThTPase}} \text{ThDP} + P_i \tag{1}$$

At least two species of this enzyme have been reported in the brain. In 1972 Hashitani and Cooper described a soluble enzyme having a pH optimum of 9.0 to 9.5 which exhibited less than 10% of optimal activity when assayed at pH 6.5. At about the same time our laboratory reported the characteristics of a membrane-associated ThTPase in rat brain which showed maximum hydrolytic activity between pH 6.5 and 7.0, with less than 20% of optimal rates being observed above pH 9.0 (8). Both enzymes require the presence of a divalent cation for maximal activity.

These two enzymes appear to represent different proteins in the rat nervous system, rather than two forms of the same enzyme. This concept is supported by the following experimental observations:

1.   The soluble enzyme shows significant substrate inhibition at levels of substrate 2 to 3 times K_m, whereas there is no evidence of similar inhibition with the membrane-associated enzyme at levels of substrate as high as 10 times K_m.

2.   The soluble enzyme is inhibited by Ca^{2+} in the 10^{-4} to 10^{-3} M range in the presence of Mg^{2+}, whereas Ca^{2+} has no such effect on the membrane ThTPase in levels as high as 3×10^{-3} M in the presence of Mg^{2+} and, indeed, is able to activate the enzyme to its full level in the absence of Mg^{2+}.

3.   The soluble enzyme is unaffected by the presence of ATP or ADP in concentrations up to 1×10^{-3} M, whereas the membrane ThTPase is strongly inhibited by those compounds at concentrations below 5×10^{-5} M.

4.   The optimal temperature for the soluble enzyme is 50°C, whereas the membrane ThTPase is rapidly inactivated at that temperature.

5.   We have been unable to solubilize the membrane ThTPase and convert it into a form active at pH 9.0; any attempt to remove the enzyme from the membrane using detergents (SDS, Na^+ dodecyl sulfate) results in complete loss of pH 6.5 activity without generation of soluble activity at pH 9.0. The soluble ThTPase, on the other hand, is activated significantly by the presence of concentrations of Na^+ dodecyl sulfate that completely eliminate the activity of the membrane-associated enzyme.

2.   Soluble Thiamine Triphosphatase

The soluble ThTPase from rat brain has been partially purified and characterized by Hashitani and Cooper (7). Their purification procedure utilized mild acid precipitation followed by cold acetone fractionation of the resultant supernatant. A late-precipitating fraction was collected and chromatographed on DEAE-cellulose to yield a final 120-fold purification in specific activity, with an overall yield of 26%. The resultant enzyme is specific for ThTP among thiamine phosphate compounds, hydrolyzing the triphosphate to ThDP and P_i. Very low rates of hydrolysis were observed when nucleoside triphosphates were substituted as substrates for the partially purified enzyme (less than 13% of control rates with ThTP), confirming the specificity of the enzyme. The authors report a Michaelis constant of 1.2×10^{-3} M for ThTP, a value confirmed in our laboratory. Progressive substrate inhibition is noted for ThTP concentrations in excess of 3×10^{-3} M; 50% inhibition is reached at approximately 6.5×10^{-3} M. The soluble enzyme has an absolute specificity for Mg^{2+} ions. At relatively low concentrations Ca^{2+} inhibits the enzyme in the presence of Mg^{2+} with a calculated K_i of 2 to 3×10^{-4} M.

A number of thiamine analogs, including oxythiamine and pyrithiamine, have been tested for inhibitory action on the soluble ThTPase, but none has proved effective. Likewise, urine from patients with SNE, which has been shown to inhibit the ThDP-ATP phosphotransferase activity of rat brain, has no effect on this triphosphatase.

3.   Membrane-Associated Thiamine Triphosphatase

The rest of this discussion will deal predominantly with the ThTPase activity associated with the subcellular membranes of rat brain. As previously indicated, this membrane-bound enzyme has a pH optimum between 6.5 and 7.2. A divalent cation is required for activation; this requirement may be satisfied by Mg^{2+}, Ca^{2+}, or Mn^{2+} within certain defined concentration ranges. All cations produce progessive inhibition of enzyme activity as their concentrations are raised above the level required for optimal activation; inhibition occurs quite rapidly with increasing concentrations with Mn^{2+}, more gradually with Ca^{2+} and Mg^{2+}. A detailed analysis of the mechanism of divalent cation activation will be given below.

Since the membrane ThTPase cannot be readily solubilized and is invariably associated with other membrane-bound enzymes such as ATPases and nonspecific nucleoside triphosphatases (NTPases) during standard subcellular fractionation procedures, it becomes important to demonstrate that the ThTPase does indeed catalyze the reaction indicated in Eq. 1 and that the enzyme is specific for ThTP and does not represent a secondary reaction of another membrane triphosphatase. The first criterion presents no major difficulty and has been satisfied by analyzing the products of the ThTPase reaction, using column chromatographic techniques. The stoichiometric disappearance of ThTP and the appearance of ThDP and P_i in equimolar concentrations can readily be demonstrated at various points over 45 minutes of reaction time, using purified membrane preparations. Only trace amounts of ThMP form during the same interval, indicating the relatively low activity of the nucleoside diphosphatase responsible for ThDP hydrolysis at this pH (optimum pH for this enzyme is 9.0); usually no correction for this second hydrolysis is necessary under the conditions of our ThTPase assay.

The second criterion is more difficult to satisfy. Substrate specificity for ThTP can be demonstrated indirectly by the use of differential inhibitors of various triphosphatase activities. The following observations have been made:

1. N-Propyltin is effective in inhibiting 70% of the membrane Mg^{2+}-ATPase activity at concentrations that have no effect on ThTP hydrolysis.

2. Both Mg^{2+}-ATPase and NTPase are less heat-labile than the ThTPase activity.

3. Membrane ThTPase is inhibited 60% by levels of Na^+ DOC that have no effect on the ATPase activity.

4. Levels of Ca^{2+} that inhibit Mg^{2+}-ATPase activity activate membrane ThTPase.

5. No activation of ThTP hydrolysis is seen in the presence of various concentrations of Na^+ or K^+ alone or in combinations that enhance ATPase activity.

4. ThMP-PCP

The strongest evidence for specificity of the active site of the membrane ThTPase, however, was obtained through the synthesis of a nonhydrolyzable analog of ThTP. This analog contains a methylene group between the β- and the γ-phosphate in the triphosphoryl side chain; the resulting molecule (ThMP-PCP) cannot be hydrolyzed between these terminal phosphates, although the structure and bond angles of the compound are nearly identical to those of the native ThTP. Thus the compound should in theory function as a specific but nonhydrolyzable substrate analog of ThTP.

The synthesis of ThMP-PCP is carried out by a modification of the method of Smith and Khorana (9) for nucleotide compounds. Modifications are necessary in light of the instability of thiamine compounds at alkaline pH.

The phosphopiperizate of thiamine monophosphate is formed by the reaction of ThMP with piperizine at pH 6.5 in aqueous solution in the presence of 1-ethyl-3(3-dimethylaminopropyl)-carbodiimide. The resultant compound, recovered as the guanidinium salt, is partially purified by gel filtration on a Sephadex G-10 column, flash-evaporated, and rendered rigorously anhydrous by repeated evaporation from absolute ethanol followed by benzene. Methylene phosphonate (Miles Laboratories, Inc.) is converted to the monotriethylammonium salt and rigorously dried as above. The two salts are then dissolved in anhydrous DMSO (Merck Company) and mixed. The reaction is allowed to proceed at 35°C with stirring for 48 hours. Formation of product is monitored by paper electrophoresis. The reaction is terminated by the addition of excess acetone, and the white precipitate is washed with acetone and ether, dissolved in water, and chromatographed on Dowex 1-X-4 anion-exchange resin. The peak corresponding to ThMP-PCP is concentrated and desalted on Sephadex G-10. The ThMP-PCP can then be crystallized out of a water-ethanol-acetone solution.

The white crystalline product is indistinguishable from ThTP by paper chromatography, paper electrophoresis, or anion-exchange chromatography. A 220 MHz NMR spectrum demonstrates a triplet at 2.1 PPM downfield, corresponding to the β-γ methyl group in the ThMP-PCP sample spectrum. The rest of the spectrum is identical to that obtained with ThTP.

The ThMP-PCP analog has no effect on the hydrolysis of ATP by membrane Mg^{2+}-ATPase, and no effect on the hydrolysis of other nucleoside triphosphates by membrane NTPase at inhibitor concentrations of up to 10 mM. The TMP-PCP, however, produces significant and progressive inhibition of the membrane ThTPase in all membrane fractions containing this activity (Fig. 1). Double reciprocal plots of enzyme activity as a function of substrate concentration in the presence of various levels of TMP-PCP, shown in Fig. 2, indicate that the mechanism of inhibition is purely competitive, as would be expected for a true substrate analog. Thus the active site for which ThTP and its structural analog, ThMP-PCP, compete is distinct from that which catalyzes the hydrolysis of ATP and other nucleoside triphosphates. Taken as a whole, the data cited above strongly support the contention that the ThTPase activity associated with the membrane fractions represents a unique and specific enzyme.

5. Tissue and Cellular Distribution of the Thiamine Triphosphatases

The membrane-associated and the soluble ThTPase are widely distributed throughout the body (Fig. 3). In all tissues examined, the total hydrolytic activity at optimum conditions of the membrane ThTPase exceeds that of the soluble ThTPase when a washed particulate pellet of a tissue homogenate is compared to a soluble extract of the same tissue; the membrane enzyme is quite labile, however, and must be assayed promptly

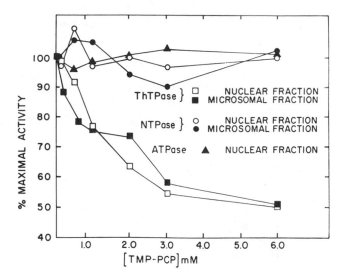

Figure 1. The effects of the substrate analog TMP-PCP on the hydrolytic activities of membrane ATPase, ThTPase, and nucleoside triphosphatase (NTPase), each assayed under optimal conditions.

to accurately evaluate activity. Specific activities of both enzymes are highest in the intestine and the kidney; activity levels in the brain are intermediate between those for these organs and for tissues such as muscle, which show lowest specific activities. In the intestine most of the membrane ThTPase is associated with the gut epithelial cells, specifically with the brush border of these cells. In the kidney the highest levels of activity are seen in the tubular epithelial cells. These observations raise the possibility of involvement of this enzyme in active transport processes.

Examination of subcellular distribution of the soluble (pH 9.0) and membrane (pH 6.5) enzymes in rat brain reveals that more than 95% of the pH 6.5 activity is associated with particulate fractions, the highest levels being found in the crude "nuclear" fraction and in the "nerve ending" fraction. On simple fractionation, however, better than 30% of the pH 9.0 activity appears in the supernatant. Much of the pH 9.0 activity associated with the particulate fractions probably represents cytoplasmic trapping in membrane-lined vesicles; thus, when the nerve ending fraction is subjected to osmotic shock and the resultant membrane fragments are washed and collected, the majority of the pH 9.0 activity is released into the supernatant, while all of the pH 6.5 activity is recovered with the membranes.

The membrane-associated ThTPase in rat kidney appears to be identical

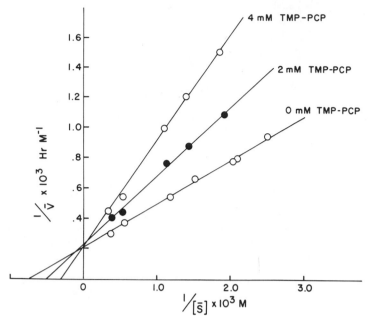

Figure 2. Double reciprocal plots of substrate versus velocity relations for ThTPase in the presence of various levels of TMP-PCP, indicating the pure competitive nature of the inhibition observed.

to that characterized in the brain. It requires divalent cations and is activated to approximately the same extent by Mg^{2+} or Ca^{2+}. This activity again demonstrates a pH optimum of 6.5 to 7.0 and is inhibited by attempts to remove it from its membrane environment. Of the enzyme activity at pH 6.5 in rat kidney, 83% is associated with the particulate fractions; the majority of this (61%) is recovered with the crude microsomes. The Mg^{2+}-ATPase in this preparation follows a similar distribution, with 51% of total activity being isolated with the crude microsomal fraction and a total of 89% in all membrane fractions.

6. Inhibition of Membrane Thiamine Triphosphatase by Nucleoside Phosphates

As previously mentioned, the membrane ThTPase is sensitive to inhibition by ATP and ADP; 50% inhibition of enzyme activity is seen in the presence of approximately 1 to 2×10^{-5} M ATP and 5 to 8×10^{-5} M ADP (Fig. 4). Other nucleoside di- and triphosphates likewise inhibit the ThTPase, but only at concentrations nearly an order of magnitude higher. For the triphosphates the sequence of inhibition is ATP > GTP > CTP > UTP; ThDP, ThMP, and free thiamine are not effective in inhibiting ThTPase activity over similar concentration ranges. The free nucleosides and the nucleoside monophosphates do not affect enzyme activity at concentrations below $1 \times 10^{-3}\ M$.

Kinetic studies on the mechanism of inhibition produced by ADP and ATP are hindered by the concurrent hydrolysis of these compounds by specific phosphatases also present in the membrane fractions containing the ThTPase. We have circumvented this difficulty by using the nonhydrolyzable methylene phosphonate analogs of ADP and ATP for kinetic studies. These compounds produce inhibition similar to that of the native ATP and ADP, although slightly higher (1.2 to 1.5-fold) concentrations are required for 50% inhibition of peak ThTPase activity. Kinetic analysis of data obtained using these analogs indicates a mixed noncompetitive inhibition, with simultaneous effects on both K_m and V_{max} for the substrate (Fig. 5). Effects on both parameters are proportional throughout the active pH range; the relationship of K_m and V_{max} to pH is not affected by either analog. Inhibition of ThTPase activity by ATP and ADP at levels within the range of physiologic intracellular concentrations

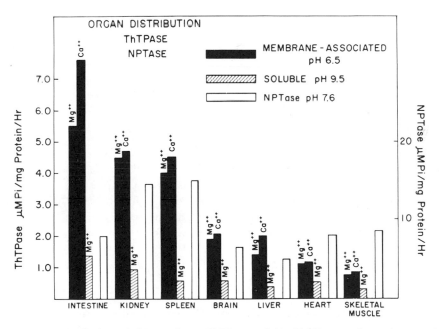

Figure 3. Distribution of the membrane ThTPase, soluble ThTPase, and membrane and nucleoside triphosphatase in various organs of the rat.

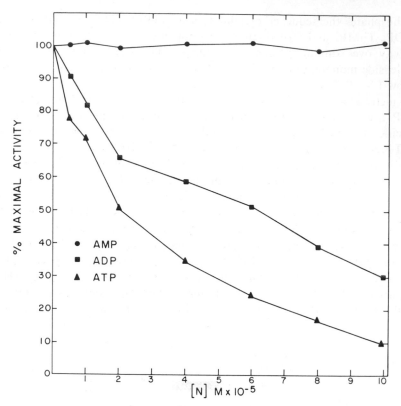

Figure 4. Inhibition of the membrane ThTPase by ATP and ADP. AMP, free adenosine, ThMP, and Th have no effect on enzyme activity in this concentration range.

suggests that these compounds may play a regulatory role in the normal functioning of the ThTPase.

Because of the possible association of ThTP hydrolysis and excitable membrane function, a number of neuroactive compounds, including acetylcholine, γ-aminobutyric acid, tetrodotoxin, 5-hydroxytryptophan, and epinephrine, were tested for specific effects on the activity of the membrane ThTPase; in no case was specific activation or inhibition observed. Likewise, enzyme activity was not affected by variations in the concentration of monovalent cations within the physiologic range.

7. Divalent Cation Activation of Membrane Thiamine Triphosphatase

Further investigation of the nature of activation of the membrane ThTPase by Mg^{2+} has led to several interesting findings concerning the nature of substrate-enzyme interaction in this system. We had initially observed that progessive addition of Mg^{2+} to a system of ThTPase and ThTP at pH 6.5 leads to increasing rates of hydrolysis up to a certain optimal concentration; above this level progressive inhibition is noted (Fig. 6). The optimal concentration of cation and the level at which 25% inhibition is observed vary as a function of the substrate (ThTP) concentration; in general, an approximate 1:1 ratio of ThTP to Mg^{2+} is required for peak activity. When the K_m of the membrane ThTPase for ThTP is determined by constructing double reciprocal plots in the presence of excess Mg^{2+} (divalent cation concentration 1 to 3×10^{-3} M, ThTP concentration 1 to 10×10^{-4} M), the experimental points and calculated values are found to coincide with those determined when the concentration of total Mg^{2+} is varied in the presence of excess ThTP. Thus the calculated enzyme affinities for Mg^{2+} and for ThTP under conditions in which the other is present in excess appear to be identical, and in each case the relationship of velocity to concentration follows the predictions of simple bimolecular kinetics. If, however, similar determinations of rates of hydrolysis as a function of the concentration of ThTP are performed in the presence of low concentrations of Mg^{2+}, marked

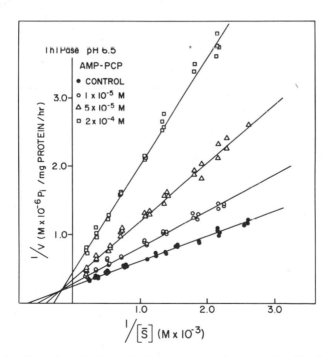

Figure 5. Double reciprocal plots of substrate versus velocity relationships for membrane ThTPase in the presence of varying levels of the nonhydrolyzable analog of ATP, AMP-PCP. A mixed noncompetitive type of inhibition is observed.

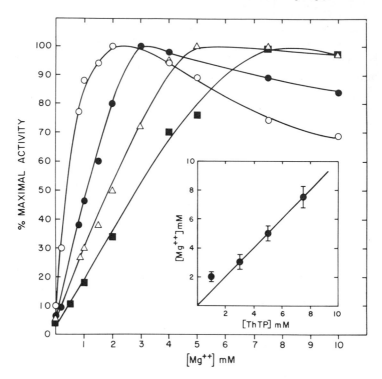

Figure 6. (*a*: Large figure) Activation of the membrane ThTPase by Mg^{2+} at four ThTP concentrations. Each point represents the average of four determinations. (*b*: Small insert) Concentration of Mg^{2+} that produces maximal activation as a function of ThTP concentration. Vertical bars indicate the range of values for full activation.

deviations from predicted kinetic behavior are found (Fig. 7). Hydrolytic activity increases along the expected hyperbolic curve for substrate concentrations below that of the Mg^{2+} present, but abruptly reaches a plateau for levels of ThTP above the ambient Mg^{2+} concentration. The point of deviation appears to vary directly with the Mg^{2+} concentration in the reaction mixture over a wide range.

The dependence of peak enzyme activity on the $ThTP/Mg^{2+}$ ratio suggests that the true substrate for the enzyme is the $ThTP \cdot Mg^{2+}$ complex. This possibility is strengthened by the observation that the Michaelis constants obtained by varying either Mg^{2+} or ThTP concentration with the other present in excess are identical. Such an observation would be expected if the dissociation constant for the substrate-metal complex relative to the concentration of Mg^{2+} or ThTP is low, and if the true substrate is the $Mg^{2+} \cdot ThTP$ complex, since with an excess of substrate the concentration of complex would very nearly equal the concentration of Mg^{2+} added, whereas with excess Mg^{2+} the same would hold true with respect to the concentration of ThTP added. If the true substrate for the membrane ThTPase is a $Mg^{2+} \cdot$ThTP complex rather than free ThTP, the deviations observed from simple kinetics might then represent merely an inaccurate evaluation of the true substrate concentration. To test this hypothesis, it is necessary to determine the dissociation constant (K_d) of the $Mg^{2+} \cdot$ThTP complex under the conditions of our assay. This value in turn makes it possible to calculate the concentration of the $Mg^{2+} \cdot$ThTP complex under experimental conditions.

For determinations of the $Mg^{2+} \cdot$ThTP dissociation constant, we employed the shift in absorption maximum of 8-hydroxyquinoline (8-OH-Q) after the addition of Mg^{2+} as an indicator of free Mg^{2+} concentration in solution. In the absence of Mg^{2+}, 8-OH-Q absorbs maximally at 305 nm; in the presence of excess Mg^{2+}, a $Mg^{2+} \cdot$8-OH-Q complex is formed which exhibits a peak absorption at 355 nm. After determining the change in absorbance at 355 nm (Δ Abs_{355}) of a known concentration of 8-OH-Q as a function of total Mg^{2+} concentration, an equation can be generated relating

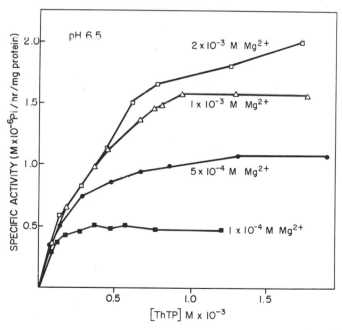

Figure 7. Determinations of the rate of hydrolysis of the membrane ThTPase as a function of substrate concentration in the presence of varying levels of Mg^{2+}. Deviation from expected hyperbolic kinetics is seen at substrate levels above that of the divalent cation.

the Δ Abs$_{355}$ of any known concentration of 8-OH-Q to the total Mg^{2+} and to the free or unbound Mg^{2+} present in the assay system.

   The presence of a second, nonabsorbing ligand in solution competing for the binding of free Mg^{2+} will reduce the amount of Mg^{2+} available for complexing with 8-OH-Q at a given total cation concentration. This will, in turn, result in a deviation in the curve of Δ Abs$_{355}$ for 8-OH-Q as a function of Mg^{2+} concentration. The difference between the expected and the observed Δ Abs$_{355}$ at any given Mg^{2+} concentration under these circumstances yields a value that can be used to calculate the amount of cation bound to the second ligand. When entire curves of Δ Abs$_{355}$ for 8-OH-Q over a Mg^{2+} concentration range between 0 and 10 mM are constructed in the presence of various levels of competing ligand, an iterative computer algorithm incorporating the equilibrium and conservation of mass equations for each binding site can be used to abstract the binding constant for the second ligand if that for the first is independently obtainable. In our system ThTP is the second ligand. Four to six separate determinations of titration curves for 8-OH-Q in the presence of each of four levels of ThTP allow a good approximation to the dissociation constant for the Mg^{2+}·ThTP complex to be reached (Fig. 8).

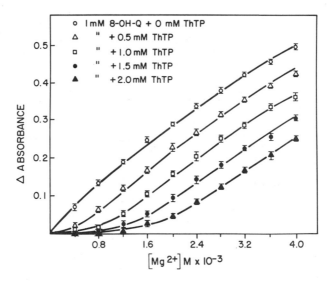

Figure 8. Change in absorption at 355 nm of a 1 mM solution of 8-OH-Q as a function of total Mg^{2+} concentration in the presence of varying levels of ThTP. Symbol and error bars indicate the mean ± S.E. for six experimental determinations at each point. Solid lines follow theoretically predicted titration curves for the equilibria described in text.

Using this approach, we find a dissociation constant of 6.5×10^{-5} M for the $Mg^{2+} \cdot ThTP$ complex in the presence of a total ionic strength of approximately 200 mM; minor deviations from this value are observed at lower ionic strengths.

Using the same techniques, we have estimated the K_d for the $Mg^{2+} \cdot ThDP$ complex to be in the range of 2 to 4×10^{-3} M, while that for the $Mg^{2+} \cdot Th$ complex is greater than 1×10^{-1} M.

After the dissociation constant for the $Mg^{2+} \cdot ThTP$ complex has been determined, the concentration of the complex under conditions of enzyme assay can be calculated. When the data from Fig. 6 are re-expressed in terms of rate of hydrolysis as a function of the $Mg^{2+} \cdot ThTP$ complex concentration, the experimental points from all ambient Mg^{2+} levels are found to fall along a single line. A double reciprocal plot of these data yields a K_m of 6×10^{-4} for the $Mg^{2+} \cdot ThTP$ complex (Fig. 9). These observations strongly support our hypothesis that the true substrate for the membrane ThTPase is the $Mg^{2+} \cdot ThTP$ complex.

8. Excess Free Substrate and Excess Free Mg²⁺

Two further points need to be considered: first, the inhibition of enzyme activity by excess Mg^{2+}; and, second, the apparent absence of similar inhibition of the enzyme by excess free thiamine.

Kinetic studies of the effects of excess free Mg^{2+} on the K_m and V_{max} of membrane ThTPase indicate little effect on either parameter for levels of free Mg^{2+} below 5 mM. At higher levels a progressive increase in K_m is observed, with no change in the maximal velocity at substrate saturation, suggesting a purely competitive pattern of inhibition. The K_i calculated for free Mg^{2+} is 7×10^{-3} M. The purely competitive nature of this inhibition suggests that Mg^{2+} is able to bind at the active site, although with relatively low affinity, and when bound prevents the subsequent attachment of the $Mg^{2+} \cdot ThTP$ complex.

Similar experiments have been done with excess free ThTP and varying concentrations of $Mg^{2+} \cdot ThTP$ complex. No sign of inhibition is seen with concentrations of free ThTP as high as 8 mM; levels above this interfere with our phosphate assay and therefore have not been studied. Although weak binding of free ThTP cannot be ruled out because of the limited range of concentrations which have been examined, there is no doubt that the enzyme has a considerably lower affinity for free ThTP than for the $Mg^{2+} \cdot ThTP$ complex.

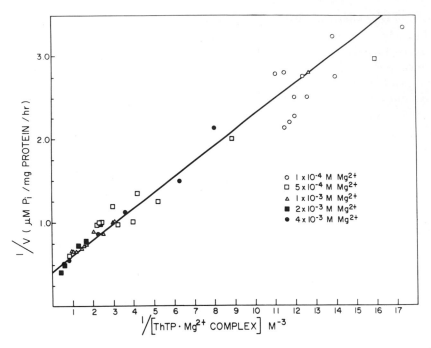

Figure 9.   Recalculation of data shown in Figure 7 in terms of the actual concentration of $Mg^{2+} \cdot ThTP$ complex. A double reciprocal plot of these data now indicates that all points fall along a single line with a calculated K_m for the complex of 6×10^{-4} M.

9. Mg^{2+} and Thiamine Triphosphate

It appears that the membrane ThTPase is specific for the $Mg^{2+} \cdot ThTP$ complex, showing relatively low affinity for free ThTP or free Mg^{2+}. Excess free Mg^{2+} is, however, able to bind, presumably at the active site, and competitively inhibit hydrolysis of the $Mg^{2+} \cdot ThTP$ complex. A possible explanation for the large difference in binding affinity of the enzyme for free ThTP and complexed ThTP may be found in the orientation of the triphosphate side chain in each case. It has been demonstrated by X-ray crystallographic techniques that in crystalline ThDP the pyrophosphate side chain is folded back over the ring portion of the molecule, presumably a conformation favored by interaction between the thiazole nitrogen formal positive charge and the negative charges on the phosphate side chain (10). Studies of ThDP and ThTP in aqueous solution have likewise indicated an interaction between the phosphate side chain and the body of the thiamine molecule (11). The strong temperature dependence of these interactions suggests that an equilibrium exists between a "folded" and an "unfolded" state, the latter with the phosphate chain extended away from the ring portion of the molecule, and that in the absence of divalent cations the folded configuration is favored. The presence of divalent cations, especially Mg^{2+}, appeared in these studies to shift the favored configuration to the "unfolded" form; this may be due to shielding of the negative charges on the side chain produced by binding of the cation between the terminal phosphates of the side chain (10). If we conceptualize the active site of the membrane ThTPase as being specific for the unfolded form of ThTP, the gross change in molecular configuration of the "folded" form of ThTP, as well as the possibility that sites necessary for binding are sterically blocked in this configuration, could easily account for the low affinity of free ThTP for the enzyme (Fig. 10). Thus the specificity of the enzyme for the $Mg^{2+} \cdot ThTP$ complex is really an expression of specificity for the unfolded configuration of the molecule.

Since the precombination of Mg^{2+} with ThTP is required to favor the "unfolded" form, it is likely that this Mg^{2+} will also provide a bridging point during attachment at the active site of the enzyme, a phenomenon observed with many other Mg^{2+}-requiring phosphatases. Saturation of this enzyme site with free Mg^{2+} would necessarily impede binding of the

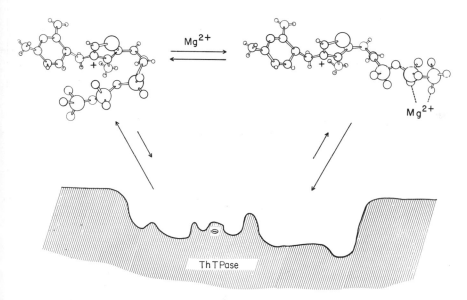

Figure 10. Conceptual representation of the folded and unfolded forms of ThTP interconverted by the presence of Mg^{2+}. The enzyme may select for the unfolded form of the substrate by the conformation of the active site.

complex, and hence account for the inhibition seen with excess divalent cation.

The membrane ThTPase is found in virtually all tissues of the body; its natural substrate ThTP enjoys a similar wide distribution. The role of this combination in cellular function, however, remains a mystery. In tissues such as the kidney, the brain, and the intestine, the correlation of enzyme activity with membranes active in transport processes suggests an association between ThTPase and active transport. The possible role of ThTP in maintaining fixed surface charge density in excitable membranes is an intriguing one and is discussed more fully in Chapter 20. It is interesting to speculate that the role of ThTP and its associated triphosphatase in most tissues lies in this direction; the question of the fate of the γ-phosphate of ThTP after hydrolysis may hold the key to our puzzle. We hope that future research will help to clarify the functional relationship of substrate, enzyme, and membrane.

References

1.   G. Rindi and L. de Guiseppe, *Biochem. J.*, **78**, 602 (1961).
2.   Y. Itokawa, R. Schulz, and J. Cooper, *Biochim. Biophys. Acta.* **266**, 293 (1972).
3.   Y. Itokawa and J. Cooper, *Biochim. Biophys. Acta,* **196**, 274 (1970).
4.   J. Pincus, Y. Itokawa, and J. Cooper, *Neurology,* **19**, 841 (1969).
5.   H. P. Gurtner, *Helv. Physiol. Acta,* Suppl. XI (1961).
6.   Y. Itokawa and J. Cooper, *Biochim. Biophys. Acta,* **158**, 180 (1968).
7.   Y. Hashitani and J. Cooper, *J. Biol. Chem.,* **247**, 2117 (1972).
8.   R. Barchi and P. Braun, *J. Biol. Chem.,* **247**, 7668 (1972).
9.   M. Smith and H. Khorana, *J. Am. Chem. Soc.,* **80**, 1141 (1958).
10.   J. Pletcher and M. Sax, *J. Am. Chem. Soc.,* **94**, 3998 (1972).
11.   A. Gallo, I. Hansen, H. Sable, and T. Swift, *J. Biol. Chem.,* **247**, 5913 (1972).

15. Some Properties of the Enzyme System Degrading Phosphorylated Thiamines in the Brain and the Effect of Chlorpromazine

H. IWATA, M.D.
A. BABA, Ph.D.
T. MATSUDA, M.S.
Z. TERASHITA

Department of Pharmacology
Faculty of Pharmaceutical Sciences
Osaka University
Osaka, Japan

1. Introduction

In 1965 we started our studies on the change in the adrenergic mechanism of the rat in thiamine deficiency. We observed a marked accumulation of catecholamine in tissues, including the brain, of the deficient rat, which is derived from an impairment of catecholamine turnover. It was further shown that these changes in the adrenergic mechanism in thiamine deficiency have a close relationship with the appearance of the polyneuritis syndrome and of disturbances in carbohydrate metabolism (1–5).

Further studies on the enzymatic degradation process of phosphorylated thiamines in the nervous system were undertaken. We reported that brain thiamine diphosphatase (ThDPase) activity was increased after the administration of physostigmine, ambenonium, or pentetrazol. Furthermore, it was observed that the brain total and phosphorylated thiamines were reduced by physostigmine (6, 7). It was shown that ThDPase is a membrane-bound enzyme (8–11). On the other hand, Hashitani and Cooper (12) and Barchi and Braun (13) reported the existence of two types of specific thiamine triphosphatase (ThTPase) in rat brain.

It seems very important to know the dynamic changes in these thiamine phosphatase activities corresponding to functional changes in the brain. However, no single factor, such as pathophysiological changes in the brain or drugs acting on the central nervous system, has been found that affects both of these enzyme activities in nerve tissue.

From these considerations we performed studies to find some neuroactive agents that would produce changes in thiamine metabolism in rat brain. The procedures for obtaining the various subcellular fractions of rat brain and the assay methods for ThDPase and ThTPase activities have already been described (11, 14). The production of thiamine diphosphate (ThDP) or monophosphate (ThMP) was found to be equimolar with the inorganic phosphate liberated. Hence we used the amount of the latter for the expression of enzyme activities in the following experiments.

2.   Results and Discussion

First we examined the *in vivo* effects of chlorpromazine (CPZ), DL-methamphetamine, reserpine, and insulin, and of thiamine deficiency and food deprivation, on ThTPase activities in rat brain and liver. DL-Methamphetamine, CPZ, and thiamine deficiency caused some changes in brain ThTPase activity (15). These changes, though statistically significant, were rather slight, and it may be said that the enzyme activity is hardly influenced by these three conditions.

In *in vitro* studies, ThTPase and ThDPase activities were not affected by various neuroactive agents, such as noradrenaline, acetylcholine, tyramine, diphenylhydantoin, and colchicine. But CPZ, which is known to affect several membrane-bound enzymes, was found to vary the activities of these thiamine phosphatases. As shown in Fig. 1, soluble and microsomal ThTPase activities were inhibited 20 to 70% by CPZ at concentrations of 0.25 to 1.0 mM. Imipramine and desipramine were also found to inhibit ThTPase activities of both fractions, but to a lesser extent than CPZ. On the other hand, microsomal ThDPase activity was markedly activated (20 to 180%) by CPZ at concentrations of 0.125 to 0.5 mM (Fig. 2).

From kinetic studies, it was found that CPZ decreased the V_{max} of ThTPase by about one half without any change in the K_m value and increased the V_{max} of ThDPase about threefold with a corresponding decrease in the K_m value.

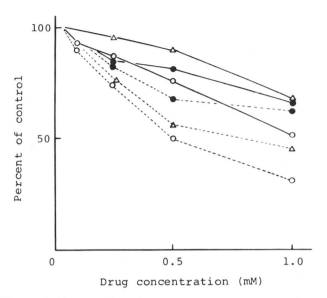

Figure 1. Effects of chlorpromazine (-O-), imipramine (-●-), and desipramine (-△-) on microsomal and soluble ThTPase activities. The reaction mixtures were as follows: for soluble ThTPase, 100 mM Tris-HCl (pH 7.5), 6 mM MgCl$_2$, 3 mM ThTP, and about 100 μg/ml of protein; for microsomal ThTPase, 100 mM Tris-maleate buffer (pH 6.5), 3 mM MgCl$_2$, 3 mM ThTP, and about 600 μg/ml of protein. Reactions were started by the addition of substrate after 5 minutes of preincubation and carried out for 30 minutes at 37°C. ——, microsomal ThTPase [control activity; 0.75 μ moles P$_i$/(mg protein)/(hr)]; ----, soluble ThTPase [control activity; 4.48μ moles P$_i$/(mg protein)/(hr)]. The control activities are taken as 100. Reproduced from H. Iwata et al., *J. Neurochem.*, **24**, 1209 (1975), with permission of Pergamon Press Ltd.

It was indicated by Barchi and Braun (13) that the hydrolysis of ThTP by the membrane-bound enzyme (ThTPase) has an absolute divalent cation requirement which is satisfied by Mg^{2+} or Ca^{2+}.

As seen in Table 1, when 3 mM Ca^{2+} was substituted for Mg^{2+}, CPZ did not cause any marked inhibition of ThTPase activity. This may indicate that the inhibitory action of this drug is quite specific.

As is well known, CPZ inhibits not only membrane-bound enzymes, such as ATPase, but also soluble ones, e.g., phosphodiestrerase (16). On the other hand, only a few enzymes are known to be activated by this drug. For instance, adenylate kinase is markedly activated by CPZ (17). When these facts are taken into consideration, our results, which show that brain ThTPase and ThDPase, both of which are vicinal membrane-bound enzymes in thiamine metabolism, are affected in an opposite manner by this drug, are very interesting.

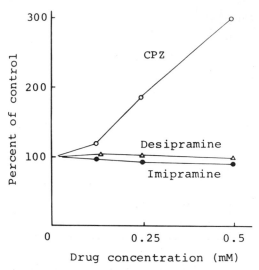

Figure 2. Effects of chlorpromazine (-O-), imipramine (-●-), and desipramine (-△-) on microsomal ThDPase activity. The standard reaction mixtures were as follows: 75 mM Tris-HCl (pH 9.0), 4 mM $CaCl_2$, 4 mM ThDP, and about 180 $\mu g/ml$ of protein. Reactions were started by the addition of substrate after 5 minutes of preincubation and carried out for 30 minutes at 37°C. The control activity [1.05 μ moles $P_i/(mg\ protein)/(hr)$] is taken as 100. Reproduced from H. Iwata et al., *J. Neurochem.*, **24,** 1209 (1975), with permission of Pergamon Press Ltd.

Table 1. Effect of Chlorpromazine on Microsomal ThTPase Activity in the Presence of Ca^{2+} [a]

Chlorpromazine, mM	Relative Activity, %	
	Mg^{2+}-Dependent Activity	Ca^{2+}-Dependent Activity
0	100	100
0.25	83	100
0.50	73	98
1.00	39	84

[a] The incubation conditions were as described for Fig. 1, except that the medium for Ca^{2+}-dependent activity contained 3 mM $CaCl_2$ as divalent cation. The control activities of Mg^{2+}-dependent ThTPase [0.80 μmoles $P_i/(mg\ protein)$ (hr)] and Ca^{2+}-dependent ThTPase [0.98 μmoles $P_i/(mg\ protein)$ (hr)] are taken as 100. Reproducted from H. Iwata *et al.*, J. Neurochem. *24*, 1209 (1975) with permission of Pergamon Press Ltd.

In the experiments described below, we studied in more detail the mechanism of action of CPZ on thiamine phosphatases and the relationships between the action of the drug and the organization of the enzymes in the microsomal fraction.

Figure 3 shows the effects of acetone treatment of microsomes on the enzyme activities and on the CPZ effect. The microsomes were extracted with acetone twice, and the resulting powder was used as the enzyme source. Acetone treatment markedly lowered the activity of ThTPase, and CPZ further inhibited this activity. In contrast to ThTPase, ThDPase activity was increased about fourfold after acetone treatment, and CPZ inhibited this activity.

From a kinetic study on ThDPase in acetone-treated microsomes, it was found that acetone treatment of the microsomes increased the V_{max} of the enzyme with a corresponding decrease in the K_m value, and that CPZ caused a competitive inhibition.

The effects of sodium deoxycholate (DOC) on ThDPase and ThTPase activities are shown in Fig. 4. At a concentration of 0.02%, DOC caused about 80% activation of ThDPase and inhibited ThTPase. However, in acetone-treated microsomes, DOC inhibited ThDPase activity (data not shown). The effects of Triton X-100 solubilization, a freezing-thawing procedure, and phospholipase C treatment on microsomal ThDPase activity were the same as the effect of acetone treatment.

As to the mechanism of the action of CPZ on the biological membrane, several authors have reported that this compound interacts with the lipid

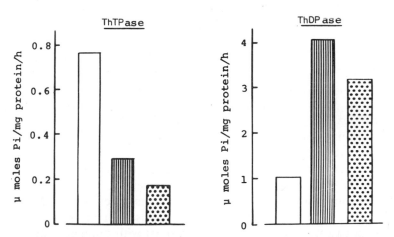

Figure 3. Effect of acetone treatment on microsomal ThTPase (left) and ThDPase (right). The incubation conditions are described for Figs. 1 and 2. □, fresh microsomes; ▥, acetone-treated microsomes; ▨, acetone-treated microsomes + chlorpromazine (0.5 mM). Reproduced from H. Iwata et al., *J. Neurochem.*, **24**, 1209 (1975), with permission of Pergamon Press Ltd.

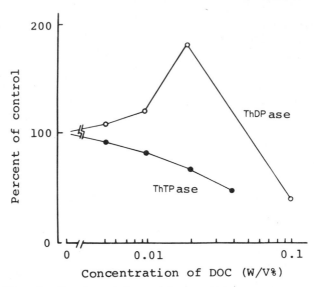

Figure 4. Effect of sodium deoxycholate on microsomal ThDPase (-O-) and ThTPase (-●-). The incubation conditions were described for Figs. 1 and 2. The control activities of ThDPase [1.05 μ moles P_i/(mg protein)/(hr)] and ThTPase [0.75 μ moles P_i/(mg protein)/(hr)] are taken as 100. Reproduced from H. Iwata et al., *J. Neurochem.*, **24**, 1209 (1975), with permission of Pergamon Press Ltd.

part of the membrane, although the possibility of protein modifications cannot be ruled out (18–20). Recently, Leterrier el al. (21) reported a mild detergent-like action of this compound on synaptosomal membrane. Our data may therefore indicate that CPZ activates microsomal ThDPase through its action on acetone-extractable materials or by modifications of the membrane structure. It was also suggested that brain microsomal ThDPase and ThTPase could be influenced in opposite manners by the changes in membrane properties. Furthermore, results suggest that ThDPase exists generally in a "latent form" and is influenced by microenvironmental changes within the membrane.

Although the concentrations of CPZ used are of the same order of magnitude as those reported to be present in the brain after therapeutic doses of this drug (22), it is difficult to correlate the effect of CPZ on thiamine phosphatases with its pharmacological actions on the central nervous system, because the changes in ThDPase and ThTPase induced by this compound were similar to those obtained with promethazine, another phenothiazine derivative with no antipsychotic effects (data not shown). However, as already shown, "Ca^{2+}-dependent ThTPase" was scarcely inhibited by this drug. Hence the fact that ThDPase and ThTPase, vicinal enzymes in thiamine metabolism, were affected in opposite directions by CPZ is interesting. The changes in these enzymes in diverse directions by the modification in membrane properties caused by CPZ, acetone, or DOC are very useful in further studies on the physiological roles of thiamine and its phosphate esters in the central nervous system.

As to the interaction of thiamine phosphate esters with membrane function, a possible relationship between phosphorylated thiamines and the sodium channel was suggested by Itokawa et al. (23). To pursue a possible role of thiamine in membrane function, we studied the effects of thiamine and its phosphate esters on rat brain microsomal ATPase activity *in vitro* in the following experiments.

The effects of thiamine, pyrithiamine, ThMP, ThDP, and ThTP on microsomal Na^+–K^+-ATPase, Mg^{2+}-ATPase, and Ca^{2+}-ATPase activities were examined. A DOC-treated microsomal fraction was obtained by the method of Heckenbergs and Kriegstein (24). It was found that 1 mM ThDP and ThTP caused about 40 and 50% inhibition, respectively, of Ca^{2+}-ATPase. On the other hand, no change was observed in Mg^{2+}-ATPase and Na^+–K^+-ATPase activities (data not shown).

Kinetic studies showed that the inhibition of Ca^{2+}-ATPase by ThTP (noncompetitive) differs from that by EGTA (competitive).

The Ca^{2+}-ATPase mentioned above, whose physiological role in the central nervous system is not clear, was activated only by high concentrations of Ca^{2+} (in our case 5 mM Ca^{2+} was used). The same experiment was performed with microsomal Mg^{2+}–Ca^{2+}-ATPase, an enzyme believed to be related to Ca^{2+} transport across the membrane.

The DOC-treated microsomes for the determination of Mg^{2+}–Ca^{2+}-ATPase activity were obtained by the method of Nakamaru and Konishi (25). In this preparation the addition of 0.1 mM Ca^{2+} caused a 50% activation of the enzyme in the presence of $1.25 \times 10^{-4} M$ of EGTA.

The effect of 10^{-6} to 10^{-3} M ThTP on Mg^{2+}–Ca^{2+}-ATPase activity is shown in Table 2. Though Mg^{2+}-dependent activity was not influenced, Ca^{2+}-dependent activity was strongly inhibited by ThTP. At concentrations of 10^{-5} to 10^{-3} M ThTP, 20 to 50% inhibition was observed. Furthermore, ThTP-induced inhibition of the Ca^{2+}-dependent activity was independent of Ca^{2+} concentration (data not shown).

Thus ThTP inhibited only "Ca^{2+}-dependent ATPases" among various ATPases, and the mechanism of the inhibition seemed to be different from that caused by EGTA, though the concentrations of ThTP required to cause inhibition were above the physiological level.

Similar results were also found with erythrocyte Mg^{2+}–Ca^{2+}-ATPase. On the other hand, ThTP did not influence the activity of Mg^{2+}–Ca^{2+}-phosphodiesterase in rat brain microsomes. Therefore the inhibitory action of ThTP seemed to be specific for ATPase.

Table 2. Effect of ThTP on Mg^{2+}–Ca^{2+}-ATPase Activity in Rat Brain Microsomes

ThTP, M	Mg^{2+}-Dependent Activity[a]		Ca^{2+}-Dependent Activity[b]	
	Specific Activity, μmoles P_i/ (mg protein) (10 min)	%	Specific Activity, μmoles P_i/ (mg protein) (10 min)	%
0	2.46	100	1.09	100
10^{-6}	2.39	97	1.00	92
10^{-5}	2.46	100	0.86	79
10^{-4}	2.44	99	0.69	63
5×10^{-4}	2.39	97	0.65	60
10^{-3}	2.31	94	0.55	50

[a] EGTA (1.25×10^{-4} M) was present.
[b] Ca^{2+} (6×10^{-5}) was added.

The interaction of phosphorylated thiamine and Ca^{2+} was next studied. Thiamine showed no chelating action, but ThTP, ThDP, and ThMP (0.7 mM), in the order named, exhibited chelating effects toward Ca^{2+} as determined by the murexide method by Ohnishi and Ebashi (26). Furthermore, the effects of thiamine compounds on the binding of Ca^{2+} to microsomes were studied using the chlortetracycline fluorescence method described by Caswell and Hutchison (27). It was found that 0.3 mM ThTP markedly inhibited the binding of Ca^{2+} to microsomes, this binding being independent of ATP.

These phenomena, together with the effect of thiamine phosphates on Ca^{2+}-ATPase, could provide a clue for further studies on the relationship between thiamine metabolism and ion fluxes in the central nervous system.

Acknowledgment

We wish to thank Pergamon Press Ltd. for the kind permission to reprint the Figures and Table 1.

References

1. H. Iwata, S. Fujimoto, T. Nishikawa, and K. Hano, *Experientia,* **24,** 378 (1968).
2. H. Iwata, T. Nishikawa, and K. Watanabe, *Experientia,* **25,** 283 (1969).
3. H. Iwata, T. Nishikawa, and S. Fujimoto, *J. Pharm. Pharmacol.,* **21,** 237 (1969).
4. H. Iwata, T. Nishikawa, and A. Baba, *Eur. J. Pharmacol.,* **12,** 253 (1970).
5. H. Iwata, A. Baba, T. Baba, and T. Nishikawa, *J. Pharm. Pharmacol.,* **26,** 707 (1974).
6. A. Inoue, S. Shim, and H. Iwata *J. Neurochem.,* **17,** 1373 (1970).
7. H. Iwata, A. Inoue, and M. Tomoi, *J. Neurochem.,* **18,** 1371 (1971).
8. L. Seijo and G. Rodriguez de Lores Arnaiz, *Biochim. Biophys. Acta,* **211,** 595 (1970).
9. J. R. Cooper and M. M. Kini, *J. Neurochem.,* **19,** 1809 (1972).
10. R. L. Barchi and P. E. Braun, *J. Neurochem.,* **18,** 1039 (1972).
11. A. Inoue and H. Iwata, *Biochim. Biophys. Acta,* **242,** 459 (1971).
12. Y. Hashitani and J. R. Cooper, *J. Biol. Chem.,* **247,** 2117 (1972).
13. R. L. Barchi and P. E. Braun, *J. Biol. Chem.,* **247,** 7668 (1972).
14. H. Iwata, A. Baba, and T. Matsuda, *Jap. J. Pharmacol.,* **24,** 817 (1974).
15. H. Iwata, A. Baba, T. Matsuda, Z. Terashita, and K. Ishii, *Jap. J. Pharmacol.,* **24,** 825 (1974).
16. F. Honda and H. Imamura, *Biochim. Biophys. Acta,* **161,** 267 (1968).
17. J. D. Robinson, J. Lowinger, and B. Bettinger, *Biochem. Pharmacol.,* **17,** 1113 (1968).
18. P. S. Guth and M. A. Spirtes, *Int. Rev. Neurobiol.,* **7,** 231 (1964).
19. W. O. Kwant and P. Seeman, *Biochim. Biophys. Acta,* **183,** 530 (1969).
20. P. Seeman, W. O. Kwant, M. Goldberg, and M. Chau-Wong, *Biochim. Biophys. Acta,* **241,** 349 (1971).
21. F. R. Leterrier, F. Rieger and J. -F. Mariaud, *Biochem. Pharmacol.,* **23,** 103 (1974).
22. N. P. Salzman and B. B. Brodie, *J. Pharmacol. Exp. Ther.,* **118,** 46 (1956).
23. Y. Itokawa, R. A. Schulz, and J. R. Cooper, *Biochim. Biophys. Acta,* **266,** 293 (1972).
24. H. Heckenbergs and J. Kriegstein, *Naunyn-Schmiedebergs Arch. Exp. Pathol. Pharmakol.,* **274,** 63 (1972).
25. Y. Nakamaru and K. Konishi, *Biochim. Biophys. Acta,* **159,** 206 (1968).
26. T. Ohnishi and S. Ebashi, *J. Biochem.* (Tokyo), **54,** 506 (1963).
27. A. H. Caswell and J. D. Hutchison, *Biochem. Biophys. Res. Commun.,* **42,** 43 (1971).

DISCUSSION

Chapters 14 and 15

Dr. Connelly. You pointed out the K_m for the membrane-bound enzyme at pH 7.2. Have you determined the K_m for the soluble enzyme at physiological pH, and if you have, does it shed any light on the possible roles of these enzymes in the physiological state?

Dr. Barchi. We determined the K_m of the enzyme at its pH optimum, which is around 9.0. I have not determined the K_m at pH 6.5 simply because there is so little activity at that point. Jack, have you done that?

Dr. Cooper. No.

Dr. Danner. I would like to direct this question to Dr. Barchi. In your study on the pH optimum effect, since you are talking about the folded versus the open form as the preferred substrate, is the pH effect an effect on substrate, rather than on enzyme, to give you the lower pH optimum for the membrane-bound form? Is the substrate, at the active site of the enzyme, sufficiently altered, either in the release form or the soluble form, to prefer the folded form of the thiamine diphosphate as substrate? Finally, would the addition of phospholipids to the soluble form of the enzyme alter the substrate further?

Dr. Barchi. Let me see whether I can answer you. There are about four questions there. The first question is, essentially, what is the pK of the substrate? There are a number of pKs for thiamine triphosphate. For instance, there is a pK for the protonation of the pyridine ring nitrogen, which is about 5.2. There are a number of pKs for the phosphate side chains, at least two of which are low, and I am not sure they have been potentiometrically determined for ThTP. If anybody has any more information on this, I would be interested in it. A series of reactions that take place in basic solution makes the structure of thiamine variable in the pH range above 8 and very different from the thiamine structure below that point. The thiazole ring may actually open at higher pH.

Dr. Danner. Then how do you explain the pH curve having an effect on the substrate?

Dr. Barchi. I would suspect that, with the activation between pH 6.5 and 7, I would not be able to assign the effect specifically to the pK of the substrate; rather I would suspect that the pK of an active group in the enzyme is involved. As far as the desirable form of enzyme is concerned, I really do not think that the soluble activity is just the same enzyme as the membrane enzyme in solubilized form. We have never been able to solubilize the membrane-associated enzyme; any attempt to do so inactivates it. The soluble enzyme is quite stable in the absence of lipids; you can dialyze it, you can do a number of things with it, and it is quite happy. As to whether it prefers the folded configuration, the soluble enzyme also requires divalent cation and is also activated by magnesium.

Dr. Danner. But it is still substrate inhibited.

Dr. Barchi. It is at higher concentrations. So the question is whether the soluble enzyme has any bonding for the folded form, and one would suspect from the kinetics that it does in that, at least to a certain extent, the active site is able to bind with the folded configuration. There is another possibility that has not been pursued—that the true substrate for the soluble enzyme may not be the magnesium-ThDP complex, but rather one of the myriad of other enzymatic mechanisms in which divalent cations are involved: either a bridging mechanism, or the formation of an enzyme-metal complex with subsequent formation of an enzyme-metal-substrate complex, or the simultaneous binding of the metal and the substrate to the active site. These are all possibilities that have not been looked into. All I can say, on the basis of the kinetics that we have, is that the picture is going to be different from what we see with the membrane-associated enzyme and that those possibilities are still open.

Dr. Cooper. Dr. Iwata, I wish to make a couple of points. I think you mentioned that you were not too impressed with the chlorpromazine activity in the sense of its being a reflection of how CPZ acts *in vivo,* and I tend to agree with that. The concentration seems to be very high, and CPZ is such a reactive molecule that it affects virtually every enzyme tested at anything higher than 10^{-4} M concentration. Therefore I do not think that the effect on TTPase is a reflection of the drug's antipsychotic effect. Have you looked in other tissues besides brain for the calcium phosphatase effect?

Dr. Iwata.   Do you mean the effect on calcium TTPase?

Dr. Cooper.   Yes. Was it present only in brain, or did you find it in other tissues?

Dr. Iwata.   Only with liver.

Dr. Cooper.   And you get the same effect in liver as you do in brain?

Dr. Iwata.   Yes, so I believe that it is not so special to brain.

Dr. Cooper.   That may be important in connection with the discussions with Dr. Barchi on the physiological role of ThTP.

Dr. Iwata.   At first I used CPZ because it is a psychoactive agent. But, as Dr. Cooper pointed out, I also think that the concentrations used are relatively high and that it is difficult to correlate the effect of this drug on ThDPase and ThTPase with its pharmacological actions on the central nervous system. I believe that the unique characteristics of thiamine phosphatases were demonstrated by this compound.

FOUR

THIAMINE AND NEUROPATHY

16. Thiamine-Deficiency Encephalopathy: Thoughts on Its Pathogenesis

PIERRE M. DREYFUS, M.D.

Department of Neurology
School of Medicine
University of California
Davis, California

T he encephalopathy caused by thiamine deficiency has been the subject of intense investigation since it was first described by Eijkman almost 100 years ago. With the constant development of new and more sophisticated ultrastructural, biochemical, biophysical, and neurophysiological research tools, an ever-increasing amount of biomedical data relevant to thiamine deficiency and its effects on the nervous system has been collected. The aims of the various investigations have been to elucidate the following:

1. The sequence of biological events which leads to neurological dysfunction and eventual tissue damage.
2. The principal underlying biochemical lesion or lesions.
3. The cause of the selective vulnerability of certain areas of the brain to the state of deficiency invariably observed, regardless of the animal species.

In general, there has been a lack of uniformity in the experimental approach to the problem. First of all, the compositions of the thiamine-deficient diets utilized have varied considerably. The methods of production of the state of deficiency have also differed; some studies have relied on dietary restriction of the vitamin, whereas others have produced a deficient state by using thiamine analogs. Investigations have also varied in terms of the acuteness versus the chronicity of the deficiency. Despite these shortcomings, a great deal of valuable and interesting information has been gleaned over the past half century. Nevertheless, a lack of unanimity regarding the interpretation of the experimental data continues to exist.

The following remarks are aimed at reviewing some of the experimental results obtained in various laboratories, including our own, in an attempt to find at least partial answers to the three fundamental questions outlined above.

A review of recent ultrastructural studies undertaken on the remarkable brain-stem lesions found in every animal species, including man, suggests that the earliest changes produced by thiamine deficiency are detected in membranous structures. Robertson et al. (1), studying the lesion in the deficient rat brain stem, have noted in the early stages a predominance of intracellular edema involving glial cells—in particular, perivascular glial foot processes. In the slightly more advanced stages of the disease, edema seems to involve myelin sheaths and the extravascular compartment. These changes presumably result in defective electrolyte transport across membranes. The lack of increased permeability to protein noted during the early stages suggests a relatively restricted pathological process. Similar observations have been made by Collins and Converse (2, 3).

More recently, Vick and Schulman (4), studying the deficient rhesus monkey brain stem, have reported intramyelinitic splitting, or "myelin blisters," at the intraperiod line, with secondary alterations of axons. These observations further suggest that defective transport mechanisms at the level of glial and myelin membranes could ensue. The ultimate destruction of all tissue elements, the resultant demyelination, and the vascular changes which heretofore have always been described as being typical of the lesions of thiamine encephalopathy probably represent secondary lesions, or the end stages of the pathological process. It appears inaccurate, therefore, to invoke thiamine deficiency as a disease entity primarily affecting myelinated structures. Whereas the ultrastructural studies undertaken to date seem to point to the elements which are most severely affected by the state of thiamine deficiency, they fail to provide an answer to the all-important question of why there is selective topographical vulnerability.

The biochemical investigations carried out over the past half century have been very productive, yielding copious and extremely useful information concerning the vitamin: its structure and its various forms; its synthesis; its degradation; its role in carbohydrate metabolism; and the specific biochemical reactions in which it is involved, which occur in many organs of the body, including the nervous system. The concept of the "biochemical lesion," first enunciated in relation to thiamine deficiency and the nervous system by Peters (5), has formed the basis for subsequent biochemical investigations.

Extensive work on abnormal pyruvate metabolism in thiamine deficiency seemed to provide a ready explanation for the dramatic neurological events and tissue changes observed in this disease state. However, more detailed scrutiny of this biochemical lesion has failed to confirm theories postulated as the result of early observations. It would appear logical to expect serious consequences resulting from faulty α-keto acid decarboxylation. Theoretically, severe thiamine deficiency, by virtue of faulty pyruvate and α-ketoglutaric acid metabolism, should impair the synthesis of lipids and acetylcholine and the generation of ATP, particularly in the most severely involved part of the brain, i. e., the brain stem. Regional concentrations of ATP have been shown to be normal or slightly elevated in thiamine deficiency (6–8). The levels of acetylcholine have been found to be normal by some investigators (9) but significantly reduced by others (10), who also reported lower levels of acetylcoenzyme A in the face of normal pyruvate dehydrogenase, choline acetyltransferase, and acetylcholine esterase activities. Acetylcholine turnover rates have not as yet been estimated.

It is generally accepted that the pentose phosphate pathway plays an important role in synthetic mechanisms by virtue of NADPH production for lipid synthesis and ribose production for nucleic acid synthesis. Although this metabolic pathway is operative in the central nervous system, there remains some controversy regarding its importance. In the adult brain it probably plays a relatively minor role, assuming greater importance in the developing (11) and chronically depleted nervous system. In severe thiamine deficiency, decreased NADPH production could impair fatty acid and nucleic acid synthesis and the conversion of oxidized glutathione to its reduced form. The latter has been shown to be reduced in the brain of symptomatic thiamine-deficient animals (7). The synthesis of RNA and, possibly, protein has been reported to be affected (12).

In order to determine whether thiamine deficiency ultimately leads to abnormal lipid and myelin metabolism, we undertook a series of studies in developing rats to investigate the deposition of brain lipids in severely depleted animals. These studies were performed on immature animals during a period when the brain is most susceptible to environmental insults. We expected that the biochemical lesion or lesions would be more severe when thiamine deficiency was induced during a critical stage of brain development, a time when myelin metabolism is at its peak. We compared the brains of thiamine-deficient animals with those of animals on either a normal or a pair-fed control diet. The latter animals were undernourished yet adequately supplied with thiamine. Dietary thiamine deficiency was initiated in the mothers on the 14th day of pregnancy, and biochemical measurements were undertaken on the brains of the mothers and their offspring from the 5th to the 25th day after birth. Brain transketolase activity was used to monitor the degree of thiamine deficiency.

The results of our studies are as follows:

1.   During normal development, whole-brain transketolase activity increased rapidly to adult levels between day 5 and day 20 after birth. Dietary thiamine deficiency initiated on the 14th day of pregnancy resulted in a marked fall in the enzyme activity of the offspring, which dropped to 25% of that of the controls at day 25. Maternal brain transketolase activity was considerably less affected, remaining at 80% of that of controls after 34 days on the deficient diet, or 25 days after parturition (see Fig. 1).

2.   Thiamine-deficient animals developed marked anorexia, paralleled by a reduction in the body and brain growth of the developing offspring. Brain DNA concentration was higher in pair-fed and deficient animals, indicative of a smaller cell size, as reflected in the lower protein/DNA ratio. The RNA levels expressed per unit DNA were significantly reduced in the same groups, as compared to controls. Neurological symptoms characteristic of thiamine deficiency were evident in the deficient group by 25 days of age (see Table 1).

3.   Whole-brain ganglioside concentration was significantly greater in the thiamine-deficient and pair-fed control groups than in the normal animals. Cholesterol levels were similar in thiamine-deficient and control groups but low in pair-fed animals. Cerebroside and total sphingolipid (minus ganglioside) concentrations in whole brain were markedly reduced in thiamine-deficient and pair-fed animals, as compared to the levels found in normal controls. Total phospholipid concentration and the distribution of individual phospholipids were similar in all three groups (see Table 2).

4.   Similar results, with minor exceptions, were noted when the lipid compositions of the brain stem, cerebellum, and diencephalon were estimated. Cerebellar ganglioside concentrations of thiamine-deficient and pair-fed control groups were similar to those found in normal control animals. Brain-stem and cerebellar cholesterol levels were lower in thiamine-deficient and pair-fed control groups than in normal controls, but diencephalon cholesterol levels were unchanged. No marked change in the distribution of individual phospholipids was apparent in the three groups.

We conclude from these experiments that immature animals are more susceptible to dietary thiamine deficiency than are adults. Using total sphingolipids and cerebroside levels as indices of the degree of myelination, it appears that this process is equally impaired in thiamine deficiency and in the plain undernutrition represented by pair-fed control animals. Thiamine

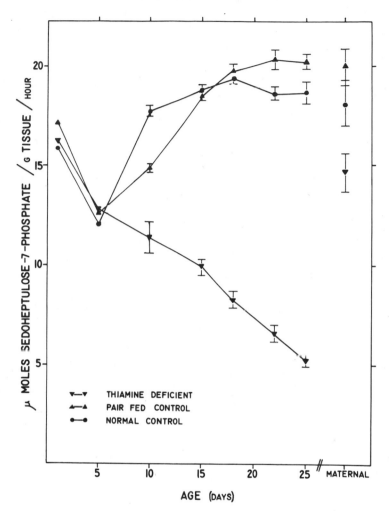

Figure 1. Whole-brain transketolase activity of thiamine-deficient and control rats during development. Points are the means for 8 to 25 animals with ± S.E.M. represented by vertical bars.

deficiency present during a period of rapid brain development does not seem to induce, in myelin lipids or other lipid components, changes which can be separated from the effects of simple undernutrition in either the whole brain or those areas most susceptible to the lack of thiamine.

On the basis of previous experiments, we had postulated that the abnormality of transketolase activity, which we had studied extensively in various parts of the brain, might be the important underlying biochemical

Table 1. Whole-Brain Protein and Nucleic Acid Concentrations of 25-Day-Old Thiamine-Deficient Rats as Compared to Controls[a]

Type of Rat	Protein, μg/mg	RNA, μg/mg	DNA, μg/mg	RNA/DNA	Protein/DNA
Normal control	84.71 ± 0.64	2.019 ± 0.014	1.838 ± 0.024	1.099 ± 0.012	46.13 ± 0.64
Thiamine-deficient	87.42 ± 0.52*[b]	2.015 ± 0.015	2.013 ± 0.029*[b]	1.003 ± 0.019†	43.51 ± 0.77*
Pair-fed control	86.75 ± 0.60*	2.074 ± 0.019	2.080 ± 0.033†	0.999 ± 0.017†	41.83 ± 0.81†

[a] Values represent means ± S.E.M. of duplicate assays from 8 to 12 animals.
[b] The asterisk ($p < .04$) and the dagger ($p < .001$) denote statistical differences from normal controls.

Table 2. Whole-Brain DNA and Lipid Compositions of 25-Day-Old Thiamine-Deficient,[a] Pair-Fed Control (Undernourished), and Normal Control rats[b,c]

	Normal Control	Thiamine-Deficient	Pair-Fed Control
DNA	1.84 ± 0.02	2.01 ± 0.03*[a]	2.03 ± 0.03*
Total lipid	69.08 ± 0.45	67.19 ± 0.39+	65.26 ± 0.96+
Ganglioside NANA	0.506 ± 0.008	0.575 ± 0.012*	0.535 ± 0.008†
Total phospholipid	45.31 ± 0.33	45.04 ± 0.47	44.68 ± 0.86
Cholesterol	13.31 ± 0.15	13.52 ± 0.13	12.27 ± 0.21*
Sphingolipid	18.90 ± 0.55	16.56 ± 0.44+	15.00 ± 0.38*
Cerebrosides	5.16 ± 0.12	4.38 ± 0.18+	3.77 ± 0.24*

[a] Thiamine deficiency induced by feeding pregnant mothers a diet containing suboptimal amounts of thiamine (0.5 mg/kg diet) from the 14th day of gestation.
[b] Values are means ± S.E.M. of replicate determinations from 8 to 10 animals.
[c] Lipid and DNA values expressed as milligrams and sphingolipid values as micromoles per gram wet tissue.
[d] Statistically significant differences (Student's t test) from normal controls denoted as follows: asterisk, $p < .001$; dagger, $p < .01$; double dagger, $p < .05$.

lesion as far as the nervous system is concerned (13). Although the enzymatic activity in different organs and the blood accurately reflects the activity of transketolase in various parts of the central nervous system, on the one hand, and neurological signs and symptoms, on the other, the true significance of this biochemical lesion remains essentially unexplained. To date the experimental evidence which points to transketolase activity as a reflection of glial cell metabolism is tenuous at best. In fact, the importance of the pentose phosphate pathway in the metabolism of the fully developed brain remains obscure.

Thiamine does not appear to be related to either the deposition or the metabolism of myelin lipids. Barchi and Braun (14) could not relate the thiamine content to the state of myelination of the nervous system of newborn animals, and we were unable to demonstrate specific alterations in lipid composition which could not be accounted for by simple undernutrition. It is therefore becoming less and less clear what the significant changes in carbohydrate metabolism engendered by thiamine deficiency mean as far as the central nervous system lesions are concerned. There is ample clinical evidence to suggest that an abnormality of carbohydrate metabolism is in some way involved in the production of neurological symptoms and signs; that is, a big carbohydrate load given to a thiamine-deficient patient may precipitate the advent of symptoms and signs of Wernicke's disease.

However, the rapidity of the clinical events, in terms of deterioration or amelioration taking place in a matter of hours, strongly suggests that extremely labile and readily reversible mechanisms are involved.

This brings us to the neurophysiological observations first made by Von Muralt (15), in part confirmed and further developed by Cooper and Itokawa (16, 17), and more recently expanded by Barchi (18), which demonstrate unequivocally that thiamine, particularly its phosphoric esters and their metabolism, is involved in the function of excitable membranes, perhaps specifically in the activation and inactivation of sodium transport. The effects of thiamine deficiency on membrane function could readily explain the dramatic evolution of the clinical events and some of the early ultrastructural changes, as well as the lack of demonstrable histological changes noted by conventional methods in at least one half of severely affected experimental animals. Repeated insults could ultimately lead to the irreversible clinical manifestations frequently observed in thiamine-deficient patients and to the permanent pathological alterations detected in their brains at the time of death. The depletion of available thiamine by a large carbohydrate load may temporarily help the enzyme systems in which thiamine is an essential cofactor at the expense of the mechanisms which require thiamine for membrane function. It is conceivable that the thiamine-deficient membrane is unable to maintain osmotic gradients and that failure of the energy-dependent component of glial-electrolyte and water transport ensues as the result of relatively acute thiamine deficiency. Chronic depletion of the vitamin may induce other irreversible physiological and histopathological changes.

The selective vulnerability of certain areas of the nervous system which is so characteristic of thiamine deficiency continues to be unexplained. It is well established that the central nervous system is not a homogeneous organ from the point of view of its histology and its biochemistry. Even in areas of the nervous system where the components appear to be fairly uniform, such as the optic nerve, there is a marked histological difference between one part and another in terms of the density, thickness, and myelination of fibers (19). Differences in the composition of the tissue undoubtedly correlate with metabolic and biochemical differences, on the one hand, and the vulnerability of the tissue to metabolic insults, on the other. It is not surprising, therefore, to detect significant biochemical differences between parts of the brain which are complex and heterogeneous in terms of their cellular compositions. As an example, we have noted significant differences in transketolase activity in various parts of the rat, cat, and human brain (see Table 3). Recently we measured differences in transketolase activity in various anatomical subdivisions of the human cerebellar cortex—a part of

Table 3. Brain Transketolase Activity[a,b]
(Normal adult)

Part of Brain	Activity, μM sedoheptulose-7-P/ (g protein) (hr)		
	Rat	Cat	Man[c]
Cerebral cortex	97.9 ± 4	173 ± 15	148.3
Caudate nucleus	107.6 ± 5	—	249.2
Brain stem	165.3 ± 5	306 ± 26	282.7
Cerebellum	151.1 ± 4	299 ± 24	241.5

[a] ± S.E. of the mean (when available).
[b] All determinations in triplicate.
[c] Brain obtained 4 hours postmortem.

the brain which displays a relative degree of histological homogeneity (see Table 4).

It is of interest to note that certain disease states that affect the cerebellar cortex do so in a highly selective manner, affecting some parts to a greater degree than others. This selectivity may be related to differences in metabolic activity. Metabolic differences and variations in enzymatic activity noted in various areas of the brain may be due to differences in vasculature; density of neurons, glial cells, and nerve fibers; and degree of myelination. The ratio of glial cells, both perineuronal and perivascular, to neurons is undoubtedly of the utmost importance in determining the metabolic vulnerability of the anatomic site. The biochemical characteristics of certain neuronal populations or specific nuclei in the brain must also play a role in the process of selective vulnerability to certain metabolic disturbances. Although we have no definite leads as to the cause of selective vulnerability in thiamine deficiency, it may well be that in the affected areas of the brain the perivascular glial cells, which seem to be responsible for the regulation of electrolyte and water transport, have an unusually high rate of oxidative activity, which renders the tissue more vulnerable to failures in transport mechanisms.

We seem to be on the verge of discovering the role of thiamine in the function of excitable membranes and the reasons why thiamine-deficient tissue ceases to function normally. It would therefore be of great interest to determine why certain parts of the brain fail before others. Perhaps at the time of our next meeting the answer will be available.

**Table 4. Transketolase Activity in Human Cerebellum[a,b]
(Normal adult)**

Part of Cerebellum	Average Activity, μM S-7-P/ (g protein) (hr)	$\pm$ S.E.
A. Superior vermis	216	28.0
B. Posterior vermis	239	19.1
C. Inferior vermis	161	15.0
D. Flocculus	266	13.3
E. Nodulus	291	44.5
F. Lateral hemisphere	276	22.3

[a] Three different subjects; all determinations done in triplicate.
[b] Significant differences between (C) and (B), (D), (E), (F), $p < .001$.

Acknowledgments

Dr. Stanley E. Geel performed all of the lipid and nucleic acid determinations. Research was supported by grant NS 08399 from the National Institute of Neurological Diseases and Stroke and by Health Sciences Achievement award RR 06138.

References

1. D. J. Robertson, S. M. Wasan, and D. B. Skinner, *Am. J. Pathol.*, **52**, 1081 (1968).
2. G. H. Collins, *Am. J. Pathol.*, **50**, 791 (1967).
3. G. H. Collins and W. K. Converse, *Am. J. Pathol.*, **58**, 219 (1970).
4. N. A. Vick and S. Schulman, *Neurology*, **24**, 362 (1974).
5. R. A. Peters, *Lancet*, **23**, 1161 (1936).
6. J. Holowach, F. Kauffman, M. G. Ikossi, C. Thomas, and D. B. McDougal, Jr., *J. Neurochem.*, **15**, 621 (1968).
7. D. W. McCandless and S. Schenker, *J. Clin. Invest.*, **47**, 2268 (1968).
8. A. Inoue, S. Shim, and H. Iwata, *J. Neurochem.*, **17**, 1373 (1970).
9. K. V. Speeg, Jr., D. Chen, D. W. McCandless, and S. Schenker, *Proc. Soc. Exp. Biol. Med.*, **134**, 1005 (1970).
10. C. P. Heinrich, H. Stadler, and H. Weiser, *J. Neurochem.*, **21**, 73 (1973).
11. F. Novello and P. McLean, *Biochem. J.*, **107**, 775 (1968).
12. H. Reinauer and S. Hollmann, *Hoppe-Seylers Z. Physiol. Chem.*, **350**, 23 (1969).

13. P. M. Dreyfus, in G. E. W. Wohlstenholme, Ed., *Thiamine Deficiency: Biochemical Lesions and Their Clinical Significance,* Little, Brown and Company, Boston, 1967.

14. R. L. Barchi and P. E. Braun, *Brain Res.,* **35,** 622 (1971).

15. A. Von Muralt, *Exp. Cell Res.,* **5,** 72 (1958).

16. J. R. Cooper, *Biochim. Biophys. Acta,* **156,** 368 (1968).

17. Y. Itokawa and J. R. Cooper, *Biochim. Biophys. Acta,* **196,** 274 (1970).

18. R. L. Barchi, Conference on Thiamine, Monterey, 1974.

19. A. M. Potts, D. Hodges, C. B. Shelam, K. J. Fritz, N. S. Levy, and Y. Mangnall, *Invest. Ophthal.,* **80,** 980 (1972).

DISCUSSION

Chapter 16

Dr. Collins.   My question is in reference to the recent report by Vick in which "myelin blisters" or blebs were found in acute deficiency. Do you feel that this represents a change that has been missed by other investigators as significant, or that it represents a nonspecific change in myelin due to a hypotonic medium?

Dr. Dreyfus.   The "myelin blisters" that were shown by Dr. Vick to occur in the brain-stem lesions of thiamine-deficient monkeys are probably not specific for that disease entity since they have also been observed by other investigators in experimental tin and hexachlorophene intoxication. Dr. David Robertson showed some years ago that the tonicity of the fixatives used could significantly alter the appearance of the myelin sheath. The changes demonstrated by Dr. Vick at the San Francisco meetings of the American Academy of Neurology seemed quite convincing. However, I hasten to add that I do not consider myself an expert in electron microscopy and will let others who work in the field be the judges. More work is surely needed in this area.

Dr. Blass.   Has anyone determined whether thiamine triphosphate falls more rapidly or more completely in the affected regions of the brain than other thiamine derivatives?

Dr. Cooper.   Dr. Pincus measured all forms of thiamine during thiamine deficiency and found that all forms of thiamine esters fell except ThTP, which, percentage-wise, increased. The impression was that the brain wants to hold onto ThTP right to the end.

Dr. Dreyfus.   The data of Pincus and Grove on the levels of thiamine esters in progessive thiamine deficiency can be interpreted in several ways. I have noted that in their experiments the standard deviations of the various determinations were rather large, and I suspect that the circumstances under which the animals were sacrificed may have determined the levels of ThDP or ThTP. The rate of exchange between these two phosphate esters and their levels may fluctuate considerably, depending on the state of the membrane.

Dr. Kark. There is evidence to suggest that transketolase activity is reduced in liver and that in combined deficiency of thiamine and magnesium activity is not restored *in vitro* simply by adding thiamine (L. Zieve, W. M. Doizaki, and L. E. Stenroos, *J. Lab. Clin. Med.,* **72,** 268, 1968). Was that the case in your studies of brain? Is so, is there reason to ask whether thiamine deficiency may affect the turnover rates or the synthesis of specific proteins?

Dr. Dreyfus. There appears to be clinical evidence to suggest that transketolase apoenzyme levels can be affected by thiamine deficiency both in human beings and in animals. We have noted that in some instances, after treatment with thiamine, it may take several weeks before the activity of blood transketolase is restored to normal levels, whereas in other cases this occurs in a matter of hours or days. Thus we have been able to separate acutely deprived from chronically deprived individuals. To the best of my knowledge, no one has had the opportunity to look specifically at the apoprotein of transketolase during progressive thiamine depletion.

We have tried on numerous occasions to restore transketolase activity of deficient liver or brain by the *in vitro* addition of thiamine alone, ThMP, or ThDP. We have even attempted to preincubate these tissues with thiamine plus ATP but were never able to restore enzymatic activity to normal levels, as we could in either erythrocytes, white cells, or whole blood.

Dr. Brin. There appears to be a very large species difference. In man, where you get improvement of neurological function such as ophthalmoplegia, obviously there is a restoration of enzyme activity. In regard to the erythrocytes in man, just as you described, there are some people who may not be restored for 2 weeks. But those who are thiamine deficient have a ThDP effect, and that ThDP effect is readily measured. In other words, you can saturate the available apoenzyme immediately. In the case of the rat you can sometimes measure a ThDP effect, showing a restoration of activity in the erythrocytes. It turns out that the asay is far better for man than for the rat. In the case of the dog you can restore activity to almost all tissues; this is unpublished information. So there is very great species variability, and one cannot assume that an observation on the ability to restore activity in one species will necessarily apply to another species.

Dr. Kark. Is the problem just technical, or might there be a defect in the synthesis of particular proteins such as apotransketolase?

Dr. Brin. A substrate protection of the apoenzyme may be involved. For instance, in the case of the rat, we administered labeled pyruvate and labeled pentose (this was published in the *Israeli Journal of Medical Sciences* some years age) to the intact animal, studied the rate of release of respiratory CO_2, and correlated that with the ability to restore tissue activity *in vitro*. It correlated very well. There was a lag in the restoration of respiratory CO_2, as there is in the ability to restore activity of the enzymes *in vitro*. This may occur simply because you have to wait until the apoenzyme is resynthesized.

There have been many attempts to use sulfhydryl reagents and all varieties of micronutrients (i.e., minerals, other vitamins, and coenzymes), all without success.

17. Calcium Deficiency as Related to Thiamine-Dependent Neuropathy in Pigeons

YOSHINORI ITOKAWA, M.D.
MOTONORI FUJIWARA, M.D.

Department of Hygiene
Faculty of Medicine
Kyoto University
Kyoto, Japan

Recently, considerable evidence has accumulated to show that thiamine has a function in nervous tissue independent of its coenzyme function. This evidence is summarized as follows.

1. Electrical stimulation of nervous tissue promotes the release of thiamine (1, 2).

2. An antimetabolite of thiamine, pyrithiamine or fern extract, blocks the action potential in the node of Ranvier of a single myelinated nerve fiber (3, 4).

3. When isolated spinal cord and sciatic nerve from frogs and rats previously injected with labeled thiamine are perfused, neuroactive agents, such as tetrodotoxin and lidocaine, cause the release of the labeled thiamine, whereas drugs that do not affect ion movements in the nerve membrane are ineffective (5–7).

4. Drug-inducible release of thiamine can be seen in broken nerve cell preparations, and this is localized in the purified membrane fraction of the cell (8, 9).

5.   The abolished action potential of ultraviolet-irradiated nerve can be restored by the addition of thiamine (10).

6.   When two breeds of pigeons were force-fed a thiamine-deficient diet, one breed developed neurological signs whereas the other did not manifest these symptoms. Nonetheless, there is no significant difference in the level of either brain α-ketoglutarate dehydrogenase or of brain transketolase between the two breeds, and it is postulated that the neurological signs of thiamine deficiency are related to factors other than the decreased activity of the enzyme systems (11).

However, the mechanisms involved in thiamine-related neural disease are still obscure. Therefore we have attempted an experiment using pigeons, as they are one of the species most sensitive to thiamine deficiency.

1.   Materials and Methods

PIGEONS

White pigeons of *Colmba livia domestica* strain weighing about 300 grams were used.

DIETS

Polished rice: Prepared by washing with distilled water several times and drying.
Calcium-mixed polished rice: 10 ml of calcium chloride solution (177 mg $CaCl_2$/ml) was mixed with 1 kg of polished rice.
Commercial pigeon diet: Purchased from Victory Company, Japan.

SUBCELLULAR FRACTIONATION

Pigeons were killed by decapitation, and portions of the telencephalon were removed and homogenized in 0.32 M sucrose. The homogenates were centrifugally separated into nuclei, crude mitochondria, microsomes, and supernatant fractions. The crude mitochondrial fraction was subsequently separated into myelin membrane, synaptosomes, and mitochondrial fractions by sucrose gradient centrifugation, as described by Itokawa and Cooper (8). The purity of the fraction was confirmed by electron microscopy (Fig. 1).

DETERMINATION OF THIAMINE CONCENTRATION

The method of Fujiwara and Matsui (12) was used.

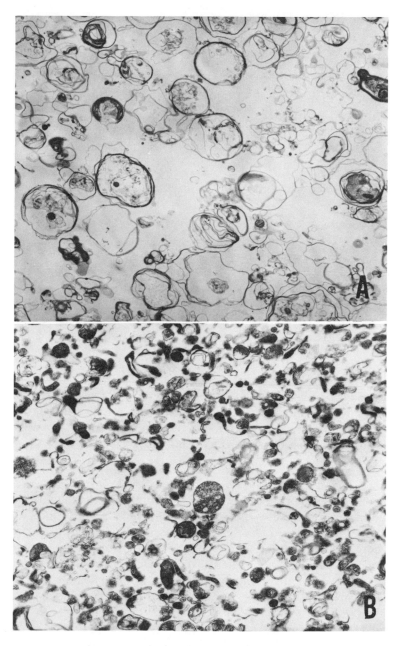

Figure 1. Electron micrographs of pigeon brain subfractions. (*a* Myelin membranes. (*b*) Synaptosomes. (*c*) Mitochondria. Dr. Y. Ago, Kansai Medical School, Japan, kindly performed the electron microscopic examination of the subfractions.

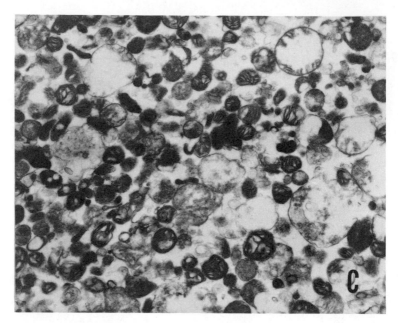

Figure 1. (*Continued*)

DETERMINATION OF CALCIUM

Tissues and subcellular fractions were digested to a nearly colorless solution with nitric acid, and digestion was completed with perchloric acid to yield a colorless solution. The concentration of calcium was then determined, using atomic absorption spectrophotometry (Shimadzu, Japan, Model AA-610).

ASSAY OF RADIOACTIVE THIAMINE

A portion of tissue, or of the subcellular fractions, which contained labeled thiamine was transferred to counting vials, to which 3 ml of NCS solution (Nuclear Chicago) was added. The contents in the vials were incubated at 40°C until the solid matter dissolved. Ten milliliters of toluene containing 8 grams of PPO and 130 mg of dimethyl POPOP per liter were then added. Samples were counted for radioactivity with a liquid scintillation counter (Nuclear Chicago, Mark II).

ASSAYS OF THIAMINE-DEPENDENT ENZYMES

Transketolase activity was assayed according to the method of Brin (13), and the sedoheptulose produced was determined according to Dische (14).

Pyruvate dehydrogenase and α-ketoglutarate dehydrogenase activities were determined by the method of Hayakawa et al. (15).

2. Results and Discussions

When white pigeons were placed on a diet of polished rice for 20 to 25 days, typical opisthotonus was observed. When very small amounts of thiamine were administered to the pigeons, they recovered quite quickly—within 2 hours—and remained in a normal state for about 2 weeks. Fifty percent of the effective dose of thiamine for these convulsive pigeons was 48.3 μg/kg of body weight, according to the method of Litchfield and Wilcoxon (16).

A dose of 50 μg of ^{14}C-thiamine (specific activity 18.9 mCi/mM) was injected intramuscularly into pigeons in convulsive states, and radioactivity was determined in various regions of nervous tissues or in subcellular fractions in the telencephalon before and after recovery from convulsion. Recovered, unrecovered, and commercial diet-fed pigeons were sacrificed 34 minutes after the injection of ^{14}C-thiamine.

The results are shown in Table 1. In the stage immediately after recovery from convulsions, ^{14}C-thiamine incorporation was most evident in the telencephalon, followed by the cerebellum, brain stem, and spinal cord. It was lowest in the sciatic nerve. By contrast, in the stage before recovery from convulsions, the increase of ^{14}C-thiamine in the central nervous system was less significant. In subcellular fractions of the telencephalon, radioactivity was highest in myelin membrane and synaptosomal fractions after recovery from convulsion.

We also tested various drugs other than thiamine for effectiveness in treating the convulsions. Two substances were found to be temporarily effective: diphenyl hydantoin (100 mg/kg, effective rate $\frac{3}{5}$ = 60%), an anticonvulsant agent, and calcium chloride (50 mg/kg, effective rate $\frac{4}{12}$ = 33.3%). However, after 5 to 10 hours, the convulsions recurred. Pincus (17) suggested that diphenyl hydantoin interacts with calcium at the nerve membrane and reduces the permeability of the membrane to calcium. It is feasible that calcium itself plays a role in preventing opisthotonus in pigeons.

Following former research procedures, we utilized polished rice as the thiamine-deficient diet. However, it was found that this diet was also deficient in calcium (thiamine and calcium levels in polished rice are 15 μg and 6.4 mg/100 g, respectively, while these values in commercial pigeon diet are 200 μg and 15.7 mg/100 g). Such being the case, we were interested in the pigeons' reaction to a diet of calcium-supplemented polished rice. The pigeons fed polished rice without the addition of calcium developed

Table 1.   Incorporation of ¹⁴C-Thiamine into Various Regions of Nervous Tissue and Subcellular Fractions of Telencephalon in Pigeons[a]

Region of Nervous Tissue	¹⁴C-Thiamine, μg/100 g		
	Normal Pigeon	Nonrecovered Pigeon	Recovered Pigeon
Telencephalon	6.2 ± 0.4	19.0 ± 2.1*[b]	51.1 ± 4.0*†[b]
Cerebellum	8.2 ± 0.5	22.1 ± 3.4*	45.7 ± 3.9*†
Brain stem	8.3 ± 0.5	24.5 ± 3.4*	42.0 ± 3.1*†
Spinal cord	6.1 ± 0.3	18.2 ± 2.9*	28.2 ± 2.9*
Sciatic nerve	4.8 ± 0.2	15.8 ± 3.0*	17.0 ± 3.0*

Subcellular Fraction of Telencephalon	¹⁴C-Thiamine, μg/100 g		
	Normal Pigeon	Nonrecovered Pigeon	Recovered Pigeon
Nuclei	1.3 ± 0.3	3.2 ± 0.3*	6.2 ± 0.4*†
Mitochondria	1.1 ± 0.3	2.9 ± 0.2*	4.6 ± 0.5*†
Synaptosomes	1.0 ± 0.2	4.9 ± 0.5*	16.9 ± 2.0*†
Myelin membranes	0.7 ± 0.2	1.9 ± 0.2*	11.6 ± 1.1*†
Microsomes	0.4 ± 0.1	0.9 ± 0.2	1.5 ± 0.2*
Supernatant	1.7 ± 0.3	5.2 ± 0.3*	10.3 ± 1.2*†

[a] Values represent mean ± S.E. for five pigeons.
[b] Asterisk indicates significant difference ($p < .05$) when compared to normal pigeon; dagger, significant difference ($p < .05$) when compared to nonrecovered pigeon.

opisthotonus. In contrast, when calcium was added, the pigeons had no convulsions.

Pigeons fed the calcium-mixed, and polished rice diets were sacrificed at the same time, and the thiamine and calcium concentrations in various regions of nervous tissue, as well as in subcellular fractions of the telencephalon, were determined.

Table 2 shows the thiamine levels in these pigeons. Thiamine concentrations in the nervous systems of pigeons fed the commercial diet showed a gradient from central nervous tissue to peripheral nervous tissue. On the thiamine-deficient diets (polished rice or calcium-mixed polished rice), the thiamine concentrations in all regions of nervous tissue were markedly decreased. The decrease of thiamine was more significant in central nervous tissue, such as telencephalon, cerebellum, and brain stem, than in peripheral nervous tissue, such as spinal cord and sciatic nerve. In subcellular fractions of the telencephalon, thiamine was decreased in all fractions in thiamine-deficient pigeons; the decrease was most marked in the myelin membrane and the synaptosomal fractions. When a comparison was made between pigeons fed polished rice and those fed calcium-mixed rice, the thiamine concentration was significantly higher in the telencephalon of calcium-mixed rice-fed pigeons than in that of polished rice-fed pigeons. No significant difference was observed in other nervous tissue. In subcellular fractions of the telencephalon, the thiamine concentrations in myelin membrane and synaptosomal fractions differed most markedly between calcium-mixed rice-fed pigeons and polished rice-fed pigeons.

Table 2. Thiamine Levels in Various Regions of the Nervous System and in Subcellular Fractions of Telencephalon of the Pigeon[a]

Region of Nervous Tissue	Thiamine, μg/100g		
	Commercial Diet-Fed Pigeon	Ca-Enriched Rice-Fed Pigeon	Polished Rice-Fed Pigeon
Telencephalon	256.3 ± 15.0	69.3 ± 5.0*[b]	38.7 ± 2.1*†[b]
Cerebellum	231.0 ± 8.8	81.2 ± 6.8*	64.1 ± 4.7*
Brain stem	222.4 ± 9.4	80.8 ± 5.4*	68.4 ± 2.9*
Spinal cord	169.6 ± 5.7	72.9 ± 7.3*	60.0 ± 2.7*
Sciatic nerve	105.6 ± 6.0	67.7 ± 6.2*	57.2 ± 2.1*

Subcellular Fraction of Telencephalon	Thiamine, μg/100g		
	Commercial Diet-Fed Pigeon	Ca-Enriched Rice-Fed Pigeon	Polished Rice-Fed Pigeon
Nuclei	34.3 ± 4.2	11.8 ± 2.2*	10.0 ± 1.9*
Mitochondria	68.6 ± 5.5	14.1 ± 3.0*	14.6 ± 3.1*
Synaptosomes	42.5 ± 3.0	17.9 ± 2.8*	3.6 ± 1.2*†
Myelin membranes	31.5 ± 3.0	12.6 ± 2.5*	3.0 ± 1.1*†
Microsomes	13.6 ± 1.3	2.6 ± 0.3*	2.6 ± 0.4*
Supernatant	68.1 ± 6.7	10.4 ± 2.5*	5.3 ± 0.8*

[a] Values represent mean ± S.E. for five pigeons.
[b] Asterisk indicates significant difference ($p < .05$) when compared to commercial diet-fed pigeon; dagger, significant difference ($p < .05$) when compared to Ca-enriched rice-fed pigeon.

Table 3. Calcium Levels in Various Regions of the Nervous System and in Subcellular Fractions of Telencephalon of the Pigeon[a]

Region of Nervous Tissue	Calcium, mg/100g		
	Commercial Diet-Fed Pigeon	Ca-Enriched Rice-Fed Pigeon	Polished Rice-Fed Pigeon
Telencephalon	2.68 ± 0.43	1.96 ± 0.47	1.28 ± 0.20*[b]
Cerebellum	3.61 ± 0.22	2.29 ± 0.50	1.99 ± 0.22*
Brain stem	3.64 ± 0.35	3.67 ± 0.63	2.94 ± 0.37
Spinal cord	5.70 ± 0.42	5.09 ± 0.54	5.97 ± 0.64
Sciatic nerve	9.73 ± 1.18	9.43 ± 1.22	9.18 ± 1.56
Subcellular Fraction of Telencephalon	Commercial Diet-Fed Pigeon	Ca-Enriched Rice-Fed Pigeon	Polished Rice-Fed Pigeon
Nuclei	0.46 ± 0.06	0.41 ± 0.06	0.29 ± 0.04
Mitochondria	0.67 ± 0.08	0.44 ± 0.08	0.33 ± 0.07*
Synaptosomes	0.59 ± 0.07	0.32 ± 0.03*	0.19 ± 0.03*†[b]
Myelin membranes	0.45 ± 0.04	0.22 ± 0.05*	0.16 ± 0.04*†
Supernatant	0.26 ± 0.03	0.25 ± 0.05	0.18 ± 0.04

[a] Values represent mean $\pm$ S.E. for five pigeons.
[b] Asterisk indicates significant difference ($p < .05$) when compared to commercial diet-fed pigeon; dagger, significant difference ($p < .05$) when compared to Ca-enriched rice-fed pigeon.

Table 3 shows the calcium levels in various regions of the nervous system and in subcellular fractions of the telencephalon of pigeons. In polished rice-fed pigeons and calcium-mixed rice-fed pigeons the calcium contents decreased significantly in the telencephalon and cerebellum. The calcium levels in telencephalon, cerebellum, and brain stem were slightly higher in calcium-mixed rice-fed pigeons than in polished rice-fed pigeons. In subcellular fractions of the telencephalon, the calcium levels in synaptosomal and myelin membrane fractions were significantly higher in calcium-mixed rice-fed pigeons than they were in polished rice-fed pigeons.

The activities of thiamine-dependent enzymes (i.e., transketolase, pyruvate dehydrogenase, and α-ketoglutarate dehydrogenase) in the brains of these pigeons are shown in Table 4. Enzyme activities in the brains of polished rice-fed pigeons showed only about a 10% decrease as compared to those of commercial diet-fed pigeons; there was no difference in activity between calcium-mixed rice-fed pigeons and polished rice-fed pigeons.

From these findings, it is assumed that the opisthotonus suffered by thiamine-deficient pigeons can be attributed to abnormalities in central nervous tissue rather than in peripheral nervous tissue. Especially, thiamine and calcium deficiency in membrane and synaptosomal fractions seem to be closely correlated with opisthotonus in pigeons. The lesion could be attributed to the deficiency in thiamine, which plays a role in the functioning of the excitable membrane. On the other hand, thiamine in cocarboxylase-dependent enzyme systems has little influence on opisthotonus in pigeons. There is a possibility that calcium plays a role in binding the protein and thiamine which is related to the sodium transport system of excitable membrane.

Table 5 shows the main nutrient intakes of various species per kilogram of body weight. In the rat diet, all nutrients are much higher than in the

Table 4. Activities of Thiamine-Dependent Enzymes in Pigeon Brain[a]

	In vitro Addition		
Enzyme	None (A)	Thiamine Diphosphate (B)	ThDP Effect $(B - A/ A \times 100)$, %
Transketolase, nmoles sedoheptulose-7-phosphate produced/(mg protein)(hr)			
Commercial diet-fed pigeon	217 ± 12	224 ± 15	3.2
Ca-enriched rice-fed pigeon	174 ± 13	198 ± 10	13.7
Polished rice-fed pigeon	189 ± 9	214 ± 12	13.2
Pyruvate dehydrogenase, nmoles pyruvate dehydrogenated/(mg protein)(hr)			
Commercial diet-fed pigeon	358 ± 65	362 ± 68	1.1
Ca-enriched rice-fed pigeon	327 ± 52	338 ± 40	3.4
Polished rice-fed pigeon	320 ± 64	341 ± 50	6.5
α-Ketoglutarate dehydrogenase, nmoles α-KG dehydrogenated/(mg protein)(hr)			
Commercial diet-fed pigeon	294 ± 48	300 ± 40	2.0
Ca-enriched rice-fed pigeon	293 ± 63	322 ± 72	9.9
Polished rice-fed pigeon	280 ± 60	295 ± 51	5.4

[a] Values represent mean ± S.E. for five pigeons.

Table 5. Comparison of Nutrient Intake in Various Species (per kilogram body weight per day)

Nutrient	Human[a]	Pigeon Polished Rice	Pigeon Normal Diet[b]	Rat[c]
Protein, grams	1.3	2.1	3.4	8.0
Fat, grams	0.7	0.3	0.8	1.8
Carbohydrate, grams	6.3	25.5	24.6	17.4
Calcium, mg	8.8	2.0	5.3	326.7
Thiamine, μg	19.5	5.0	66.6	570.8

[a] From the National Nutrition Survey (Japan, 1970).
[b] Commercial pigeon diet (Victory Co., Japan).
[c] Commercial rat diet (Oriental Co., Japan).

human diet. In contrast, the composition of commercial pigeon diet resembles that of human diets, except that it contains more thiamine. Polished rice is deficient in thiamine, calcium, and lipids. When attempting to elucidate differences in neurological manifestations of thiamine deficiency in different species, the fact that there are dietary deficiencies other than an insufficiency of thiamine should not be overlooked.

Figure 2 shows the annual number of deaths from beriberi in Japan. The death rate was very high in the years 1915 to 1930, showing a peak of 46.5 per 100,000 population in 1924. Since rice is cheap and easily obtained in Japan, the older generation eats much rice and tends to avoid other

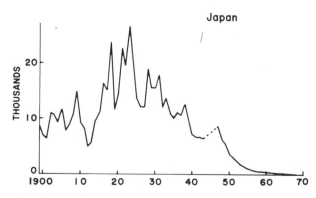

Figure 2.   Annual deaths from beriberi (Japan).

subsidiary foods. A national survey in 1926 revealed that the rice consumption was about 500 grams per person daily. Calcium deficiency coupled with thiamine deficiency probably plays a role in causing beriberi. However, the nutritional status of the Japanese has improved, the intake of calcium and thiamine has increased, and cases of beriberi have been very rare in recent years in Japan.

References

1. H. P. Gurtner, *Helv. Physiol. Pharmacol. Acta,* Suppl. XI, 1 (1961).
2. J. R. Cooper, R. H. Roth, and M. M. Kini, *Nature* (London), **199,** 609 (1963).
3. S. F. Petropulos, *J. Cell. Comp. Physiol.,* **56,** 7 (1960).
4. Von H. A. Kunz, *Helv. Physiol. Acta,* **14,** 411 (1956).
5. Y. Itokawa and J. R. Cooper, *Biochem. Pharmacol.,* **18,** 545 (1968).
6. Y. Itokawa and J. R. Cooper, *Science,* **166,** 759 (1969).
7. Y. Itokawa and J. R. Cooper, *Biochem. Pharmacol.,* **19,** 985 (1970).
8. Y. Itokawa and J. R. Cooper, *Biochim. Biophys. Acta,* **196,** 274 (1970).
9. Y. Itokawa, R. A. Schulz, and J. R. Cooper, *Biochim. Biophys. Acta,* **266,** 293 (1972).
10. J. Eichenbaum and J. R. Cooper, *Brain Res.,* **32,** 258 (1971).
11. H. B. Lofland, H. O. Goodman, T. B. Clarkson, and R. W. Pritchard, *J. Nutr.,* **79,** 188 (1963).
12. M. Fujiwara and K. Matsui, *Anal. Chem.,* **25,** 810 (1953).
13. M. Brin, *J. Nutr.,* **78,** 179 (1962).
14. Z. Dische, *J. Biol. Chem.,* **204,** 983 (1953).
15. T. Hayakawa, M. Hirashima, S. Ide, M. Hamada, K. Okabe, and M. Koike, *J. Biol. Chem.,* **241,** 4694 (1966).
16. J. T. Litchfield, Jr., and F. Wilcoxon, *J. Pharmacol.,* **96,** 99 (1949).
17. J. H. Pincus, *Arch. Neurol.,* **26,** 4 (1972).

DISCUSSION

Chapter 17

Dr. Dreyfus. Thank you very much, Dr. Itokawa, for this most interesting paper. As you know, the early work on thiamine deficiency began with experiments on chickens and pigeons. Since then, experimental deficiency has been produced in a variety of species, including primates. Perhaps, however, the pigeon is the ideal animal to use since thiamine deficiency is so easily and reproducibly achieved. It is particularly interesting that most of the changes seemed to occur in synaptosomes and membranous structures rather than other organelles. I was rather disappointed, however, to note that the brain stem was not the part of the brain which was most involved, particularly since this area of the brain is uniformly involved in the thiamine-deficient pigeon. Histological observations by Alexander, Prickett, and Swank and, more recently, by Terry and others all show spectacular brain-stem lesions in deficient pigeons. These seem to correlate best with the symptoms observed, namely, opisthotonus and the biochemical observations made by Peters and his colleagues. Have you any explanations for this discrepancy?

Dr. Itokawa. Although we did not determine thiamine and calcium levels in membrane and synaptosomal fractions of brain stem, thiamine and calcium levels in the brain stem decreased in convulsing pigeons. This was not the part of brain in which the decrease was greatest, but the functioning of the brain stem may be affected by a decrease in thiamine and calcium. However, I do not know at this moment whether opisthotonus is attributed to abnormalities in the brain stem or in some other part of the brain.

257

Since there is no marked difference in thiamine-dependent enzyme activities between convulsing pigeons and normal pigeons, opisthotonus observed in thiamine-deficient pigeons may not be attributable to a defect in thiamine-dependent enzymes, and I think that the decrease in oxygen uptake in an *in vitro* system is a secondary effect of thiamine deficiency.

Dr. Gubler. I noticed in your illustrations that you observed very little change in the pyruvate dehydrogenase activity in these animals. Is that usual? I thought that back in Peters' day they usually showed a drop.

Dr. Dreyfus. The difference, Dr. Gubler, is that in the early days the methods were different. The methods measured oxygen uptake, and other things besides just one reaction may have been measured.

Dr. Gubler. Yes.

Dr. Blass. Actually, Peters himself has pointed out that those measurements were difficult to reproduce over the years. They were reproducible, but I believe that even in his own laboratory he had to mash brain tissue with a spatula at room temperature (R. A. Peters, in G. W. E. Wolstenholme, Ed., *Thiamine Deficiency,* J. & A. Churchill Ltd., London, 1967).

Dr. Gubler. But at the Ciba Symposium Dr. Peters was going over my old data, and he was surprised that I did not report a decrease in pyruvate dehydrogenase activity. When I went back to the data, I did find a significant decrease that I had not noticed before.

Dr. Collins. In these cases we may be dealing with a biochemical lesion that is responsible for the production of symptoms, but not for the production of the tissue lesion. Might not the enzymatic composition of the tissue be different if tissue damage is present?

Dr. Blass. One very reproducible observation has been the accumulation of lactate in the brain stem of the thiamine-deficient pigeon (R. A. Peters, in G. W. E. Wolstenholme, Ed., *Thiamin Deficiency,* J. & A. Churchill Ltd., London, 1967). That has to be explained. Also, we are talking about morphological changes. Are these closely related? Are the episodes in fact seizures? Where in the brain do they originate?

Dr. Dreyfus. Dr. Itokawa specifically stated that these were not seizures but rather opisthotonus, which is a manifestation of brain-stem dysfunction.

Dr. Kark. Are there electrophysiological data on which part of the nervous system or specific neurons generate the arched posture?

Dr. Dreyfus. I believe that the abnormal postures that have been observed in both thiamine-deficient pigeons and rats are indicative of brain-stem or, more specifically, vestibular dysfunction. There is little to suggest that the animals lose consciousness.

Dr. Gubler. What got me into thiamine research in the beginning was the observation that the symptoms of poisoning from manganese, copper, arsenic, and various other heavy metals resemble in many respects the neurological symptoms of thiamine deficiency. This brings us back to the question, What are these heavy metals affecting? Do they affect what we originally thought was the dehydrogenase, i.e., pyruvate and α-ketoglutarate dehydrogenase, or do they affect something entirely different? They certainly do not bind to the thiamine, thiamine diphosphate, or thiamine triphosphate.

Dr. Dreyfus. Which specific heavy metals are you talking about? Clinically, heavy-metal intoxication in man is really different from thiamine deficiency.

Dr. Gubler. There are many biochemical similarities between them, at least from my reading on arsenic, manganese, and copper.

Dr. Kark. The only definite similarities I happen to be aware of between thiamine deficiency and mercury poisoning are that both cause cerebellar disease in man and that, for both, the group in Oxford under Professor Peters described inhibition of pyruvate oxidase as a possible biochemical lesion (R. A. Peters, *Lancet,* **230,** 1161, 1936; R. H. S. Thompson and V. P. Whittaker, *Biochem. J.,* **41,** 342, 1947). The various mercurials inhibit a number of other biochemical mechanisms (T. W. Clarkson, *Ann. Rev. Pharm.,* **12,** 375, 1972; B. L. Vallee and D. D. Ulmer, *Ann. Rev. Biochem.,* **41,** 91, 1972). One has to ask whether it is possible in principle to define a single biochemical lesion as the sole pathogenic site for an exogenous toxin with widespread effects such as mercury.

Dr. Gubler. It seems to me that what originally led Peters to the idea that pyruvate metabolism was affected was his studies of the arsenical war gases, where the symptoms had such a marked resemblance to those of thiamine deficiency.

Dr. Warnock. What Dr. Gubler is saying about arsenicals was stated by Dr. Peters years ago. He noted that there was a disulfide link somehow in pyruvic oxidation, which Dr. Reed later showed us to be lipoic acid.

18. The Morphology of Myelin Degeneration in Thiamine Deficiency

GEORGE H. COLLINS, M.D.

Department of Pathology
State University of New York
Syracuse, New York

Myelin degeneration has been regarded as one of the characteristic central nervous tissue alterations occurring as a result of thiamine deficiency. Early studies on the central nervous system have, for the most part, demonstrated this change (1–3). On the other hand, studies of peripheral nerve have not been convincing in regard to myelin change (4, 5), and difficulties have been encountered in producing any lesion in the periphery by means of thiamine deprivation. Continuing studies on the central nervous system have consolidated earlier observations to the extent that a reliable and reproducible model involving the lateral pontine tegmentum has been developed, and refinements in the understanding of tissue mechanisms have been introduced. Since continuing investigation of chronic lesions make pathogenetic inferences difficult, acute lesions have been studied recently. The position of myelin degeneration as a primary or secondary tissue change in thiamine deficiency is still uncertain, however, and the sequence of tissue mechanisms responsible for its occurrence remains in doubt.

Abnormalities that may be seen in the lateral vestibular nucleus of chronically depleted animals include not only myelin degeneration but also vesicular changes in the neuronal cell body, membrane and vesicular changes in neuronal processes, vascular and fibrillar changes in glial cells,

261

tissue edema, and pericapillary basement membrane degeneration. Analysis of such a lesion led us to suggest (6) that a primary glial cell abnormality represented the basic changes and that oligodendroglial dysfunction was the cause of myelin degeneration. Since we had previously published some evidence of remyelination in similar lesions (7), it could as easily have been concluded that the myelinating system was intact, requiring only adequate axons to re-establish a myelin sheath. However, since a return of axons would presumably require a replenishment of tissue thiamine, which at the same time could restore the myelinating capability of the oligodendrocyte, the problems in such analysis became apparent. Thus, although studies of chronic nervous system lesion by light and electron microscopy suggest primary glial changes and repeatedly demonstrate myelin degeneration, no definite conclusions can be reached.

More recently, several investigators have studied the electron microscopy of tissue changes in the acutely deprived animal. In these experiments, in contrast to the months of repeated bouts of acute depletion which the chronic experiment requires, the animal is exposed to a thiamine-deficient diet for 25 to 60 days, within which period acute manifestations of thiamine deficiency develop. The results, as reported by Tellez and Terry (8), Robertson et al. (9), and Pena and Felter (10), are in agreement that myelin degeneration does not occur in this early lesion in the lateral vestibular nucleus of the rat and that terminal axonal changes can be seen, as reported earlier by Swank and Prados (11). Pena and Felter (10) found changes only in the presynaptic boutons and axons with no evidence for glial or vascular changes. The findings of Tellez and Terry (8) were similar, but extracellular edema and mild intracellular edema of the oligodendrocytes were also noted. Robertson et al. (9), on the other hand, found an initial swelling of glial cytoplasm, followed later by extracellular edema and fluid accumulation in the myelin sheath. They considered the early defect to be in energy metabolism of the glial cell with resultant abnormalities in fluid and electrolyte transport. Except for this fluid accumulation in the myelin sheath, no myelin abnormalities were reported in these acute studies. Further studies of the acute lesion by Robertson and Manz (12, 13) have clearly shown increased permeability of the vasculature to fluorescein, Evans blue, and horseradish peroxidase.

Peripheral nerve studies have been less productive but lead, nevertheless, to the same conclusions. Our experiments on chronic changes (4) produced alterations similar to those of starvation controls and consisted of membranous changes in the axoplasm with rare myelin breakdown. More recently, Prineas (14) demonstrated in acute deficiency experiments collections of membrane-bound sacs in the axons of interosseous muscles and the fasciculus gracilis. There were no myelin changes and no abnormalities in dorsal root ganglion or anterior horn cells. Thus myelin changes in mammalian peripheral nerve occur rarely, if at all, but axonal changes are seen, particularly in the terminals.

Tissue culture studies by Yonezawa and Iwanami (15) of newborn cerebellum and fetal spinal ganglia of rat and mouse treated with the thiamine antimetabolites, pyrithiamine and oxythiamine, produced some interesting information. In the central nervous system a chronic myelin degeneration occurred without apparent neuronal damage, whereas, acutely, damage of neurons, oligodendroglia, axons, and myelin was shown, with myelin breakdown preceding the axonal degeneration. In the peripheral tissue, chronic and acute changes were similar. Treatment of other cultures with cocarboxylase in addition to the antimetabolites prevented any of these degenerative changes. These studies suggested to the investigators that the acute changes caused by higher levels of antagonists were due to interference with both the tricarboxylic acid cycle and the hexose monophosphate shunt, whereas the chronic changes, which consisted mainly of myelin degeneration, were due only to hexose monophosphate shunt blockage. Although the reason for the discrepancy between these findings and those from *in vivo* studies is not apparent, the variation in technique and the use by Yonezawa and Iwanami of immature tissue may be factors. The latter possibility is supported by their own observation that older cultures were less susceptible.

From these studies it is apparent that myelin degeneration may be a feature of chronic lesions in both central and peripheral nervous tissue *in vivo* and in cultures of newborn and fetal tissue. In the peripheral nerve such changes may or may not be specific, whereas the central changes occur in a lesion of the brain stem that has repeatedly been shown to be thiamine specific. In acute lesions, however, myelin degeneration was essentially absent, not only indicating that myelin is not the earliest tissue element to change but also raising serious questions regarding the mechanism whereby the myelin change occurs in the chronic state.

Our studies on thiamine deficiency have been limited primarily to the chronic lesion, though some acute studies were involved (Table 1). Most of the peripheral nerve studies are unpublished because of negative results. These consisted of dietary restriction of thiamine and the administration of oxythiamine and pyrithiamine during the fetal stage, continued during suckling and in some cases in the weanling and young adult. No central nervous system studies were done on these animals, and peripheral nerve endings were not examined. Chronic central nervous system lesions, in which typical lesions occurred in the rat brain stem (Fig. 1), were studied in collaboration with Dr. Pierre Dreyfus. The histopathology consists of loss of myelin (Fig. 2) and breakdown of most of the tissue elements but with

Table 1. Thiamine Deficiency Study: Methods of Study

	Central Nervous System		Peripheral Nervous System	
	Light Microscopy	Electron Microscopy	Light Microscopy	Electron Microscopy
Dietary restriction (chronic)	67	29	32	12
Administration of pyrithiamine	—	12	—	10
Administration of oxythiamine	—	16	—	12

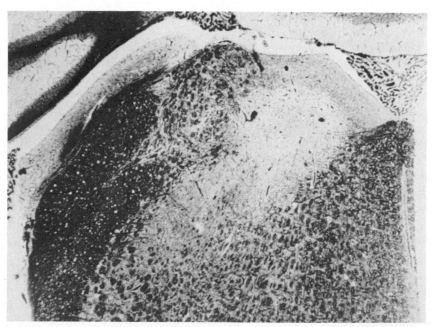

Figure 1. This photomicrograph of the rat brain stem at the upper medulla level contains an area of pallor with prominent blood vessels involving the principal and lateral vestibular nuclei. This is a characteristic appearance of this lesion. (Weigert method for myelin. ×10.)

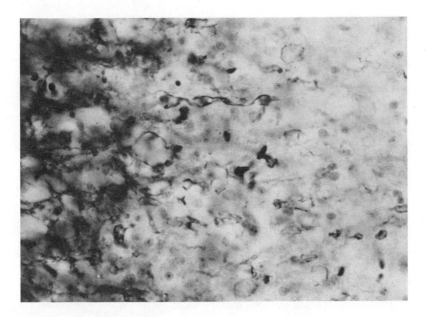

Figure 2. At the edge of a fully developed lesion an abrupt loss of myelin can be demonstrated. (Weigert method for myelin. ×480.)

preservation of the neuronal cell body. The glial cells frequently have enlarged pale nuclei, and with phase microscopy cytoplasmic swelling of these cells can also be seen (Fig. 3). Axonal changes are of two basic types. The first consists of a collection of tubules, vesicles, and other fragments (Fig. 4). The second type consists of simple and complex membranous collections and crystalloid structures with repeating subunits. These were reported by Tellez and Terry (8) but were subsequently shown by Sotelo and Palay (16) to occur also in normal animals and are thought to be characteristic of nonspecific axonal degeneration. The axon may finally become a dense amorphous mass, and it is only in association with these changes that myelin degeneration occurs (Fig. 5).

Any attempt to identify at the present time a meaningful tissue mechanism for myelin breakdown must involve, therefore, the features of the chronic central nervous system lesion. The potential complexity of this analysis becomes apparent when the possible explanations for the observed changes are considered. The data seem to demonstrate that myelin degeneration occurs secondarily to axonal changes. It would appear equally possible, however, that the myelin breakdown may require a combination of axonal and glial defects, that the glial and axonal changes occur

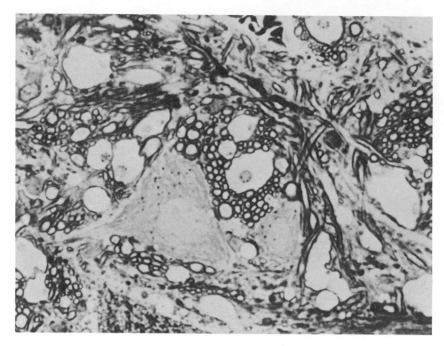

Figure 3. In this phase micrograph of the lateral vestibular nucleus the early change in glial cells is shown. A marked watery swelling of the cytoplasm of these cells is noted, with some nuclear abnormality. Random axons many also be swollen. (Osmium tetroxide. 120×.)

simultaneously in response to a deficiency of thiamine, or that the axonal change occurs secondarily to glial failure, which also causes myelin degeneration. Support for such possibilities from other studies is scanty and comes mainly from peripheral nerve, where such events have been closely examined. It has been shown, for example, in lead neuropathy (17), which causes primarily segmental change, that direct axonal damage seems to occur, suggesting an effect on both Schwann cell and axon. It would seem possible, therefore, that thiamine deficiency could be exerting a simultaneous effect on both of these tissue elements. At the same time, there is apparently no known precedent for the simultaneous occurrence of a defect that acts synergistically to cause myelin breakdown, but neither has such a possibility been ruled out. The final possibility to be considered is axonal change secondary to glial failure. In peripheral nerve studies it has been shown by Singer and Salpeter (18) that labeled histidine is transported through the Schwann cell to the axon, suggesting a metabolic support role for this cell. It has been suggested that in degenerating lesions degeneration of two to three consecutive internodal segments will promote axonal

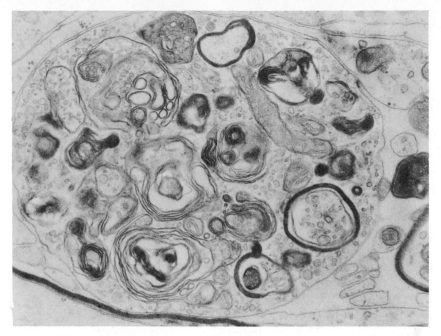

Figure 4. This electron micrograph demonstrates the collection of membranous structures, myelin figures, dark bodies, and other organelles which are frequently seen in the axons within the lesion. (×28,000.)

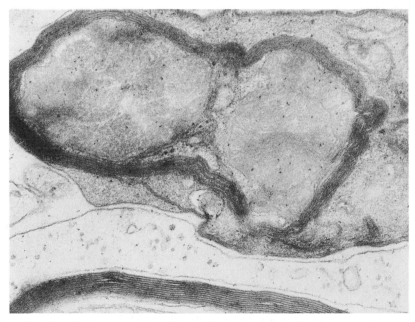

Figure 5. The relative preservation of the myelin sheath associated with an amorphous axonal structure is shown in this electron micrograph. (×35,000.)

267

degeneration, which again points to an essential support role for the Schwann cell. In the central nervous system, demyelinating lesions gradually spare the axon, but this is not absolute. Although the reason for occasional axonal degeneration is not known, it is quite possible that loss of oligodendroglial support may contribute. Within the total context of these studies, however, it seems most reasonable, since further morphologic analysis is not likely to be fruitful, to accept the occurrence of primary axonal change and to leave open the possibility that a superimposed and concurrent oligodendroglial dysfunction may contribute to myelin abnormality.

From the acute lesion we not only learn that myelin degeneration is lacking but also realize that by its absence it cannot be related to the occurrence of the acute symptomatology. It should be noted, nonetheless, that acute biochemical changes which fail to correlate with the symptomatology may still be important in the causation of other tissue changes such as myelin degeneration. This point, which is far from settled, is significant in a consideration of myelin degeneration only insofar as it emphasizes the fact that a potential role exists for any of the known biochemical defects. Unfortunately, the morphologic data do not lend significant support to any of the biochemical mechanisms suggested, since the tissue changes are far from conclusive in regard to the mechanism for myelin degeneration.

References

1. H. R. Street, H. M. Zimmerman, G. R. Cowgill, H. E. Hoff, and J. C. Fox, *Yale J. Biol. Med.,* **13,** 293 (1941).

2. J. F. Rinehart, M. Friedmann, and L. D. Greenberg, *Arch Pathol.,* **48,** 129 (1949).

3. K. V. Juff, L. Z. Saunders, and H. V. Coats, *J. Comp. Pathol.,* **66,** 217 (1956).

4. G. H. Collins, H. deF. Webster, and M. Victor, *Acta Neuropathol.,* **3,** 511 (1964).

5. J. D. K. North and H. M. Sinclair, *Arch. Pathol.,* **62** 341 (1956).

6. G. H. Collins, *Am. J. Pathol.,* **50,** 791 (1967).

7. G. H. Collins, *Am. J. Pathol.,* **48,** 259 (1966).

8. I. Tellez and R. D. Terry, *Am. J. Pathol.,* **52,** 777 (1968).

9. D. M. Robertson, S. M. Wasan, and D. B. Skinner, *Am. J. Pathol.,* **52,** 1081 (1968).

10. C. E. Pena and R. Felter, *Z. Neurol.,* **204,** 263 (1973).

11. R. L. Swank and M. Prados, *Arch. Neurol. Psychiat.,* **47,** 97 (1942).

12. D. M. Robertson and H. J. Manz, *Am. J. Pathol.,* **63,** 393 (1971).

13. H. J. Manz and D. M. Robertson, *Am. J. Pathol.,* **66,** 565 (1972).

14. J. Prineas, *Arch. Neurol., ***23,** 541 (1970).

15. T. Yonezawa and H. Iwanami, *J. Neuropathol. Exp. Neurol., ***25,** 362 (1966).

16. C. Sotelo and S. L. Palay, *Lab. Invest., ***25,** 653 (1971).

17. P. M. Fullerton, *J. Neuropathol. Exp. Neurol., ***25,** 214 (1966).

18. M. Singer and M. M. Salpeter, *J. Morphol., ***120,** 281 (1966).

DISCUSSION

Chapter 18

Dr. Henderson. Would you care to comment on the nuclear changes that you saw and the possible mechanisms of these changes? Is it true that you did not observe any neuronal involvement but just saw changes in glial cells?

Dr. Collins. In this early stage the only abnormality is in the glial nuclei. This type of change is seen in a variety of metabolic encephalopathies, such as those associated with liver disease, hypoglycemia, and, less frequently, anoxia.

Dr. Henderson. It cannot really be related to a specific mechanism?

Dr. Collins. I do not know of any real specific mechanism that has been identified in this abnormality. In liver disease, ammonia intoxication is most frequently considered, but a nuclear mechanism has not been implicated. Dr. Lowell Lapham has made a concerted effort to understand these cells and believes that they represent a reactive change and not a degenerative one. As far as identifying a mechanism is concerned, I am not aware that this has been done.

I have had much less experience with pyrithiamine, but I think that the clinical picture for this antimetabolite differs from that for dietary restriction of thiamine. The tissue lesions seem to be less frequently seen.

Dr. Gubler. I have wondered quite a few times whether the neurological symptoms obtained in thiamine deprivation are the same as those seen with pyrithiamine. I have worked almost entirely with rats, and I have seldom seen a neurological symptom in deficient rats. They occasionally show ataxia and some other mild signs, but normally under our conditions we do not see neurological symptoms. I depend mostly on pyrithiamine for studying the neurological symptoms. Do both of these show basically the same type of neurological symptomatology?

Dr. Dreyfus. The composition of the diet used to produce the thiamine-deficient state is extremely important in terms of the production of neurological manifestations. Autoclaved yeast diets, used many years ago, were unsatisfactory since they were deficient in other essential vitamins besides thiamine. Synthetic diets, in which the composition can be carefully controlled, have proved to be very satisfactory. Some years ago we noted that the advent of neurological manifestations was dependent on the carbohydrate and thiamine content of the diet. A high carbohydrate concentration tended to hasten the onset of clinical symptoms and death. The clinical manifestations seemed to be telescoped to the point where no neurological abnormalities could be observed before demise. When the carbohydrate content was decreased and a small amount of thiamine was added, the animals began to show severe neurological symptoms only after 3 to 5 weeks. A total absence of thiamine in the diet on the other hand, seemed to lead to a rapid demise. I believe that Dr. Collins has had ample opportunities to observe the classical neurological manifestations of thiamine deficiency in rats. Am I correct?

Dr. Collins. Yes. If I understand Dr. Gubler's question, I think that pyrithiamine produces classical neurological signs less frequently and the tissue lesions seem to occur with even more rarity in comparison to dietary thiamine deficiency.

Dr. Gubler. I am wondering whether that is true. It seems as though it would be better to use pyrithiamine. An acute state of deficiency would ensue, neurological symptoms might occur rapidly, and the animals might die before they lost much weight. Inanition would thus be eliminated.

19. Reversible Impairment of Cerebral DNA Synthesis in Diet-Induced Thiamine Deficiency*

G. I. HENDERSON, Ph.D.
S. SCHENKER, M.D.

Departments of Pharmacology and Medicine (Gastroenterology)
Vanderbilt University School of Medicine
and Veterans Administration Hospital
Nashville, Tennessee

Thiamine deficiency is a common finding in chronic alcoholics. Severe depletion of this vitamin may lead to central nervous system abnormalities (Wernicke's or Korsakoff's encephalopathy), peripheral neuropathy, and beriberi heart disease. The cause of the neurologic dysfunction associated with major thiamine deficiency is, as yet, unknown. Current theories concerning the neurologic dysfunction have invoked a neurophysiologic or a metabolic disorder. This report presents a new metabolic abnormality in thiamine-deficient brain.

Figure 1 shows schematically the known sites of impaired enzyme activity induced by severe thiamine deficiency in various organs, including the brain. Thiamine in its diphosphate form is a known cofactor of three enzymes involved in carbohydrate metabolism. These three enzymes (transketolase, pyruvate decarboxylase, and α-ketoglutarate dehydrogenase) and their respective locations in the metabolic pathways are shown in Fig. 1. As indicated by the bar at the top of the figure, thiamine deficiency inhibits the activity of transketolase (1), which is an important step in the pentose

* These studies are being reported in detail in *The Journal of Laboratory and Clinical Medicine* (**86:** 77, 1975).

273

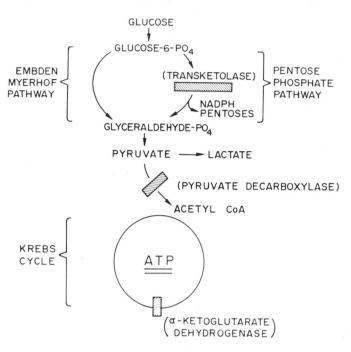

Figure 1. Schematic representation of the biochemical sites at which thiamine diphosphate acts as a coenzyme. These sites are indicated by the hatched bars. Some key products of the metabolic pathways are indicated adjacent to their origin.

phosphate pathway. This pathway is primarily responsible for the synthesis of NADPH and pentoses. As shown by the bottom two bars, thiamine deficiency also impairs pyruvate decarboxylase and, to a lesser extent, α-ketoglutarate dehydrogenase (1, 2). These enzymes in turn are relevant to the operation of the Krebs cycle, a major source of energy in the form of ATP. Prior studies have shown that cerebral regional net ATP levels remain normal in thiamine deficiency (1, 3), but ATP turnover and its subcellular pools in the brain have not been investigated. The effects of cerebral transketolase depression in thiamine deficiency on the synthesis of NADPH or pentoses or, for that matter, on the overall pentose cycle activity have also not been studied. Since ATP, pentoses, and possibly NADPH are required for nucleotide synthesis, the effect of severe thiamine deficiency on brain DNA synthesis was investigated, and the results are the basis of this report.

The animal model used in this study consisted of sets of three littermates—one fed a thiamine-deficient diet, one pair-fed a thiamine-complete diet, and a third reserved as an *ad libitum* control on a thiamine-

Figure 2. Schematic representation of brain areas obtained for analysis. The numbers denote the anatomic areas analyzed: (1) cerebral cortex, (2) brain stem, (3) cerebellum, and (4) residual subcortical white matter (see experimental procedure). The location of the cannula in the lateral brain ventricle is indicated. (Reproduced with permission—J. Lab. Clin. Med. 86: 77, 1975)

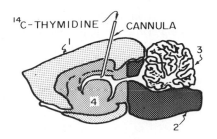

complete diet. The study was begun when the rats were 30 days old (about 70 grams in weight). Approximately 3 days before sacrifice, a polyethylene cannula was inserted into the left lateral brain ventricle. When the animals were ready to be sacrificed, 10 μl of ^{14}C-thymidine was injected into the lateral ventricle of the brain.

The rats were sacrificed by decapitation, and the brains were dissected into four areas as shown in Fig. 2. The four areas are cortex (1), brain stem (2), cerebellum (3), and subcortex (4).

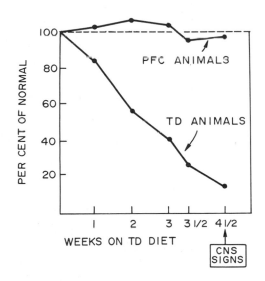

Figure 3. Brain thiamine levels in progressive thiamine deficiency. Total brain thiamine was determined at weekly intervals (horizontal axis) in seven sets of thiamine-deprived rats and their pair-fed controls. Overt neurological signs were apparent by 4½ weeks on the diet, as indicated by the arrow. Brain thiamine levels are expressed as percentages of those for seven normal controls fed *ad libitum* (vertical axis). These levels were 3.72 ± 0.08 μg/g tissue. Statistical significance was determined by the paired t test. Values at 2, 3, and 3.5 weeks and during the symptomatic stage were significantly depressed ($p < .001$). Pair-fed control brain thiamine levels remained normal ($p > 0.05$) throughout the study. (Modified with permission, J. Clin. Invest. 47: 2268, 1968

To extract DNA, five sets of brains were pooled for each animal group per experiment. The brains were extracted in cold perchloric acid and washed in cold ethanol and ether-ethanol, the RNA was removed by treatment with NaOH, and the DNA was solubilized in hydrochloric acid at 70°C. The DNA was assayed by the Burton modification of the diphenylamine method, the RNA by the orcinol reaction, and protein by the Lowry technique. The DNA assay gave recoveries of close to 100%, and the recovered DNA (labeled and unlabeled) was fully hydrolyzed by DNAase. The ^{14}C-thymidine incorporation into DNA is expressed as disintegrations per minute per microgram DNA.

Figure 3 shows the effect of progressive dietary thiamine deficiency on brain thiamine levels. Controls fed *ad libitum* had brain thiamine levels of 3.7 μg/g tissue. As indicated by this figure, pair-fed controls had normal brain thiamine levels. However, with progressive thiamine deprivation the brain thiamine levels fell dramatically in the thiamine-deficient rats. At $4\frac{1}{2}$

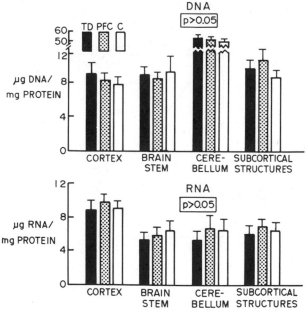

Figure 4. Cerebral regional DNA and RNA concentrations in thiamine deficiency. The studies in thiamine-deficient rats were carried out at the time of development of neurologic signs. Controls were sacrificed at comparable times. Abbreviations: TD, thiamine-deficient rats; PFC, pair-fed controls; C, control rats fed *ad libitum*. Each bar refers to the mean ± S.E. of 70 rats. The DNA and RNA concentrations in each brain area of thiamine-deficient rats were comparable ($p > .05$) to the appropriate control values. (Reproduced with permission, J. Lab. Clin. Med. 86: 77, 1975)

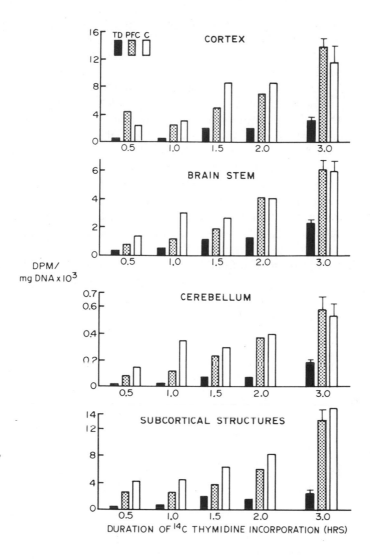

Figure 5. Regional cerebral DNA synthesis in severe thiamine deficiency. For each brain area, the incorporation of ^{14}C-thymidine into DNA on the vertical axis is plotted versus time after injection of the thymidine. Abbreviations: TD, thiamine-deficient rats sacrificed at the onset of overt neurologic signs; PFC, pair-fed controls; C, controls fed *ad libitum* and sacrificed at a comparable time. Each bar at all time intervals (except 3 hours) represents a single assay of five pooled brains. The 3-hour bars refer to the mean ± S.E. of four sets of five pooled brains each. There was a major decrease in DNA labeling in each brain area of TD rats, as compared to either control group ($p < .05$). DNA labeling in both control groups was comparable in each brain area ($p > .05$). (Reproduced with permission, J. Lab. Clin. Med. 86: 77, 1975)

weeks of thiamine deprivation, the brain thiamine level was reduced to 17% of control values, at which time neurologic signs developed.

Net levels of regional brain DNA and RNA were unaffected by thiamine deficiency, as shown in Fig. 4.

Figure 5 illustrates the effect of severe thiamine deficiency (occurrence of overt neurologic signs) on the incorporation of ^{14}C-thymidine (^{14}CdT) into cerebral DNA. The data are shown as a function of time between injection of thymidine and sacrifice of the animals for DNA analysis. These data clearly show a decrease in labeling of extracted DNA in all of the four brain areas studied. A statistical difference was confirmed both by regression analysis of the experimental and control slopes for the whole time curve and by comparison of the data at 3 hours alone. At 3 hours the thymidine incorporation in the thiamine-deficient rats was only 22, 37, 31, and 19% of the pair-fed control (PFC) values in cortex, brain stem, cerebellum, and subcortical structures, respectively.

The effect of progressive thiamine deficiency on cerebral DNA synthesis is shown in Fig. 6. It is evident that the degree of depression of ^{14}CdT

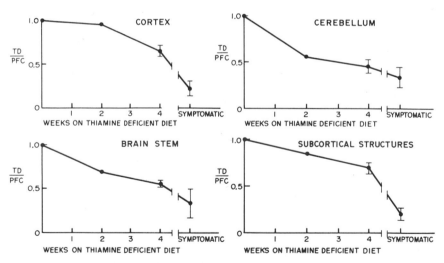

Figure 6. The effect of progressive thiamine deficiency on regional cerebral DNA synthesis. The DNA labeling is plotted on the vertical axis as a ratio of thiamine-deficient (TD)/pair-fed control (PFC) rats. The duration of thiamine-free dietary intake is plotted along the horizontal axis. The 2-week data consist of one set of five pooled brains, the 4-week data of three sets each of five pooled brains, and the symptomatic data of four sets of five pooled brains. Where appropriate, the data are given as mean ± S.E. All data were obtained 3 hours after thymidine injection. Statistics are given in the text. (Reproduced with permission, J. Lab. Clin. Med. 86: 77, 1975)

incorporation into cerebral DNA is related to the progressive depletion of brain thiamine. Some evidence of reduced DNA labeling was apparent after 2 weeks on the thiamine-deficient diet, and by 4 weeks labeling had declined to 65, 54, 46, and 68% of PFC values in cortex, brain stem, cerebellum, and subcortical structures, respectively. Thiamine-deficient (TD) brain thiamine levels at 4 weeks were 25% of PFC values (1).

As previously mentioned, overt neurologic signs were completely reversed within 6 hours of a single IP injection of 500 μg thiamine. Figure 7 illustrates DNA labeling patterns at various time intervals after thiamine supplementation. The depression in DNA labeling was partially reversed within 6 hours, and by 24 hours DNA synthesis was normal in all brain areas except the cerebellum, which required 48 hours for normal labeling. Within 72 hours of thiamine supplementation, DNA synthesis rates were completely reversed and were, in fact, 124, 236, 270, and 155% of PFC values in cortex, brain stem, cerebellum, and subcortical structures, respectively.

In summary, (a) severe diet-induced thiamine deficiency caused a major decrease in ^{14}C-thymidine incorporation into brain DNA, while total net DNA levels remain normal; (b) this effect was seen in all brain areas studied; and (c) the effect is rapidly reversible with thiamine administration. There are several variables other than DNA synthesis that could yield false results in these experiments. First, thiamine deficiency could cause an increase in endogenous thymidine levels which would dilute the added isotope, resulting in a decrease in ^{14}C incorporation into DNA without a depressed DNA synthesis. Current studies in this laboratory have shown, however, that endogenous free and combined phosphorylated thymidine pools are normal in the whole brain of TD rats. Second, added thymidine may not enter cerebral tissues in TD rats with the same efficiency as in controls. This possibility has likewise been eliminated since the uptake of ^{14}CdT from the ventricle is comparable in TD and control rat brain. Third, a concurrent hypothermia is found in TD rats; thus the apparent reduced DNA synthesis could be caused by a nonspecific hypothermic effect and not directly by a lack of thiamine. This factor has also been eliminated by current experiments in which TD rats warmed to normal body temperatures still exhibited a profound depression in ^{14}CdT incorporation into cerebral DNA. It thus appears that the presence of thiamine is, in some as yet unknown manner, necessary for normal cerebral DNA synthesis. The mechanism of the above disorder and the DNA species involved are the objects of future investigations.

Several mechanisms for impaired brain DNA synthesis in thiamine deficiency are possible. First, we have not excluded fully the possibility that some cellular or subcellular precursor pool of thymidine or its

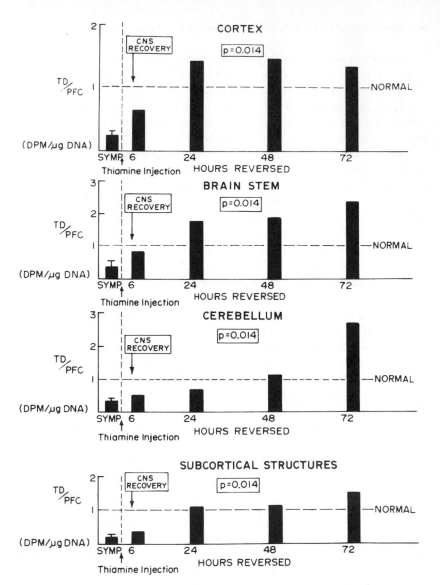

Figure 7. The effect of reversal of neurologic signs of thiamine deficiency with parenteral thiamine on regional cerebral DNA synthesis. The data are plotted on the vertical axis as a ratio of DNA labeling in thiamine-deficient (TD)/pair-fed control (PFC) rats. The term "symp" refers to overtly thiamine-deficient symptomatic rats with neurologic signs studied 3 hours after thymidine injection (see Fig. 5). Thiamine injection consisted of an intraperitoneal dose of 500 μg thiamine hydrochloride, which was repeated at 24-hour intervals (not shown). "CNS recovery" refers to major resolution of neurologic signs. Each bar following the first thiamine injection refers to one set of five pooled brains (and matched pair-fed tissue). Analysis of the combined data over 72 hours for each brain area revealed a significant increase of DNA labeling after thiamine administration as compared to the symptomatic rats ($p = .014$). (Reproduced with permission, J. Lab. Clin. Med. 86: 77, 1975).

phosphorylated derivative may be increased in the brain of TD rats, resulting in a dilution of the labeled thymidine administered. Second, although absorption of the labeled thymidine from the ventricles of TD rats was normal, we cannot rule out the possibility of binding of the administered thymidine to some component of the TD brain, thus making the labeled precursor less available to the DNA-synthesizing machinery. Third, we have considered the possibility that decreased food intake or zinc deficiency may have caused the decreased DNA labeling in the TD rats; fasting and zinc deficiency are known to depress DNA synthesis. These possibilities are unlikely since (*a*) the PFC rats failed to exhibit a significant depression of brain DNA labeling, (*b*) increased food intake in PFC rats, after reversal of thiamine deficiency, over 24 hours did not increase their brain DNA labeling, (*c*) TD rats exhibited an increase in brain DNA synthesis within 6 hours of thiamine administration, and (*d*) brain zinc levels in all animal groups were comparable. We cannot rule out, however, the possibility that decreased food assimilation or utilization in the TD rats could have contributed, at least in part, to impaired DNA synthesis. Further studies in this area are needed. Finally, it is known that glucocorticoids may depress tissue DNA synthesis (4), and there are data which suggest that corticosteroid levels in various experimental thiamine deficiency states may be increased (5). Further investigations in this area may lead to a better understanding of our observations.

Acknowledgment

These studies were supported by grant 5R01AA00267-04 from the National Institutes of Health and Veterans Administration research funds.

References

1. D. W. McCandless and S. Schenker, *J. Clin. Invest.*, **47**, 2268 (1968).
2. P. M. Dreyfus and G. Hauser, *Biochim. Biophys. Acta*, **104**, 78 (1965).
3. J. Holawach, F. Kauffman, M. G. Ikasse, et al., *J. Neurochem.*, **15**, 621 (1968).
4. R. Balazs and M. Cotterrell, *Nature*, **236**, 348 (1972).
5. R. A. Bitter, C. J. Gubler, and R. W. Heninger, *J. Nutr.*, **98**, 147 (1969).

20. The Nonmetabolic Role of Thiamine in Excitable Membrane Function

ROBERT L. BARCHI, M.D., Ph.D.

Departments of Neurology and Biochemistry
University of Pennsylvania School of Medicine
Philadelphia, Pennsylvania

Thiamine deficiency syndromes affecting the nervous system form a major part of the neurologic complications associated with alcoholism and nutritional deprivation in the adult, and are entities frequently seen in the receiving ward of any major urban medical center. In spite of the ubiquity of these disorders, however, the nature of the relationship between excitable membrane function and thiamine remains a perplexing mystery.

Considerable effort has been directed at uncovering a possible causal relationship between deficits in the thiamine diphosphate-dependent enzymes of intermediary metabolism and the pathophysiology of these thiamine-deficient states. To date, however, such studies have been unrewarding. Early reports indicated that thiamine-requiring enzymes were progressively reduced in specific activity in many peripheral tissues under conditions of thiamine deprivation. Indeed, the erythrocyte transketolase stimulation index developed as a result of these observations remains one of the most sensitive indicators of early thiamine deficiency. Measurements of pyruvate and α-ketoglutarate dehydrogenase activities in brain, however, indicate that these enzymes maintain full activity well past the time at which neurologic symptoms become apparent (1). Levels of transketolase have been noted to fall earlier in the course of thiamine depletion, but there is no selective decline in the areas found to be pathologically affected at autopsy, and even after severe depletion levels 60% of control are usually maintained (2). In light of these and other data, it appears unlikely that neurological defects seen in thiamine deficiency are due directly to alterations in the known thiamine-requiring enzymes of intermediary metabolism, and many workers have suggested the existence of a special role for thiamine in the function of excitable membranes.

The suggestion that thiamine compounds play a part in excitable membrane function independent of their well-recognized role as coenzymes in intermediary metabolism is not a new one. As early as 1941, Von Muralt had postulated such a function on the basis of his observation that thiamine was released from nerves when they were stimulated electrically (3). It was later observed that ultraviolet light of the wavelengths specifically absorbed by thiamine was capable of inactivating nerve fibers, and this was taken as further circumstantial evidence for the direct involvement of thiamine in the generation of the action potential. At about the same time evidence was obtained indicating that thiamine compounds were released into the heart during vagal stimulation in a manner analogous to acetylcholine (Ach) (4).

Further pharmacologic evidence bearing on the involvement of thiamine compounds has been provided by the recent work of Itokawa and Cooper. These authors labeled the thiamine pools of frogs and rat by the repetitive administration of ^{35}S-thiamine and subsequently isolated and perfused preparations of spinal cord and sciatic nerve in such a way that the effluent could be monitored for the presence of trace amounts of thiamine compounds (5). It was demonstrated that the exposure of these preparations to physiologic concentrations of neuroactive agents (Ach 10^{-6} M, tetrodotoxin 3×10^{-8} M, ouabain 10^{-6} M, LSD 1.5×10^{-7} M) produced dose-related release of thiamine compounds. Thiamine and its three phosphate esters were characterized both in the neural tissue before stimulation and in the perfusate after stimulation. The released material appeared to be in the form of thiamine and thiamine monophosphate (ThMP), while 80% of the material originally present in the nerve was in the form of thiamine diphosphate (ThDP) and thiamine triphosphate (ThTP).

Itokawa and Cooper also demonstrated a similar release of thiamine compounds by neuroactive agents from the subcellular membrane isolated from previously labeled neuronal tissue (6). Furthermore, this release was seen predominantly in the membrane fractions believed to contain axonal membranes, while no release was observed in those containing predominantly mitochondria, although a major proportion of the total thiamine was found there. The composition of the subcellular fractions was confirmed by electron microscopy. Analysis of the thiamine phosphate compounds present in the various subcellular fractions revealed a significantly higher percentage of ThTP in the neural membrane fractions than in the mitochondrial fraction. After treatment with neuroactive agents, the ThTP levels fell to 30% of the control values, while the released compounds identified in the perfusion medium were again predominantly thiamine and ThMP, with no ThTP detectable.

1. Thiamine Triphosphate

Investigation of subacute necrotizing encephalomyelopathy, a rare, fatal disease of infancy that pathologically resembles the thiamine-deficiency state, has raised the possibility that the form of thiamine specifically involved in nerve membrane function is not cocarboxylase (ThDP) but rather ThTP. Biochemical studies have shown that the brains of infants affected by this hereditary disease contain normal concentrations of thiamine, ThMP, and ThDP. Thiamine triphosphate, which usually comprises 5 to 9% of the total central nervous system thiamine pool, is either completely absent or is present in levels below the limits of detection by the usual analytical techniques (7).

Fox and Duppel have recently reported an important observation of the effects of thiamine phosphate compounds on the slow decline of ionic currents normally observed with time in the single-node preparation from *Xenopus laevis* (8). These authors had previously described a consistent exponential decline with time in the peak sodium and potassium currents from a single node under voltage clamp conditions, a phenomenon usually referred to as "run-down." The rate of decline varies from preparation to preparation, but is always present; the absolute rate appears to be strongly dependent on the ambient temperature. A Q_{10} of approximately 3.0 is observed, suggesting the involvement of a chemical reaction in the decay process. The process also appears to depend on the potential at which the nodal membrane is held during voltage clamp; hyperpolarizing voltages reduce the decay rate, whereas depolarizing voltages enhance it. These authors concluded from these and other data that the exponential decay represented a progressive decrease in the effective electrical field across the excitable membrane. Since the total transmembrane potential was held constant by the voltage clamp system, such a reduction in field felt by the membrane would imply a change in the fixed surface charges of the membrane.

In experiments directed at controlling the rate of exponential decay, Fox and Duppel found that thiamine compounds applied to the inner surface of the membrane by diffusion from the cut ends of the axon produced significant effects. After an initial control period of sufficient duration to allow the projection of the expected exponential decay rate for the peak sodium and potassium current in a given fiber, thiamine, ThMP, ThDP, or ThTP was allowed to diffuse through the axoplasm to the inner surface of the nodal membrane. Thiamine significantly reduced the rate at which this decline progressed after a delay period of 5 to 10 minutes. Application of ThDP resulted in more pronounced reductions in decay rate with shorter lag periods. Thiamine triphosphate was able to eliminate completely the decay in ionic currents with a minimal lag period between application and onset of action. When applied to the outside of the single node, ThDP and ThTP, compounds considered by most authors to be impermeable to the intact membrane, had no effect on the exponential decline in membrane ionic currents. The magnitudes of these effects are shown by calculating the ratio of the time constant for exponential decay during the control periods to that determined after exposure to the thiamine compound; thiamine produced a ratio of 3.16 ± 0.86, ThDP a ratio of 6.0 ± 0.64, and ThTP a ratio of 12.2 ± 5.9 in a limited number of experiments.

Fox and Duppel briefly suggest that the beneficial effects of thiamine phosphate compounds seen in their experiments may relate to an involvement of these compounds in the maintenance of fixed negative charges on the membrane inner surface and hence to a preservation of the effective field across the excitable membrane. This possible function of ThTP will be discussed more fully in a later section of this chapter.

2. Thiamine Analogs

During the 1950s a number of analogs of thiamine were developed which proved unable to function as effective catalysts in thiamine-requiring enzymatic reactions in spite of close structural relationships to their parent compound. Some of these analogs were subsequently shown in animal studies to produce the clinical symptoms of thiamine deficiency in the nervous system even in the presence of daily quantities of thiamine known to be sufficient for the maintenance of normal function in otherwise healthy animals. The specific effects of two of these compounds on the excitable membrane of the isolated single node of Ranvier were studied by Kunz in 1956 (9). Pyrithiamine (PTh), a thiamine analog in which the thiazole ring is replaced by a pyridine ring, was shown to inhibit the action potential at concentrations in the range of 2 to 5×10^{-3} M. This effect was characterized by a dramatic drop in the maximum rate of rise of the action potential, coupled with a 300 to 400% prolongation of the mean depolarization time. These effects were maximal within 15 minutes of the addition of the PTh to the solution bathing the external surface of a single node. Analysis of differentiated action potentials at various levels of membrane depolarization was interpreted as indicating a reduction of available sodium influx channels in the presence of PTh. Oxythiamine (OTh), a thiamine analog previously shown in chronic animal experiments to produce the systemic effects of thiamine deficiency but not the neurologic symptoms, had no effect on the action potential of the same preparation.

The actions of PTh and OTh have been further investigated by Armett and Cooper in the rabbit vagus nerve, a preparation containing mostly unmyelinated fibers. These authors observed a persistent increase in the amplitude and the integrated area of the compound action potential recorded from this nerve after exposure to PTh in concentrations of 1 to 5×10^{-3} M (10). Oxythiamine in similar concentrations produced no effect. Parallel biochemical experiments showed that after incubation of the vagus nerve under physiologic conditions with these analogs all measurable OTh was found in the soluble tissue fraction, while more than 25% of the PTh was associated with the membrane fractions. Cooper later demonstrated a release of thiamine from the vagus nerve during incubation with PTh but not OTh, suggesting that the observed effects of the former were due to the displacement of active thiamine from a functional site within the membrane.

3. Current and Voltage Clamp Studies of Thiamine Analogs in the Single Node of Ranvier

We have extended the studies of Kunz, Armett and Cooper, and others by examining the effects of a number of thiamine analogs on the single node of Ranvier under current clamp and voltage clamp conditions. Single nodes were exposed cyclically to various concentrations of PTh and four other thiamine analogs by a continuous superfusion technique. The nodes were maintained under voltage clamp conditions, using a chamber similar to that described by Nonner in conjunction with solid-state feedback amplifiers for current control and voltage control (11).

Each of the thiamine analogs used contain alterations in the thiazole ring that affect the ability of the C_2 carbon to form a carbanion, thus interfering with the accepted coenzymatic function of thiamine. In addition, some analogs have substitutions that affect the size or relative lipid solubility of the molecule (Fig. 1).

All of the analogs that we have studied produced qualitatively similar effects on the action potential of the single node; however, there were variations between analogs in regard to (a) the minimum concentration required to produce a specific effect, (b) the temporal characteristics of the development of these effects, and (c) the extent and time course of the recovery of the node from these effects. In view of the qualitative similarity

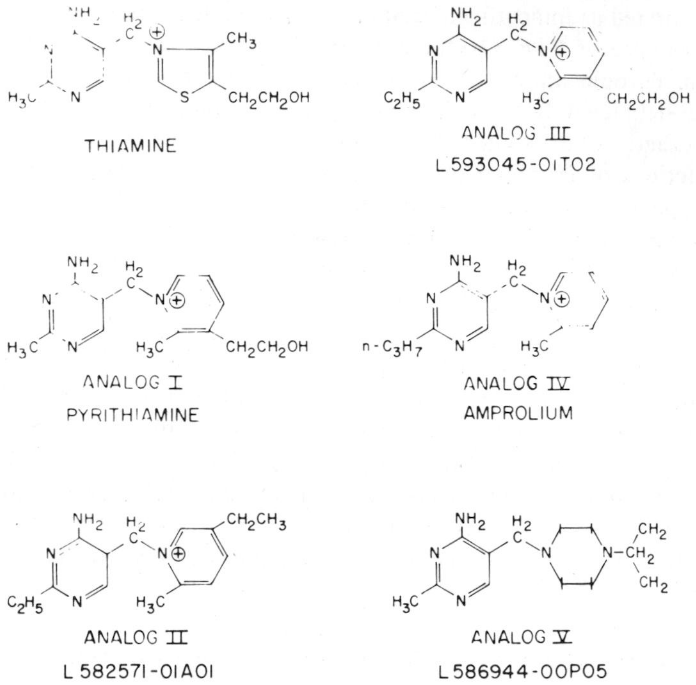

Figure 1. Structural diagrams of thiamine analogs used in current clamp and voltage clamp studies.

in the actions of these analogs, the main characteristics of their effects on the single node will be described in detail for PTh. The quantitative aspects of this response will then be considered for each of the analogs tested.

CURRENT CLAMP

When the single node of Ranvier is exposed to concentrations of PTh between 2 and 5 mM at pH 7.4, the initial effect observed is a slight increase in the minimal stimulus current necessary to produce an action potential. The action potentials recorded from the node then undergo a progessive and characteristic widening as exposure time increases. A prominent depolarizing after-potential concurrently develops. The time necessary for the maximal development of these effects varies directly with the analog concentrations but is relatively constant from experiment to experiment for a given concentration. In the presence of 3 mM PTh, the effects reach a maximum after 20 to 30 minutes of exposure.

Changing the superfusion medium back to control Ringer's solution results in a progessive reversal of this sequence of events; after exposure of a single node to 3 mM PTh, the action potential gradually returns to within a few percent of its initial state after 20 to 30 minutes of washout with normal Ringer's solution. Cyclic exposure and washout periods can be repeated 2 or 3 times on a given nodal preparation before other factors make termination of the experiment necessary. The pattern of progressive development and regression of variations in the action potential is essentially unchanged from cycle to cycle.

With our preparation, the fully developed PTh effect is characterized by an action potential with a stimulus threshold about 25% above control values, a peak amplitude 5 to 10 mV below control level, and a mean depolarization time of 2.0 to 2.5 msec, as opposed to 0.7 to 1.0 msec during control periods. The prolonged action potential has a depolarizing phase with a decreased maximal rate of rise (700 V·sec as opposed to 1200 V·sec for control action potentials). Repolarization is characterized by a slowly falling phase lasting about 60% of the total depolarization time, followed by a short, rapid drop ending in a long depolarizing after-potential. This after-potential usually continues for an additional 2 to 4 msec.

Representative action potentials recorded during control periods, during exposure to an analog after maximal effects have developed, and after various periods of washout for each of the analogs reported are shown in Fig. 2. The qualitative similarity of the actions of these analogs is immediately apparent. Two points should be emphasized. First, with the pyridine analogs (analogs I to IV) reported here, the peak height of the action potential fell only 5 to 10 mV during the exposure period, even in the presence of a 200 to 300% increase in the mean depolarization time. Nodes exposed to high levels of analog V, however, routinely generated action potentials with peak heights 15 to 20 mV below control levels when maximal effects developed. Second, the effects of all these analogs on the single node were completely reversible by returning the node for varying periods to normal Ringer's solution.

Exposure of single nodes to thiamine or thiamine diphosphate in concentrations as high as 15 mM had no effect on the threshold, the waveform of the action potentials, or the duration of depolarization.

To characterize the time course for development and reversal of the effects produced by thiamine analogs, an arbitrary parameter was abstracted from sequences of action potentials recorded during exposure and washout cycles. This parameter, the time from depolarization to -10 mV during the rising phase to repolarization to -10 mV during the falling phase of the action potential, was determined as a relative measure of the depolarization time. During exposure to a constant concentration of each of

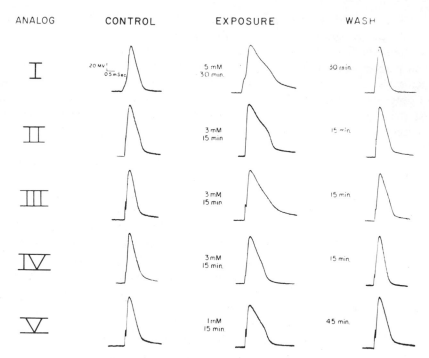

Figure 2. Representative action potentials from single nodes of Ranvier, recorded before and during exposure to various thiamine analogs, and after washout with control Ringer's solution. The qualitative similarity of the effects of each analog is apparent.

the analogs tested, the mean depolarization time described an exponential increase with time after an initial lag period of variable duration. During washout this parameter reverted to its control level, again following an approximately exponential time course; in the washout phase, however, no lag period was observed. In general, exposing a node to increasing concentrations of a given analog in subsequent cycles resulted in shortening the observed lag period and reducing the half-time of the exponential increase in the mean depolarization time. The kinetics of the washout period for a particular analog varied only slightly with increase in concentration during exposure.

Representative plots of mean depolarization time of the action potential versus duration of exposure and washout for each of the analogs are given in Fig. 3. The half-times for the development of effects were nearly equal to the corresponding washout times for pyrithiamine and for analogs I through IV. Analog V was remarkable in that it produced the fastest onset of effects on the single node and also had the slowest washout time course. Often nodes exposed to this analog required more than 1 hour of washing before their action potentials returned to control levels. In all cases when the nerve was not otherwise damaged, however, the effects of each of the analogs could be reversed with sufficient washout periods.

The effects of PTh on the refractory period of the single node were also studied. In four fibers exposed to 3 to 5 mM PTh, absolute and relative refractory periods were determined. The average control absolute refractory

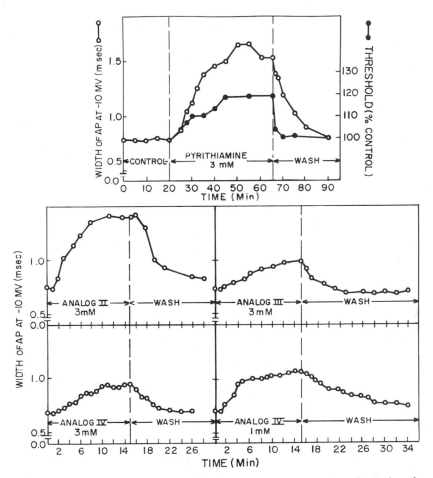

Figure 3. The time course of development and reversal of analog action in the single node as expressed by the prolongation of depolarization during the action potential. Values plotted represent the elapsed time between depolarization to −10 mV on the rising phase of the action potential and repolarization to −10 mV during the recovery phase.

period in these fibers was 1.5 ± 2 msec. Exposure of the node to PTh resulted in a progressive lengthening of the absolute refractory period which paralleled the change in mean depolarization time. In two fibers exposed to 5 mM PTH, the absolute refractory period reached maxima of 3.5 and 3.2 msec. Again, this effect was completely reversible after washing the node with control Ringer's solution.

The quantitative effects of each analog at a given concentration were quite reproducible from cycle to cycle on a given nodal preparation. In general, these effects were also quantitatively similar from preparation to preparation. We have, however, observed a number of fibers in which the response to a given concentration of an analog was far smaller than expected; this was observed most often with analogs I and II. In all cases, however, the qualitative nature of the effects remained constant.

VOLTAGE CLAMP

Further information concerning the site of action of the thiamine analogs has been sought in some preliminary voltage clamp studies. Two analogs were chosen for use in these studies: analog V because of its rapid onset of action and its more extensive effects on the action potential, and pyrithiamine as a prototype of the remaining four pyridine-substituted analogs.

Axons exposed to analog V at a holding potential of −70 mV showed no alteration from normal membrane currents in response to depolarizing pulses between 10 and 100 mV during the first 1 to 2 minutes of perfusion. With further exposure two effects progessively appeared: (a) a decrease in the peak inward sodium currents at all depolarizing steps, and (b) a decrease in the rate of development and decay of the early sodium current (Fig. 4). Both effects became more pronounced with continued exposure, and neither was readily reversible with washing within the time scale of the voltage clamp experiments (usually 15 to 30 minutes).

The amplitude of the sustained outward potassium current did not appear to be affected by exposure to analog V at any depolarizing step; the time course of activation of the potassium current during depolarization clamps to the sodium equilibrium potential was similarly unchanged by exposure to this analog. The absence of effects on potassium currents is further suggested by two experiments in which nodes were exposed to analog V in the presence of 10^{-6} M tetrodotoxin to eliminate the early sodium currents. In these experiments no significant changes were observed in the residual membrane currents to any depolarizing voltage after exposure to this analog.

In the limited number of axons we have studied, no alteration in the

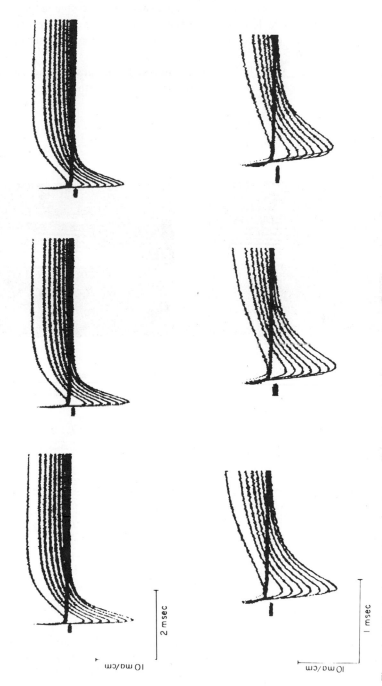

Figure 4. Effects of analog V on membrane currents from the single node. Note the reduction in peak inward sodium current and the decrease in the rate of development and decay of this current with continued exposure to the analog. Delayed currents do not appear to be significantly affected.

293

relationship of delayed current to voltage with progressive exposure to analog V was observed. The early currents, however, were symmetrically decreased at all voltages. The cross-over potential for the early current was not affected by analog V.

Axons superfused with PTh showed marked changes in the rates of development and decay of the early sodium currents, similar to those seen

CONTROL   ANALOG II   3mM   5 MIN

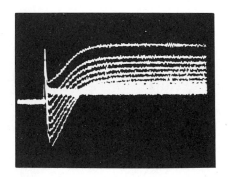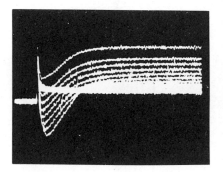

(a)

THEORETICAL IONIC CURRENTS - SINGLE NODE OF RANVIER

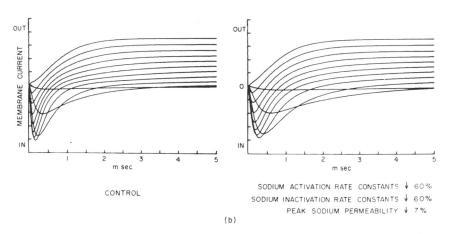

CONTROL

SODIUM ACTIVATION RATE CONSTANTS ↓ 60%
SODIUM INACTIVATION RATE CONSTANTS ↓ 60%
PEAK SODIUM PERMEABILITY ↓ 7%

(b)

Figure 5. (*a*) Membrane currents of a single node before and after exposure to pyrithiamine. The effects are similar to those seen in Fig. 4. (*b*) Computer-generated voltage clamp curves iteratively fit these experimental data. The best approximation was obtained with simultaneous reduction in sodium activation and inactivation rate constants.

with analog V. The peak inward sodium currents, however, decreased only slightly—often by no more than is seen with time in control nodes during voltage clamp experiments (see below). The time course for the development of PTh action was 2 to 3 times longer than for analog V, as would be anticipated from current clamp studies.

Rate constants and peak conductances for the sodium and potassium systems during control periods and during exposure to PTh were estimated from the current curves of two nodes, using an iterative curve-fitting computer routine in conjunction with a mathematical model of the single node after that of Frankenhaeuser and Huxley. In two experiments analyzed in this manner, the forward and reverse rate constants for the sodium activation parameter (m) and the sodium inactivation parameter (h) were found to be progressively reduced during PTh exposure. Furthermore, the extent of reduction appeared to be the same for all four rate constants at each time point within the limits of resolution of the analysis (about $\pm 10\%$). After 15 minutes of exposure to PTh, these rate constants were decreased by 52 and 60%, whereas the peak sodium conductance was reduced only 12 and 7% (Fig. 5). Rate parameters for potassium activation and peak potassium conductance appeared to be unchanged during PTh exposure with this method of analysis.

4. Reconstructed Action Potentials

By means of a mathematical model of the single-node excitable membrane at 22°C based on the equations of Frankenhaeuser and Huxley, the possible contributions of the effects of pyrithiamine and analog V noted in voltage clamp experiments to the configuration of the current-clamp action potential were evaluated. An experimental action potential recorded after 20 minutes of perfusion with PTh was chosen for comparison. Action potentials calculated with reductions in either sodium activation rate constants or sodium inactivation rate constants alone cannot duplicate the values recorded experimentally. Reduction of both activation and inactivation rate constants produces action potentials closer in configuration to those actually recorded; a nearly perfect fit is obtained only when the forward and reverse rate constants for sodium activation and inactivation are all reduced by the same amount. Small changes in the peak height of the action potential can be duplicated by additionally decreasing the maximal sodium conductance. Thus, at least at selected points, action potentials recorded after exposure to pyrithiamine can be duplicated using the mathematical model when the sodium activation and inactivation rate constants are all reduced in a uniform manner.

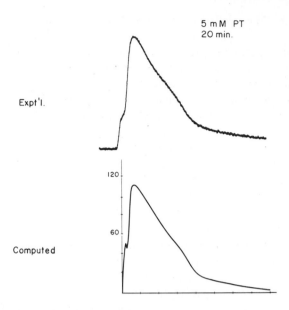

Figure 6. Comparison of experimentally recorded current-clamped action potential from a single node after exposure to pyrithiamine and a computer-generated action potential based on a mathematical model of this node (see text). For the computer action potential, all rate constants, maximal conductances, etc., are unchanged from control values with the exception of uniform decreases in the forward and reverse rate constants for sodium activation and inactivation.

Figure 6 indicates a comparison between computed and observed action potentials. The action potential recorded in axon 23 after 20 minutes of exposure to 5 mM PTh is shown in Fig. 6a; Fig. 6b indicates a computed action potential in which all values for rate constants, maximal conductances, and so forth are unchanged from the control values with the exception of α_m, α_h, β_m, β_h. These four rates have been reduced by the same percentage value (47%). It can be seen that the predicted action potential is in good qualitative agreement with the experimentally recorded tracing.

These preliminary simulations indicated to us that the effects of PTh did not represent simple blockage of either sodium or potassium pores, as is the case with tetrodotoxin or tetraethylammonium ion. Rather, these data suggested a specific lowering of the rate constants for sodium activation and inactivation as the mechanism of action of thiamine analogs in excitable membranes.

5. Models for the Role of Thiamine in the Function of the Excitable Membrane

A number of hypotheses for the role of thiamine in excitable membrane function can be proposed that will account for at least a part of the experimental data presented in the preceding sections. Two such hypotheses will be discussed below and analyzed in terms of their ability to unify the available data and to predict future avenues of research.

The first hypothesis to be examined is that thiamine or one of its phosphate esters is intimately involved in the molecular mechanisms which vary the permeability of the excitable membrane to sodium ions during the action potential. The thiamine compound is presumed to act as a catalytic cofactor in this voltage-dependent reaction and, as such, is not turned over during each membrane transition.

If thiamine is considered to be acting catalytically in the control of sodium permeability, and if the theoretical peak permeability, $\bar{p}_{na}$, remains constant, the effects of such catalysis would be expected to be expressed most directly in the rates at which inactive and active forms of the sodium translocation site can be interconverted. In this thesis such an effect would be reflected in α_m and β_m, the forward and reverse rate constants for sodium activation. If thiamine is assumed to act as a true catalyst, the α_m and β_m must be equally affected. If sodium inactivation is actually a further reaction of this site, then its forward and reverse rate constants, α_h and β_h, would be similarly related to thiamine catalysis.

A computer model of the excitable membrane can be constructed that incorporates this concept. The mathematical description of the time and voltage dependences of the sodium, potassium, and leak currents used is that of Frankenhaeuser and Huxley, based on the voltage clamp data of Frankenhaeuser for the single node of Ranvier from *Xenopus*. The reader is referred to their paper for a complete description of the formulations involved. In the model a thiamine compound catalyzes the voltage-dependent transitions in membrane sodium conductance by action at a specific membrane active site. The thiamine analogs are considered to compete with thiamine compounds for binding sites in the active region of the membrane. This competition can be programmed into the model of the nodal system by defining a constant K_T:

$$K_T = \frac{\text{binding sites occupied by thiamine}}{\text{total possible binding sites for thiamine}}$$

The value of K_T will then vary between 1.0 for the totally thiamine-saturated control membrane and zero for a hypothetical membrane in which all the thiamine sites have been occupied by pyrithiamine molecules. All functions evaluating the α's and β's for the sodium system may then be multiplied by this single constant to reflect the number of active sites occupied by functional thiamine molecules.

In a system progressively exposed to an analog competing with the native compound for specific membrane catalytic sites, the value of K_T would be expected to decrease as a function of time. If thiamine does act in the capacity postulated, the simultaneous solution of a monotonic function relating K_T to time (indicating the degree of replacement of thiamine compounds by PTh) and of the entire set of membrane equations will yield a series of progressively changing action potentials which should duplicate those recorded from isolated nodes during exposure to PTh.

We have incorporated this model into a computer routine that solves the necessary differential equations by an iterative predictor-corrector algorithm for numerical integration. The predicted effects of thiamine analog competition were compared with selected runs from the experimental data presented in the previous section for detailed analysis.

Since initial values for nonspecific leakage current and for voltage dependences of the various α and β parameters varied slightly from axon to axon, control action potentials from several selected nodes were modeled as closely as possible to set specific values in each case. These values were then held constant for the rest of the simulations.

By use of the initial values determined in this manner, a sequence of action potentials for each experimental axon was simulated by progressively changing the value of K_T in a stepwise manner from 1.0 to 0.30. These series were then compared with action potentials recorded from these axons during PTh exposure. Curves that fit to within $+5\%$ in their voltage versus time characteristics were then associated with their appropriate time points, and their K_T values noted. From these values a continuous function of $K_T = F(T, x)$, where x is a constant concentration of PTh, was constructed for each axon (Fig. 7).

These $K_T = F(T, x)$ curves were then used to generate a complete sequence of action potentials, following the same time scale as the original experiments. Selected time points from the simulated sequence and corresponding points from the experimental sequence are shown in Fig. 8 for axon 23. It can be seen that there is essentially complete agreement.

As a further evaluation of this hypothesis, appropriate values of K_T from the curve derived from axon 23 were then used to generate computer-simulated refractory periods which were compared to those actually obtained from this nerve for corresponding time points after initiation of pyrithiamine superfusion. A control refractory period and a series of curves simulating 30 minutes of PTh treatment are shown in Fig. 9. These may be compared with the experimentally recorded refractory periods obtained at these time points shown in the same figure. Again, the predicted values agree with the

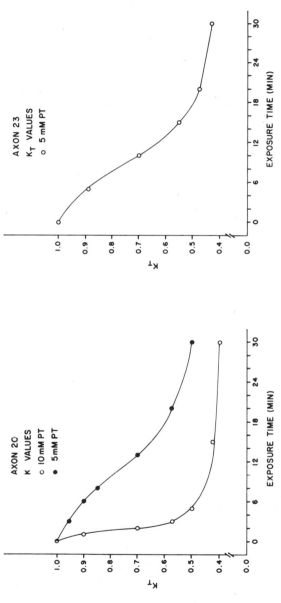

Figure 7. Values of K_T calculated by computer modeling of action potentials recorded after varying periods of exposure to pyrithiamine of two concentrations. In all cases a smooth double exponential function of K_T versus time is obtained. Increasing the concentration of pyrithiamine increases the rate at which K_T approaches its new equilibrium state.

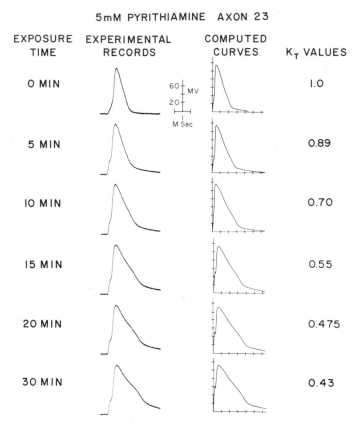

Figure 8. Action potentials recorded experimentally from a single node at various times after exposure to pyrithiamine are compared to computer-generated action potentials in which K_T has been changed by the amount indicated in Fig. 7 for each time point. All other computational parameters are held constant. The observed and computer progressions in action potential configuration are in close agreement.

experimental records for the time points examined to within ±0.2 msec.

This hypothesis provides an adequate, although not unique, explanation for the observed effects of thiamine analogs on the nodal action potential. There are several reservations, however. Action potentials generated by the mathematical model are relatively insensitive in general configuration to significant changes in K^+ rate constants. Hence a good test is not provided for exclusion of the K^+ system from the effects of the analogs. Also, the mechanism by which thiamine moderates the sodium system is not specified, and no theoretical preference can be given for one phosphate compound over another.

A second hypothesis for the role of thiamine compounds in excitable membrane function is mentioned by Fox and Duppel (8) in their analysis of the effects of thiamine phosphates on the time-dependent decay of currents in the single node. As has been previously stated, their data suggest that the exponential decline in membrane currents seen in this system is the result of a progressive decrease in the fixed negative charges on the inner surface of the axon membrane. Since the addition of thiamine phosphates, especially ThTP, to the axoplasm results in cessation of this decline, it can be postulated that ThTP in some way acts to maintain the fixed negative charges of the membrane inner surface. This could be accomplished if ThTP were involved in a reaction that resulted in the transfer of its terminal

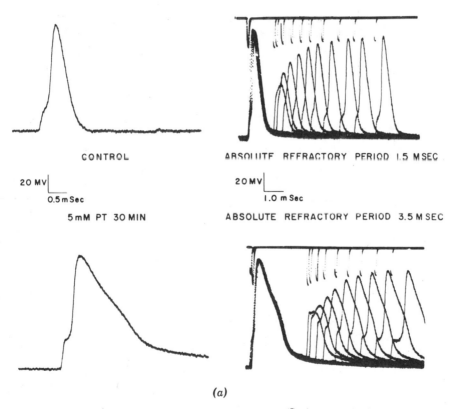

CONTROL   ABSOLUTE REFRACTORY PERIOD 1.5 MSEC

20 MV   20 MV

0.5 m Sec   1.0 m Sec

5 mM PT 30 MIN   ABSOLUTE REFRACTORY PERIOD 3.5 M SEC

(a)

Figure 9. (*a*) Refractory periods recorded experimentally before and after exposure to pyrithiamine (5 mm, 30 minutes). Note prolongation of absolute and relative refractory periods. (*b*) Computed action potentials and refractory periods in which the postexposure action potentials are simulated by an appropriate reduction in K_T, other variables remaining unchanged. Agreement in duration of refractory periods between experimental and simulated sequences is again apparent.

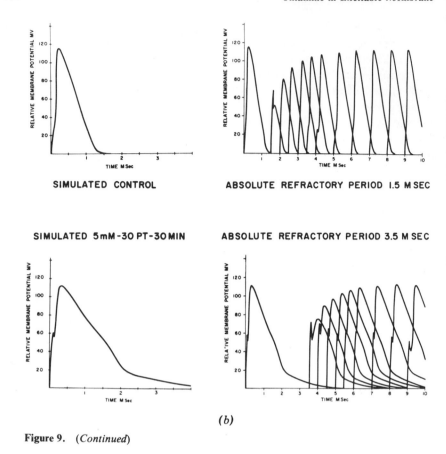

Figure 9. (*Continued*)

phosphate group to a membrane structural component, thus producing a net increase in fixed negative surface charge of the membrane.

What is the effect on membrane currents of changes in fixed negative charge density? A schematic representation of the electrical potential gradient across a voltage-clamped membrane is shown in Fig. 10. The potential difference between the bulk aqueous phases is determined by the voltage clamp (or by the distribution of electrolytes and their relative permeabilities in the unclamped membrane). The actual potential gradient appearing across the inner portion of the membrane, however, will depend on the contributions to the local field generated by fixed surface charges. In the squid axon, for example, there are considerably more fixed negative charges on the membrane outer surface than on the inner surface. These surface charges tend to make the membrane near the outer surface more negative than would be expected in a simple linear field. A similar phenomenon is seen at the inner surface but to a lesser extent. The net result as calculated for the squid axon is that, although the potential difference measured between cytoplasm and extracellular fluid is 70 mV, only approximately 55 mV of this potential actually appears across the active membrane.

Changes in the fixed charge density of the membrane inner surface can now be examined in the light of these concepts. Increasing negative charge density will serve to increase the local field gradient at the membrane inner surface and thereby increase the effective field across the membrane interior. Conversely, decreasing the density of fixed negative surface charges will reduce the local field between membrane and bulk aqueous phase. On the assumption that the density of outer surface negative charges is unchanged, this will act to decrease the potential difference measured within the membrane from one side to the other. Reducing inner membrane surface negative charges will thus produce an effect analogous to depolarizing the otherwise unaltered axon (see Fig. 10).

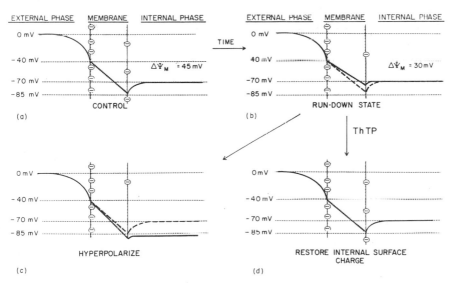

Figure 10. (a) Voltage profile across a cell membrane between two bulk aqueous phases when fixed negative charges are present on the membrane surface. If the negative charge density is higher on the outer surface than on the inner, the actual potential difference across the inner membrane will be less than that measured between bulk phases. (b) If internal surface charges are hydrolyzed or neutralized with time, the internal membrane potential will fall although the measured potential between bulk phases remains unchanged. This decay can be reversed by either (c) increasing the total potential difference between bulk phases, or (d) restoring the fixed negative charges to the membrane inner surface.

In preventing the exponential decline of membrane currents in the single node, ThTP behaves in a manner analogous to increasing the effective potential difference across the excitable membrane, an effect shown above to be consistent with increasing the density of fixed negative charges on the membrane inner surface. We have described in recent publications the existence of a membrane-associated thiamine triphosphatase whose activity appears to be controlled by the ambient levels of ATP and ADP. It is possible that this membrane-bound activity represents a phosphotransferase which results in the transfer of the γ-phosphate from ThTP to a membrane structural component and that a secondary phosphatase results in the degradation of this product, the sum of the two reactions producing the observed triphosphatase activity:

$$ \text{ThTP} + \text{membrane} \xrightarrow{\text{ThTPase}} \text{ThDP} + \text{membrane} - \text{P} $$

$$ \text{Membrane} - \text{P} \xrightarrow{\text{P'tase}} \text{membrane} + \text{P}_i $$

Such a system with suitable control mechanisms can be postulated to regulate the fixed negative charge density of the membrane inner surface. Thus, in the absence of ThTP, the slow hydrolysis of phosphate groups from the membrane would produce an exponential decline in charge density if it is assumed that degradative enzyme activity remains constant. This hydrolysis would in turn produce a decrease in effective potential across the active membrane, leading to a progressive inactivation of sodium conductance and to alterations in all membrane rate constants that are functions of the membrane potential. Replacement of ThTP would allow rephosphorylation of the membrane and prevent further degradation in excitability.

The actions of thiamine analogs can be examined in the light of this mechanism. It is possible that the thiamine analogs discussed earlier act partly or entirely by inhibiting such a ThTP-requiring phosphotransferase. Since the rate constants for sodium activation and inactivation are all complex functions of the effective potential difference across the membrane, the observed effects on sodium rate constants could reflect an indirect action resulting from an alteration in local fields dependent on fixed surface negative charges.

The experimental data available to date do not allow a choice to be made between the two mechanisms presented or others which might also satisfactorily explain the available observations. The postulation of a role for ThTP in maintaining membrane negative surface charge density is intriguing in that it suggests a possible function for the membrane-associated ThTPase; it also suggests a reason for the relatively high levels of

ThTP and membrane ThTPase in cells specializing in active transport processes, since these functions too are sensitive to the transmembrane potential. The hypothesis of a catalytic function for thiamine in the sodium permeability mechanism, however, is unusually effective in reproducing the experimental observations on the actions of thiamine analogs. Further experiments must be designed to evaluate these hypotheses. Hopefully the results of such studies will lead to a clearer understanding of the true role of thiamine compounds in nerve membrane function.

References

1. P. Dreyfus and G. Hauser, *Biochim. Biophys. Acta,* **104,** 78 (1964).
2. J. Pincus and K. Wells, *Expt. Neurol.,* **37,** 495 (1972).
3. A. von Muralt, in R. Harris and K. Thimann, Eds., *Vitamins and Hormones,* Vol. 5, Academic Press, New York, 1947, p. 93.
4. F. Wyss and A. von Muralt, *Helv. Physiol. Acta,* **2,** C-61 (1944).
5. Y. Itokawa and J. Cooper, *Biochem. Pharmacol.,* **18,** 545 (1969).
6. Y. Itokawa and J. Cooper, *Biochim. Biophys. Acta,* **196,** 274 (1970).
7. J. Pincus, Y. Itokawa, and J. Cooper, *Neurology,* **19,** 985 (1969).
8. J. Fox and W. Duppel, *Pflügers Arch.* (in press).
9. H. Kunz, *Helv. Physiol. Acta,* **14,** 411 (1956).
10. C. Armett and J. Cooper. *J. Pharm. Exp. Ther.,* **148,** 137 (1965).
11. W. Nonner, Pflü*gers Arch.,* **49,** 175 (1969).

DISCUSSION

Chapters 19 and 20

Dr. Cooper. First of all, I should emphasize that I am not a neurophysiologist, so I cannot engage in any real discussion of this topic. However, I have Dan Goldberg in my laboratory, who, for the past year, has been working along somewhat similar lines, using some other analogs than the ones you have mentioned. He has also used fern extract, which has been shown to affect conduction. What he has done is to use two preparations; one is the circumesophageal connectives of the lobster, which can be penetrated with microelectrodes, and the other is the giant axon of the squid, which can be voltage clamped. Now Goldberg found that in the lobster preparation there were three or four effects, depending on the antimetabolite. First, usually there was a decrease in the resting potential, and this varied from about 15 to 20%, depending on the antimetabolite. Second, there was a decrease in the rate of rise of the action potential, and, third, there was a prolonged after-potential somewhat similar to what Dr. Barchi showed, except that with these particular analogs the effect was much more pronounced. On occasion, repetitive firing was also observed. The effects on the rate of rise, on the amplitude, and on the rate of repolarization were all reversible when the antimetabolite was removed and the preparation was washed with seawater, but the effects on the resting potential were not generally reversible. With the fern extract preparation, effects somewhat similar to those obtained with the antimetabolites, but generally a little more pronounced, were observed. There was obviously an effect on sodium conduction, and since with the lobster preparation one could not determine whether this phenomenon was due to sodium or potassium, Goldberg did some work on the voltage-clamped squid axon.

There he could show that the antimetabolites affected both sodium and potassium conduction. This obviously was different from what Von Muralt and the people in his laboratory had found. They postulated a specific effect on the sodium conductance mechanism.

I should mention at this point that these effects that we observed with antimetabolites and fern extract were, in a sense, not dissimilar from the effects that can be seen with a variety of local anesthetics; lidocaine would be an example. You get essentially the same phenomena. So it is conceivable that these effects that we are seeing with antimetabolites have nothing to do with thiamine. They may be effects of compounds that, curiously, happen to be somewhat similar in structure to thiamine but may in fact have nothing to do with thiamine at all.

We were also interested in determining whether thiamine is specifically localized in nerve membranes. Dr. Itokawa, using a brain preparation, had done a little work in our laboratory on this problem, but here one does not have any idea of what kind of membrane one isolates from a brain preparation. It could be a mixture of plasma membrane, endoplasmic reticulum, mitochondrial membrane, and so forth. What Goldberg did was to take the walking nerve of the lobster and develop sucrose density gradient preparations of the homogenate of the axon, where one could separate a fairly pure axolemma from Schwann lemma, and then assay each of these preparations for endogenous thiamine. We increased the specificity of this assay, not only by looking at the activation and fluorescent maxima of the material in the preparations but also by using thiaminase to destroy thiamine. It turned out that thiamine was endogenously present in both axolemma and Schwann lemma, about 10 pM thiamine/mg protein. Curiously, this concentration corresponds closely to the number of sodium channels that one finds there, using tetrodotoxin binding as an indicator of sodium channels. This was very interesting to us because of the experience we had had with tetrodotoxin in terms of this agent being the most potent drug we could find for releasing thiamine from nerve membranes.

At any rate, the fact that we could find thiamine in both axolemma and Schwann lemma, coupled with the fact that these analogs seemed to affect both sodium and potassium conductances, made us think again about a more general role of thiamine. It is involved not only in conduction and excitable tissue but perhaps also, in a sense, in all tissues that have a transmembrane potential. What we are thinking of, at least this week, is that thiamine may have a function in the intramembranous regulation of ATP. Recently there has been some evidence to suggest that purified membrane fractions contain glycolytic enzymes, particularly those involved in ATP synthesis, such as phosphoglycerate kinase. Maybe there is an intramembranous synthesis of ATP, which is involved in pump activity and which is different from the ATP that is involved in whole-cell intermediary metabolism. The theory that we are working on now is that perhaps a thiamine phosphate has something to do with the generation in the membrane itself of ATP which is involved in pump activity. And then this, of course, brings us to the calcium effects that Dr. Ogawa and Dr. Itokawa have shown, and perhaps it would also explain some of the effects we have observed with pyrithiamine on the vagus, where we found a marked effect on posttetanic hyperpolarization, which does involve sodium pump activity. This is essentially what we are thinking of now: that thiamine has an effect not only on nervous tissue but on all cells.

Dr. Barchi. Let me make just a few initial comments. First, we also see a decrease in the rate of rise of the action potentials, which I am sure you observe if you look closely at Fig. 2. We do not get the prolongation much beyond this sort of effect under any circumstances in the node, and I do not think anybody else has shown that in the node it ever gets prolonged much beyond this. Second, I agree with your cynicism about the direct function of thiamine in the channel; the reason why these data have been withheld so long actually is that some experiments we did in trying to demonstrate competition of the pyrithiamine effect with free thiamine and thiamine monophosphate did not work.

Dr. Cooper. That is right. They do not work in the lobster, either.

Dr. Barchi. It was questionable as to whether they did not work because we were not getting the thiamine into the right spot. I feel much more in favor of the concept of inner membrane surface charge, fixed negative charge, as a general mechanism for ThTP function. It would certainly explain everything we have seen. I think it would also explain most of the things you have described which you see in the squid axon that we really do not see here, and it would explain observations in other tissues and give us a potential mechanism to explore a possible function of thiamine in other tissues that have active transport phenomena, as well as providing a reason why ThTP and thiamine triphosphatase are present in practically all tissues. Thiamine is especially high in tissues that are involved in active transport. The difficulty with implicating thiamine on a one-to-one basis with each sodium channel is not only a theoretical but also an experimental one.

Dr. Cooper. Yes, we cannot reverse the effect of antimetabolites on the lobster axon, but this may again be a problem of the penetration of thiamine internally where it should be. With the fern extract experiments, however, when we took a fern extract and pretreated it with thiamine, it lost its potency; in addition, we could show a correlation between the potency of the fern extract and the potency *in vitro* in destroying thiamine in the test tube. So, with the fern extract, there may in fact be some indication of interrelationship with thiamine, but we could not show this with the antimetabolites. One final experiment I should mention, which is a very preliminary one, was with the squid axon. Unfortunately, we were able to do only one experiment before Dr. Goldberg had to leave. What he did was to perfuse a squid axon internally with thiaminase, and this wiped out the action potential. Now obviously, if one could repeat this, it would be quite interesting and would be the first indication of thiamine being involved in conduction.

Dr. Barchi. Specifically in the node preparation Dr. Fox has done several experiments to test these hypotheses. He cannot demonstrate any interaction between tetrodotoxin and thiamine. This is not at all surprising, however, because tetrodotoxin, as we know, binds in the outer surface of the membrane in a selective filter area that is very close to the outer surface and is not the same area that is involved in the sodium gating mechanisms. The m gate and the h gate are internal mechanisms that are removed from the selectivity filter, and the site of interaction of tetrodotoxin is not the same as the sites of the gates. I would be surprised if there was a really direct competitive effect. If the thiamine is actually acting at the internal surface, there would be no reason to expect such interaction.

Dr. Blass. Is there an exchange between the phosphate groups of ThTP, notably the terminal phosphate and proteins or phosphoproteins in the membrane?

Dr. Barchi. Would I like to know the answer to that! We are presently studying that question using gamma-labeled ThTP.

21. Histochemical and Biochemical Approaches to Axoplasmic Transport of Thiamine

CHIKAKO TANAKA, M.D.
SEISUKI TANAKA, M.D.
YOSHINORI ITOKAWA, M.D.

Departments of Pharmacology, Orthopaedic Surgery, and Hygiene
Faculty of Medicine
Kyoto University
Kyoto, Japan

Many researchers have reported that various substances stream proximal to distal or distal to proximal in axoplasm of the peripheral nerve fiber (1–7). However, the axonal transport of vitamins has not been reported. In the present report, axoplasmic transport of thiamine in the rat sciatic nerve is described.

Male Sprague-Dawley rats weighing 250 to 300 grams were used. Under ether anesthesia the sciatic nerve was ligated with a silk suture at about 5 cm distal to the spinal ganglion. The rats were sacrificed by decapitation 48 hours after surgery. The normal and ligated sciatic nerves were dissected and divided into several pieces at various distances from the spinal ganglion, as shown in Fig. 1.

Histochemical analysis was performed by the method of Tanaka and Cooper (8) with several modifications. Pieces of sciatic nerve were frozen in isopentane chilled by liquid nitrogen. After freeze-drying for 24 to 48 hours, the samples were embedded in paraffin *in vacuo*, sectioned at 5 to 8 μ, and deparaffinized by careful addition of a drop of xylene. Subsequently, the preparations were exposed to cyanogen bromide vapor for 15 minutes at 35

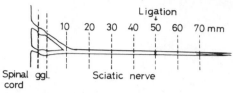

Figure 1. Schematic illustration of the ligated rat sciatic nerve.

to 40°C and then to ammonia to convert thiamine into thiochrome (fluorescent substance). The preparations were mounted in either xylene or mineral oil and then observed through a Zeiss fluorescence microscope. The light source was an Osram HBO-200 high-pressure mercury lamp with a Schott BG-12 exciter filter and a Zeiss 41 barrier.

Attention must be paid to the following points when using this technique.

1. The preparation must not be moistened at any step of the histochemical procedure. Even a small amount of water can cause diffusion artifacts.

2. The cyanogen bromide gas was prepared from cyanogen bromide crystals at 35 to 40°C in a closed reaction vessel. The cyanogen bromide gas must not be mixed with ammonia gas, since thiochrome is not formed in alkaline medium. Instead, thiamine breaks down to thiamine anhydride, and hence no fluorescent product is formed (9).

For the biochemical assay of thiamine, the fluorometric method of Fujiwara and Matsui (10) for milligram quantities of tissues was used. The

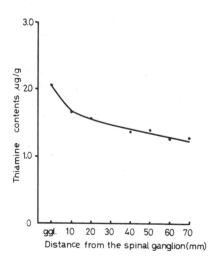

Figure 2. Thiamine content in the normal sciatic nerve.

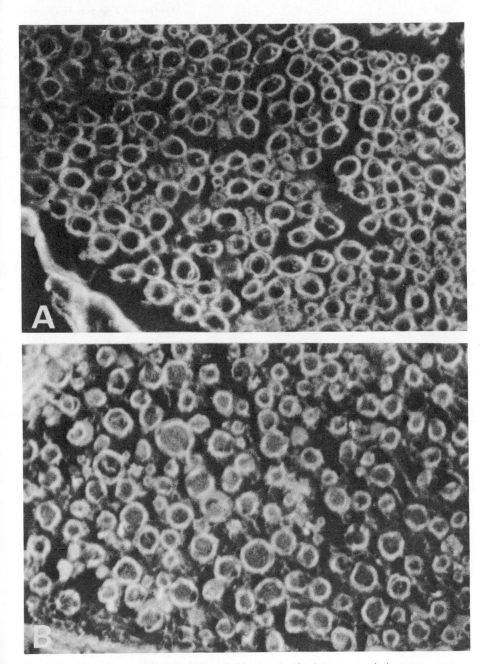

Figure 3. Histochemical demonstration of thiamine in the intact rat sciatic nerve: cross section of bundles of fibers. 380× (*A*) Distal part of the nerve: white-blue fluorescence of thiochrome can be seen in the myelin regions rather than in the axoplasm. (*B*) Proximal part of the nerve: fluorescence can be observed in both the myelin regions and the axoplasm.

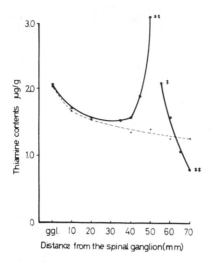

Figure 4. Thiamine content in the ligated sciatic nerve: * $p < .05$, ** $p < .01$; significant difference as compared with values for the normal nerve (dotted line).

sensitivity of the chemical assay for thiamine is sufficient to measure 5 ng of thiamine.

In the sciatic nerve, the thiamine content exhibited a proximodistal gradient, as shown in Fig. 2.

In cross sections of fibers in the distal part of the nerve, (3A) the white-blue fluorescence of thiochrome was observed in membrane structures, including myelin sheath, rather than in axoplasm. There was some fluorescent material, not only in the membrane structure, but also in the axoplasm of the proximal part of the sciatic nerve (Fig. 3B).

Occlusion of axonal flow by ligation produced histochemical and biochemical changes in thiamine distribution near the site of the lesion. The thiamine content had almost doubled in the control nerve on the adjacent proximal site of ligation 48 hours after surgery, as shown in Fig. 4.

Accumulation of thiamine was clearly visible histochemically in the highly swollen and bulgy axon just above the lesion (Fig. 5). Some accumulation of fluorescent material was also seen just below the lesion. This fluorescence revealed spectral characteristics of thiochrome and was sensitive to irradiation with ultraviolet light.

An accumulation of mitochondria, granules, and vesicles has been demonstrated in the axon above the site of constriction or cut of the peripheral nerve (3). Most of the thiamine in structural particles of the sciatic nerve was observed in the mitochondrial fraction (11). From these data, coupled with our present findings, it is assumed that the bulk of accumulated thiamine in the nerve is contained in the mitochondria, and

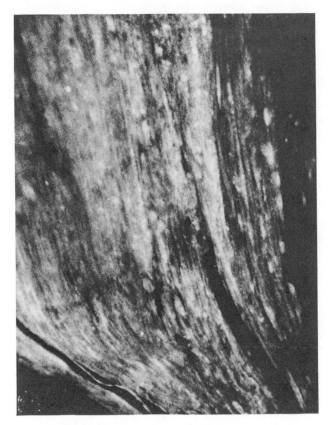

Figure 5. Histochemical demonstration of the accumulation of thiamine in the ligated sciatic nerve of a rat 48 hours after surgery. Longitudinal section of bundles of fibers. The swollen and bulgy appearance of the axons with accumulation of strongly fluorescent material is clearly visible in the nerve just above the ligation. ×160.

axoplasmic flow could be one of the routes supplying thiamine to the axon membrane and nerve endings.

References

1. C. H. Sawyer, *Am. J. Physiol.*, **146,** 246 (1946).
2. R. L. Friede, *Exp. Neurol.*, **1,** 441 (1959).
3. W. Wechsler and H. Hager, *Acta Neuropathol.*, **1,** 486 (1962).

4. P. Weiss, A. C. Taylor, and P. A. Pillai, *Science*, **136**, 330 (1962).
5. J. Zelena and L. Lubińska, *Physiol. Bohemoslov.*, **11**, 261 (1962).
6. G. Kreutzberg, *Naturwissenshaften*, **50**, 96 (1963).
7. A. Dahlström and K. Fuxe, *Z. Zellforsch. Mikrosk. Anat.*, **62**, 602 (1964).
8. C. Tanaka and J. R. Cooper, *J. Histochem. Cytochem.*, **16**, 362 (1968).
9. K. Kawasaki and T. Itoh, *Vitamins* (Japan), **13**, 391 (1957).
10. M. Fujiwara and K. Matsui, *Anal. Chem.*, **25**, 810 (1953).
11. Y. Itokawa and J. R. Cooper, *Science*, **166**, 759 (1969).

DISCUSSION

Chapter 21

Dr. Dreyfus. I think that this is a very interesting and important paper which raises a number of questions. Dr. Barchi, would you like to make some comments?

Dr. Barchi. Do you feel that the fluorescence really represents thiamine in the myelin?

Dr. Itokawa. Yes, in the myelin membrane.

Dr. Barchi. There seems to be a difficulty with that kind of technique in that you convert thiamine into a thiochrome derivative which is very lipid soluble, and the question always arises as to whether or not there is diffusion into myelin; this is why we did the experiments Dr. Dreyfus referred to before with myelination. I think it is interesting that thiamine travels down the axon and seems involved in axoplasmic flow. The question arises whether the thiamine in the myelin is really in the myelin before one starts the procedure.

Dr. Cooper. I do not really think it is in the myelin; I think it is probably in the Schwann cell.

Dr. Barchi. Yes, from the developmental studies it clearly does not concentrate in myelin or myelin-synthesizing cells.

FIVE

THIAMINE-RELATED HEREDITARY METABOLIC DISEASES

22. Pyruvate Decarboxylase Deficiency

JOHN P. BLASS, M.D., Ph.D.
GARY E. GIBSON, Ph.D.
R. A. PIETER KARK, M.D.

Departments of Psychiatry, Biological Chemistry and Neurology
and Mental Retardation Research Center
Neuropsychiatric Institute and
School of Medicine
University of California
Los Angeles, California

1. Identification of the Syndrome

In 1968 Dr. Derek Lonsdale described a child who had elevated levels of lactic and pyruvic acids and of alanine in his urine and who suffered from intermittent bouts of incoordination (1, 2). The abnormal movements were of a type called cerebellar ataxia, since they are recognized clinically typically to involve cerebellar systems. Shortly thereafter, a young man who proved to have the same syndrome came to the National Institutes of Health. Clinical studies of that patient, *in vitro* studies of his cultured skin fibroblasts and white blood cells, and a muscle biopsy were consistent with an inherited defect of pyruvate oxidation and specifically of the thiamine-dependent first enzyme of the pyruvate dehydrogenase complex (PDH). The most critical experiment was the measurement of the oxidation of [1-^{14}C]pyruvate by disrupted fibroblasts, incubated at pH 6.0 with $K_3Fe(CN)_6$ as an electron acceptor. Similar results were obtained using cell extracts from our patient and from the two affected boys in Lonsdale's family. Values for the parents were at or below the lower limit for controls, indicating a primary, recessively inherited defect. These observations have been described in detail elsewhere (3–6).

Since then, the syndrome of intermittent ataxia with abnormal pyruvate metabolism has been noted in at least five other patients from three families, including two girls (6). Biochemical studies of these patients are less extensive.

2. The Site of the Enzyme Defect

The syndrome was called pyruvate decarboxylase deficiency, because the $Fe(CN)_6{}^{3-}$-linked assay we devised was a radiochemical modification of the method of Reed and Willms (7) for yeast pyruvate decarboxylase (2-oxoacid carboxy-lyase, EC 4.1.1.1). The analogous mammalian enzyme is the thiamine-dependent first enzyme of the pyruvate dehydrogenase complex, correctly called pyruvate dehydrogenase [pyruvate:lipoate oxidoreductase (acceptor-acetylating), EC 1.2.4.1] and abbreviated PDC. Calling the syndrome "PDC deficiency" skirts our misnomer.

The $Fe(CN)_6{}^{3-}$-linked assay appears to measure PDC activity in sonicated human fibroblasts. Cofactor requirements are appropriate. Both

Table 1.   Cofactor Requirements in the Assay for PDC

The complete reaction mixture contained 0.1 M potassium phosphate, pH 6.0, 4 mM $MgCl_2$, 25 mM $K_3Fe(CN)_6$, 0.15 mM TPP, 0.1 mM sodium [1-^{14}C]pyruvate, and, when added, 0.12 mM NAD^+ and 0.05 mM CoA (3, 9). The $^{14}CO_2$ liberated by cell-free extracts of fibroblasts was determined as described previously (3). Values are means ± S.E.M. for three preparations, two from clinically normal subjects and one from a patient with a spinocerebellar disorder. The absolute activity was 40.5 ± 18.4 picomoles/(min) (mg protein).

	Activity, % of control
Control	(100)
− ThDP	65.9 ± 8.0
− $K_3Fe(CN)_6$	49.7 ± 10.0
− ThDP and $K_3Fe(CN)_6$	34.5 ± 8.8
+ CoA	96.6 ± 14.6
+ CoA and NAD^+, − $K_3Fe(CN)_6$	59.8 ± 23.1

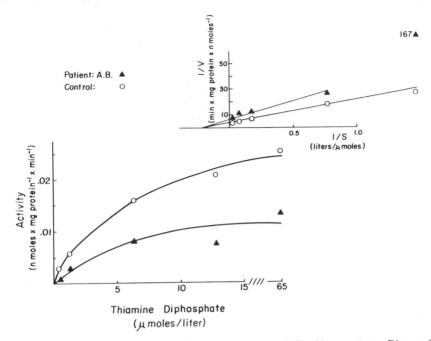

Figure 1. Apparent K_m for thiamine diphosphate in treated fibroblast extracts. Disrupted fibroblasts which had been treated with alkaline $(NH_4)_2SO_4$ at least 3 times (8) were assayed with the $K_3Fe(CN)_6$-linked assay for PDC at pH 6.0 (3) in varying concentrations of ThDP. For the extracts illustrated, the requirement for ThDP was more than 90%. Patient A. B. has a spinocerebellar disorder and apparently no PDC deficiency (48).

thiamin diphosphate (ThDP) and $Fe(CN)_6^{3-}$ are needed for full activity; CoA and NAD^+ do not stimulate PDC activity (Table 1). Repeated precipitation of the fibroblast protein from alkaline buffer with $(NH_4)_2SO_4$, a standard technique for removing ThDP from purified PDC (8), could increase the ThDP requirement to > 90% (Fig. 1). The apparent K_m for ThDP was 1 to 5 μM in such extracts of human fibroblasts, studied by the $Fe(CN)_6^{3-}$-linked assay. This value is comparable to that for purified PDC from other mammalian species (8). Cells that appeared deficient in PDC, by the $Fe(CN)_6^{3-}$-linked assay, also appeared deficient in overall PDH, as would be expected if the $Fe(CN)_6^{3-}$-linked assay were measuring the activity of the first enzyme of the complex (Table 2). The activity of the whole PDH complex was estimated radiochemically, with NAD^+ and CoA as acceptors, at pH 7.4, as described elsewhere (9). Note that the $Fe(CN)_6^{3-}$ and NAD^+-linked assays are not equivalent. Disrupted cells from two other children, with a different clinical syndrome called congenital lactic acidosis, were deficient by the NAD^+-linked assay for the overall PDH complex but had

Table 2. Enzyme Activities in Cell-free Extracts of Fibroblasts

Activities of PDC and of the overall PDH and KGDH complexes were measured as discussed in the text and described in detail elsewhere (3, 9, 49). Values are mean picomoles per minute per milligram protein, ± S.E.M. Numbers in parentheses indicate the number of control lines. At least three separate cultures were studied for each individual, patient or control. An asterisk indicates a statistically significant difference from controls ($p < .001$). The value for the KGDH complex for Patient B was within the range for controls. N.D.: not determined.

	Pyruvate Decarboxylase	Pyruvate Dehydrogenase Complex	Oxoglutarate Dehydrogenase Complex
Controls (number)	66 ± 6 (10)	389 ± 35 (18)	183 ± 34 (11)
Intermittent ataxia	11 ± 1*	68 ± 30*	101
Patient B	14 ± 5	44 ± 18	101 ± 4
Patient J	9 ± 7	32 ± 15	N.D.
Patient T	11 ± 9	128 ± 36	N.D.
Lactic acidosis	45 ± 9	53 ± 16*	265 ± 78
Patient E	40 ± 18	59 ± 16	132 ± 13
Patient JB	50 ± 12	47 ± 23	398 ± 12

activities within the lower end of the normal range in the $Fe(CN)_6^{3-}$-linked assay for PDC. The oxoglutarate dehydrogenase (KGDH) activity of all these lines was not significantly different from that of the controls. Extensive studies have shown that the purified third enzyme is the same protein in the PDH and the KGDH complexes (10).

The data are therefore consistent with a deficiency of the first enzyme of the complex in the three patients with intermittent ataxia and of the second enzyme in the two patients with lactic acidosis. Furthermore, $Fe(CN)_6^{3-}$ did not support the production of acetyl-CoA by partially purified PDH from beef brain or kidney, whereas NAD^+ did (Fig. 2). Finally, incubation with 10 mM Mg^{2+} and 0.5 mM Ca^{2+} did not increase PDH activity consistently in extracts of cells from 8 controls and one patient with lactic acidosis: PDH activity with high Mg^{2+} and Ca^{2+} was 96 ± 4% (S. E. M.) of that without them in extracts from 14 controls, and 99 ± 23% (S. E. M.) in extracts from four cultures from a patient with lactic acidosis. Nor did the addition of purified pig heart phosphatase with Mg^{2+} and Ca^{2+} increase activity in extracts of two other cell lines. Incubation of the crude extracts with 5 mM ATP usually did lower activities, by at least 50%. We have not studied the activation-inactivation system for PDH in cultured cells in greater detail.

3. Mechanisms of Brain Damage

The syndrome of PDC deficiency with intermittent ataxia differs in several ways from most of the known metabolic errors that affect the nervous system. It is a partial deficiency. It affects a major pathway of carbohydrate utilization. In three patients it was associated with a single prominent neurological sign. The clinical disorder is intermittent, typically precipitated by metabolic stresses. As pointed out elsewhere (4), PDC deficiency might be a model for other conditions in which there is a genetic predisposition to the development of particular symptoms of brain disease. We have attempted, by posing discrete experimental questions, to understand better the mechanisms by which a partial deficiency of PDC impairs the function of the nervous system.

QUALITATIVE COMPARISONS OF PDH FROM BRAIN AND OTHER TISSUES

The first question was whether there were qualitatively different forms of PDC in different tissues and cell types. Extensive studies of purified PDH by Reed and his co-workers have not provided evidence of isoenzymes (12). Dr. Burgett in Dr. Reed's laboratory found purified PDH from bovine brain

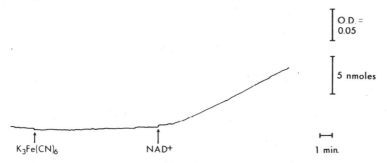

Figure 2.   Production of acetyl-CoA by partially purified pyruvate dehydrogenase complex from beef kidney. Upward deflection on the spectrophotometer tracing represents acetyl-CoA produced by a preparation of the PDH complex from beef kidney (8). Similar results were obtained with another preparation from beef kidney and one from beef brain. The coupled assay with arylamine acetyltransferase (EC 2.3.1.5) was used (11). Addition of 5 mM $K_3Fe(CN)_6$ after NAD^+ did not significantly alter the rate of acetyl-CoA production under the conditions used.

to be similar to that from other tissues (13). We found no significant kinetic differences between partially purified PDH from beef brain and that from beef kidney (8, 14). Siess *et al.* (15) found no kinetic differences between partially purified PDH from rat brain and that from other rat tissues. Furthermore, Farrell and his co-workers (16) have found PDH to be deficient in each of the three tissues they examined from a patient who died of lactic acidosis: namely, brain, liver, and cultured fibroblasts. The lack of evidence for tissue-specific isoenzymes suggests that we can continue to draw conclusions about the PDH in the brain from the study of more accessible tissues such as cultured skin fibroblasts, but it prevents our invoking cell-specific isoenzymes to account for the relative specificity of the neurological abnormalities in certain patients with PDC deficiency.

QUANTITATIVE COMPARISON OF PDH ACTIVITY AND PYRUVATE FLUX

The activity of PDH in brain appears to be low relative to the flux of pyruvate. Values for PDH in whole adult rat brain are about 100 to 225 μMoles/(g tissue) (hr), determined by a number of different techniques in laboratories from Germany to California (17–21). The pyruvate flux appears to be about 70 to 140 μMoles/(g rat brain) (hr), whether calculated from O_2 uptake (22) or from isotope fluxes (23). Since there appears to be, at most, a threefold excess of PDH, an anomaly that reduced PDH activity to less than one third of normal might be expected to impair the flux of pyruvate to acetyl-CoA, in whole rat brain. Furthermore, PDH activity appears to be relatively low in some parts of the brain as compared to others (24, 25). In cats the highest activity was in caudate nuclei and the lowest in an area of anterior cerebellar vermis, whether expressed per unit wet weight, per unit protein, or per unit DNA (Fig. 3). The ratio of PDH to three other mitochondrial activities was also lowest in the anterior cerebellar vermis. These other mitochondrial activities were those of two enzymes, succinate dehydrogenase (EC 1.3.99.1) and cytochrome oxidase (EC 1.9.3.1), and the O_2 uptake (25).

Previous work by others has shown that homogenates of whole rat cerebella oxidized pyruvate more slowly than did homogenates of various other parts of rat brain (20, 21). Pyruvate oxidation was more sensitive to inhibition by acetaldehyde (26) and to thiamine deficiency in preparations of rat cerebella (21) than in preparations from other parts of rat brain. The area of cerebellum studied was chosen to be analogous to an area of frequent damage in thiamine-deficient alcoholics (27). Cerebellar ataxia was the most prominent symptom in the first three children with inherited PDC deficiency. In at least two of them, the earliest sign of an attack was ataxia of the lower limbs, and clinical-pathological correlations suggest that the

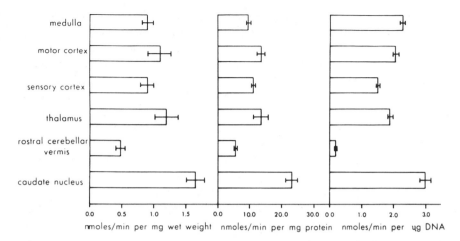

medulla

motor cortex

sensory cortex

thalamus

rostral cerebellar
vermis

caudate nucleus

0.0   0.5   1.0   1.5   0.0   10.0   20.0   30.0 0.0   1.0   2.0   3.0

nmoles/min per mg wet weight   nmoles/min per mg protein   nmoles/min per µg DNA

Figure 3.   Pyruvate dehydrogenase activity in areas of cat brain gray matter. Data are from Reynolds et al. (24, 25). Activity of PDH was measured radiochemically in pieces of cat brain that had been homogenized in saturated $(NH_4)_2SO_4$ to disrupt mitochondria (24, 25). The relative distributions were approximately similar when expressed as ratios to the activities of succinate dehydrogenase (EC 1.3.99.1) or cytochrome oxidase (EC 1.9.3.1), or to oxygen uptake by homogenates of similar pieces of brain (6, 24, 25).

anterior vermis is involved in the coordination of the hind limbs (28). Together, these data allow a hypothesis that partial deficiencies of PDH may impair the flux of pyruvate to acetyl-CoA in certain cells of the cerebellum without limiting metabolic flux in other parts of the brain.

EFFECTS OF IMPAIRED PYRUVATE FLUX

Another question involves the effects of impaired pyruvate flux. The oxidation of pyruvate to acetyl-CoA is a key, central step in metabolism. Indeed, except during prolonged fasting, adult mammalian brain has a minute-to-minute dependence on the oxidation of pyruvate derived from blood glucose (22). The acetyl-CoA produced can be burned in the tricarboxylic acid cycle, or incorporated into brain constituents such as amino acids, lipids, and the acetyl group of acetylcholine (ACh). It has often been assumed that impaired production of acetyl-CoA would lead to impaired production of energy in the form of ATP, but studies from at least three laboratories have shown that, if the brain is deprived of adequate glucose or oxygen, its electrical activity can be permanently abolished without a permanent reduction of the concentration of ATP or the ratio of ATP to ADP and AMP (29–31).

It is interesting, in considering the effects of impaired pyruvate oxidation, that PDH activity was relatively highest in the area of cat brain with highest choline acetyltransferase (EC 2.3.1.6) and lowest in the area lowest in that enzyme (which is of course a marker for cholinergic structures). The electric organ of the eel *Electrophorus electricus* is a highly cholinergic structure, and it also had high PDH activity in relation to other eel tissues (24, 25). The electric organ was not relatively enriched in succinic dehydrogenase or in cytochrome oxidase. The *ratio* of the activity of PDH to that of either of these other mitochondrial markers was strikingly higher in the electric organ than in other eel tissues, including the brain (Table 3). The adrenal medulla, which concentrates epinephrine, had relatively high PDH activity as well. The ratio of PDH to succinic dehydrogenase activity was ten- to twentyfold higher in pig adrenal medulla than in pig liver or kidney (24, 25). Patel and Koenig (32) have shown that impairment of carbohydrate oxidation by fluorocitrate alters the metabolism of another neurotransmitter, GABA. Mitochondria from rat brain synaptosomal fractions oxidized pyruvate more slowly, if anything, than did mitochondria from other rat brain fractions, suggesting that the ability to metabolize pyruvate rapidly is not a necessary property of structures which produce and store neurohormones (25). Balasz *et al.* (33) have suggested that pyruvate metabolism is particularly rapid in a nerve-ending compartment, and Tucek and Cheng (34) that it is critical for the synthesis of ACh (33).

Table 3. Ratio of Pyruvate Dehydrogenase to Succinate Dehydrogenase Activity in Tissues from Pig and from *Electrophorus electricus*

The activities of the PDH complex and of succinate dehydrogenase were measured as described elsewhere (24, 25). The ratios were calculated from the means of a total of 4 to 12 determinations for each tissue. The S.E.M. values were 5 to 25%. N.D.: not determined.

	Pyruvate Dehydrogenase/ Succinate Dehydrogenase	
	Electric Eel	Pig
Liver	0.065	0.042
Kidney	0.059	0.021
Brain	0.160	N.D.
Adrenal medulla	N.D.	0.423
Electric organ	0.639	N.D.

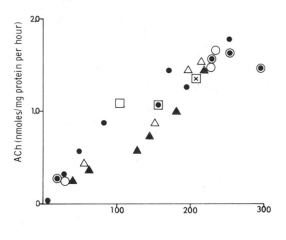

Figure 4. Inhibition of conversion of [2-¹⁴C] pyruvic acid to acetylcholine and to ¹⁴CO₂ in rat brain minces. Minced rat brain was incubated in a modified Krebs-Ringer solution containing 31 mM K⁺ and 5 mM sodium [2-¹⁴C]pyruvate, and radioactive acetylcholine and ¹⁴CO₂ were collected and measured as described by Gibson et al. (35, 36). Each value is the mean of at least two experiments done in triplicate. The inhibitors were as follows: ●, bromopyruvic acid; ▲, 2-oxobutyrate; ○, pentobarbital; ⊙, amobarbital; □, 2-oxo-3-methylpentanoic acid; △, 2-oxo-4-methylpentonoic acid; ⊡, 2-oxo-3-methylbutanoic acid; ⊠, leucine.

Dr. Gary Gibson and Dr. Richard Jope have directly examined the effects of decreased PDH activity on the metabolism of rat brain, by adding various inhibitors to minced brains respiring in buffered salines (Fig. 4). One remarkable finding was a direct relationship between the inhibition of pyruvate oxidation and that of ACh synthesis (35, 36). For instance, a concentration of bromopyruvate that inhibited pyruvate oxidation by 5% reduced ACh synthesis by 7%, even though less than 1% of the pyruvate metabolized went to ACh. This relationship has held persistently whether ACh was measured radiochemically or by gas-liquid chromatography–mass spectrometry; whether CO₂ production was followed from [1-¹⁴C]pyruvate, [2-¹⁴C]pyruvate, or [U-¹⁴C]glucose; and whether oxidation was inhibited by bromopyruvate—an irreversible inhibitor of PDH (37), by 2-oxobutyric acid—a competitive inhibitor and alternate substrate of PDH (8, 38), or in a variety of other and less direct ways (35, 36). Gibson and Jope have now tested more than 15 inhibitors, and these observations are being extended to more physiological systems. Over the last 30 years, there have been a variety of studies showing ACh synthesis and/or cholinergic transmission to be particularly sensitive to impairment of carbohydrate oxidation in various species, *in vivo* and *in vitro,* by chemical and by physiological measurements (39–44). Studies of PDC deficiency have thus led to the general question of the relationship of abnormal carbohydrate metabolism to brain disease. This problem, which was investigated decades ago, is now being re-examined in many laboratories (28, 45, 46).

4. Other Thiamine-Requiring Enzymes

Finally, it is of interest that inherited anomalies have been described in other thiamine-requiring enzymes. Anomalies of the system synthesizing thiamine triphosphate are discussed by Dr. Cooper in Chapter 24 and those of branched-chain decarboxylases by Dr. Elsas in Chapter 23. We have observed low activity of another thiamine-requiring system, KGDH, in white blood cells from a girl with spinocerebellar disease and cortical atrophy [28 ± 11 pMoles/(min) (mg protein) for 4 samples from the patient, and 173 ± 23 for 19 controls; means ± S. E. M.]. In studies done with Prof. H. McIlwain and Dr. D. Leigh, the activity of transketolase was found to be lower, on the average, in red blood cells from 5 patients with well-treated Korsakoff psychosis than in 21 controls [1.58 ± 0.21 *vs.* 2.77 ± 0.23 nMoles/ (min) (mg protein); mean ± S. E. M.]. In these studies, a spectrophotometric assay for transketolase was used, which gave values about tenfold higher than those recorded previously for human red blood cells. Individual values for the controls and the patients overlapped. Kinetic comparisons may indicate whether or not there is a constitutional abnormality in the transketolase of some patients with Wernicke-Korsakoff syndrome. Variations in transketolase among different individuals would be in accord with the genetic heterogeneity of other proteins (47).

5. Implications and Summary

Presumably, a constitutional abnormality in a particular thiamine-requiring enzyme could predispose to the development of thiamine deficiency. To use an older terminology, such an anomaly would be a molecular *locus minoris resistentiae, i.e.,* a site of least resistance (4). Genetic variations in thiamine-requiring reactions could also alter the physiological effects of thiamine deficiency among different individuals, strains, or species, and be relevant to the general problem of thiamine deficiency.

In summary, this review of PDC deficiency has attempted to document four points. First, there is such a disorder. Second, the enzyme deficiency is in the thiamine-dependent first enzyme of the pyruvate dehydrogenase complex. Third, the pathophysiology of the disorder can be accounted for, in part, in terms of animal experiments on the effects of partial deficiencies of PDC on metabolism both in the whole brain and in specific parts of the brain. In particular, impaired carbohydrate utilization appears to impair the metabolism of at least one neurotransmitter. Finally, there is evidence for anomalies affecting each of the thiamine-requiring enzyme systems. Such anomalies could influence the effects of dietary thiamine deficiency in individual patients or in groups of animals.

References

1. D. Lonsdale, *New Engl. J. Med.,* **278,** 1235 (1968).
2. D. Lonsdale, W. R. Faulkner, J. W. Price, and R. R. Smeby, *Pediatrics,* **43,** 1025 (1969).
3. J. P. Blass, J. Avigan, and B. W. Uhlendorf, *J. Clin. Invest.,* **48,** 1033 (1970).
4. J. P. Blass, R. A. P. Kark, and W. K. Engel, *Arch. Neurol.,* **24,** 449 (1971).
5. J. P. Blass, *Int. J. Neurosci.,* **4,** 65 (1972).
6. J. P. Blass, S. D. Cederbaum, and G. E. Gibson, in F. A. Hommes and C. J. Van den Berg, Eds., *Disorders of Energy Metabolism,* John Wiley and Sons, London (in press).
7. L. J. Reed and C. R. Willms, in W. A. Wood, Ed., *Methods Enzymol.,* **9,** 258 (1966).
8. J. P. Blass and C. A. Lewis, *Biochem. J.,* **131,** 31 (1973).
9. J. P. Blass, J. D. Schulman, D. S. Young, and E. Hom, *J. Clin. Invest.,* **51,** 1845 (1972).
10. Y. Sakurai, *Seikagaku,* **42,** 726 (1970).
11. R. M. Denton, H. S. Coore, B. R. Martin, and P. J. Randle, *Nature New Biol.,* **231,** 115 (1971).
12. C. R. Barrera, G. Namahira, L. Hamilton, P. Munk, M. H. Eley, T. C. Linn, and L. J. Reed, *Arch. Biochem. Biophys.,* **148,** 343 (1972).
13. M. Burgett, "Studies on the Regulation of the Mammalian Pyruvate Dehydrogenase Complex," Ph.D. Thesis, University of Texas at Austin (Ann Arbor, Mich., University Microfilms 73-7519), 1972.
14. J. P. Blass and C. A. Lewis, *Biochem. J.,* **131,** 415 (1973).
15. E. Siess, J. Wittman, and O. Wieland, *Z. Physiol. Chem.,* **352,** 447 (1971).
16. D. F. Farrell, A. F. Clark, C. R. Scott, and R. P. Wennberg, *Science* (in press, 1974).
17. J. E. Cremer and H. M. Teal, *FEBS Lett.,* **39,** 17 (1974).
18. J. Land and J. Clark, personal communication.
19. R. S. Jope and J. P. Blass, *Biochem. J.,* **150,** 397 (1975).
20. P. M. Dreyfus and G. Hauser, *Biochim. Biophys. Acta,* **104,** 78 (1965).
21. D. W. McCandless and S. Schenker, *J. Clin. Invest.,* **47,** 2268 (1968).
22. H. McIlwain and H. S. Bachelard, *Biochemistry and the Central Nervous System,* Churchill Livingstone, London, 1971, pp. 125–150.
23. M. K. Gaitonde, *Biochem. J.,* **95,** 803 (1965).
24. S. F. Reynolds, R. Jope, and J. P. Blass, *Proc. Int. Soc. Neurochem.,* **4,** 146 (1973); and article in preparation.

25. S. F. Reynolds, Ph.D. Thesis, Department of Biological Chemistry, UCLA Medical School (in press for *Dissertation Abstracts*).

26. K. H. Kiessling, *Exp. Cell Res.*, **27**, 367 (1962).

27. M. Victor, R. D. Adams, and G. H. Collins, *The Wernicke-Korsakoff Syndrome*, F. A. Davis Company, Philadelphia, 1971.

28. M. Victor, R. D. Adams, and E. L. Mancall, *Arch. Neurol.*, **1**, 579 (1959).

29. B. Ljunggren, K. Norberg, and B. K. Siesjo, *Brain Res.*, **77**, 173 (1974).

30. L. R. Drewes and D. D. Gilboe, *J. Biol. Chem.*, **248**, 2489 (1973).

31. F. M. Yatsu and C. L. Liao, *Trans. Am. Soc. Neurochem.*, **5**, 88 (1974).

32. A. Patel and H. Koenig, *J. Neurochem.*, **18**, 621 (1971).

33. R. Balasz, Y. Michiyama, B. J. Hammond, T. Julian, and D. Richter, *Biochem. J.*, **116**, 445 (1970).

34. S. Tucek and S.-C. Cheng, *J. Neurochem.*, **22**, 893 (1974).

35. G. E. Gibson, R. Jope, and J. P. Blass, *Trans. Am. Soc. Neurochem.*, **5**, 124 (1974).

36. G. E. Gibson, R. Jope, and J. P. Blass, *Biochem. J.*, **148**, 17 (1975).

37. M. E. Maldodano, K.-J. Oh, and P. E. Frey, *J. Biol. Chem.*, **247**, 2711 (1971).

38. T. Kanzaki, T. Hayakawa, M. Hamada, Y. Fukuyoshi, and M. Koike, *J. Biol. Chem.*, **244**, 1183 (1969).

39. V. Perri, O. Sacchi, and C. Casella, *J. Exp. Physiol.*, **55**, 25 (1970).

40. P. LeFresne, P. Guyenet, and J. Glowinski, *J. Neurochem.*, **20**, 1083 (1973).

41. E. T. Browning and M. P. Schulman, *J. Neurochem.*, **15**, 1391 (1968).

42. D. S. Grewaal and J. H. Quastel, *J. Biochem.*, **132**, 1 (1973).

43. P. Guyenet, P. LeFresne, J. Rossiter, J. C. Beaujouan, and J. Glowinski, *Mol. Pharmacol.*, **9**, 63 (1973).

44. M. Dolivo, *Fed. Proc.*, **33**, 1043 (1974).

45. J. Risberg and D. H. Ingvar, *Brain*, **96**, 737 (1973).

46. Unsigned editorial, *Lancet*, **1**, 440 (1974).

47. H. Harris, *Brit. Med. Bull.*, **25**, 5 (1969).

48. R. A. P. Kark, J. P. Blass, and W. K. Engel, *Neurology*, **24**, 964 (1974).

DISCUSSION

Chapter 22

Dr. Fujiwara. I have two questions. First of all, I don't think that there are such patients in Japan. Do you think this is only an inherited disease? Can you tell us the life span of these patients?

Dr. Blass. In answer to the first question, I believe that there are acquired diseases which affect the same enzyme, although we have not shown that clearly yet. One can get inhibition of the enzyme at concentrations of materials that do accumulate in certain times in certain patients, so there may be acquired causes as well. In the patients discussed here, however, the defects appear to be inherited. Dr. Tada in Tohoku University was one of the first to describe a defect in pyruvate carboxylase, another enzyme of pyruvate metabolism. I would not be surprised if patients with PDC deficiency were to be identified in Japan as they are, with increasing frequency, in Europe.

The life span of the children appears to depend on the severity of the enzyme defect. Until 3 years ago, I would have said that they all appear to be living quite happily, but I have just been told about a child with an almost complete deficiency of PDC who died in the first two months of life. If we put together all the patients that we have seen, all that we have been told about, and all that I have heard about vaguely, there are still only 10 or 12 individuals. It is very hard to make generalizations. The young man who came to the National Institutes of Health at the age of 8 is doing extremely well and is in an advanced class in the San Diego schools. One would love to know about the neuropathology in his brain, but only after he has enjoyed a long and happy life. The available data do not indicate what is likely to happen.

Dr. Warnock. Lipids have been said to spare thiamine. Does this therapy have any effect on such patients?

Dr. Blass. Maybe, particularly in patients with what we call lactic acidosis (J. P. Blass, J. D. Schulman, D. S. Young, and E. Hom, *J. Clin. Invest.,* **51,** 1845, 1972). The first patient we saw with that condition was the daughter of a doctor and a nurse. They maintained her on calves' brains, which was a home remedy for brain disease in their ethnic community. On a normal diet, she became even more acidotic. She has died. A second patient was given a 60% carbohydrate diet in preparation for a glucose tolerance test. Over the following 36 hours, he excreted 7 grams of lactate into his urine; his blood pH dropped to just above 7. The sodium bicarbonate required to bring him back into balance made him hypernatremic. He is still active (S. D. Cederbaum, J. P. Blass, and M. E. Cotton, *Clin. Res.,* **21,** 261, 1973; J. P. Blass, S. D. Cederbaum, and G. E. Gibson, in F. A. Hommes and C. J. van den Berg, Eds., *Disorders of Energy Metabolism,* John Wiley and Sons, London, 1975, in press). The third is a patient of Dr. Ron Scott in Seattle. When the child was born, he was put on a low-fat diet and changed from a floppy baby to a crying baby. A ketogenic diet is certainly no panacea; the autopsy studies and the biochemistry on that patient are now in press in *Science.* But it may help some of them.

23. Effect of Thiamine on Normal and Mutant Human Branched-Chain α-Ketoacid Dehydrogenase

LOUIS J. ELSAS, II, M.D.
DEAN J. DANNER, Ph.D.
BARRY L. ROGERS, B.A.

Division of Medical Genetics
Department of Pediatrics
Emory University School of Medicine
Atlanta, Georgia

Organization of the branched-chain α-ketoacid dehydrogenase complex of mammalian systems is based on the Reed-Koike models of mammalian pyruvate and α-ketoglutarate dehydrogenases (1–3). This multienzyme complex occupies an important position in man for the catabolism of the branched-chain amino acids isoleucine, leucine, and valine. The pathway includes first a pyridoxal phosphate-dependent reversible transamination of the L-branched-chain amino acids to their respective α-keto acids. Various degrees of impairment in their subsequent decarboxylation and acylation produce a group of diseases known collectively as maple syrup urine disease, so called for the fragrance produced when the hydroxy derivatives of the branched-chain α-keto acids are present in urine (4–6). It is presumed, on the basis of indirect evidence from Ruediger and Namba, that the coenzymes involved in this reaction include thiamine diphosphate (ThDP), Mg^{2+}, CoASH, NAD^+, lipoic acid, and FAD (7, 8). It is also presumed that three proteins are present: a decarboxylase, which initiates the decarboxylating reaction aided by magnesium and ThDP and accepts the acyl group of the decarboxylated keto acid; a transacylase with covalently bound lipoate, which transfers the acyl group from ThDP to CoA, reducing lipoate; and lipoamide oxidoreductase, a flavoprotein that oxidizes reduced lipoate and uses NAD^+ as the terminal electron acceptor. To date this model has only indirect support in mammalian systems (7).

Debate exists with respect to the presence of a single complex for the three keto acids versus a different complex for each branched-chain keto acid substrate (9). Since all variants of maple syrup urine disease affect decarboxylation of all three substrates, and since they are characterized by an autosomal recessive pattern of transmission, it is presumed that a single mutant gene produces at least one polypeptide which is aberrant and common to the complex for all three substrates (5, 10).

This discussion concerns two children affected by Maple Syrup Urine disease, their *in vivo* response to pharmacologic amounts of oral thiamine, the cofactor requirements and subcellular localization of this enzyme function in cultured skin fibroblasts and hepatic tissue, and a hypothesis for the mechanism by which this thiamine response occurred. The children affected by this disease are currently 8- and 4½-year-old black brothers. The older child is quadriparetic and trainably mentally retarded. He was not diagnosed until aged 7 weeks. His younger brother was diagnosed at birth, placed on an artificial diet restricted in the branched-chain amino acids, and has developed normally (11). He is currently in a public school kindergarten and is learning to read. Skin cultures from both parents and the children were tested *in vitro,* as shown in Table 1, for their ability to convert isoleucine, leucine, and valine to CO_2. Techniques of this culture, harvest,

Table 1. **Branched-Chain Amino Acid Decarboxylation by Cultured Fibroblasts**[a]

Patient	[U-^{14}C] L-Isoleucine,	[1-^{14}C] L-Leucine,	[1-^{14}C] L-Valine,
	dpm $^{14}CO_2$ formed/(90 min) (μg protein)		
Mother	66.4 (6)	118.4 (3)	83.7 (6)
Father	57.3 (6)	102.2 (3)	38.9 (9)
Older brother	2.3 (3)	5.9 (3)	2.6 (3)
Younger brother	2.2 (3)	7.5 (3)	3.2 (3)
Normal	81.6 ± 6.1 (16)	101.0 ± 8.3 (20)	75.5 ± 8.3 (25)

[a] Skin fibroblasts were obtained and assayed from Pedigree Car in February 1971 at from 4 to 20 population doublings in culture.

Table 2.   Reduction in Urinary Branched-Chain α-Keto Acid Excretion in Older Brother after Oral Thiamine Administration

Oral Thiamine, mg/day	Urinary α-Keto Acids, mg/24 hr	
	KIC	KMV
Base line	199 ± 80 (3)	194 ± 18 (3)
50	81 ± 21 (3)	79 ± 20 (3)
100	66 ± 38 (3)	79 ± 36 (3)
150	34 ± 19 (3)	42 ± 19 (3)

and assay system have been described previously (10). Cells from both affected brothers had 2 to 7% of normal decarboxylating activity for all three amino acids. There was no consistent impairment of branched-chain amino acid decarboxylation in cell lines derived from the parents. Thus heterozygotes in this family were not discriminated from controls by these methods.

Scriver et al. demonstrated that another patient with the intermediate variant of this disorder who had approximately 50% of normal activity was responsive to pharmacologic doses of thiamine (12). We decided to evaluate thiamine responsivity in these two affected brothers. The children were admitted to the Clinical Research Unit at Emory University, where several *in vivo* parameters of the disorder were monitored while the patients were maintained on their branched-chain amino acid restricted diet. This diet contains 2.4 mg thiamine/day. They were given increasing doses of thiamine over a 1-month period, as shown in Table 2. Each dose was maintained for 1 week. Results are depicted as the mean and standard deviations of three 24-hour urine specimens obtained during each condition from the older brother. The branched-chain α-keto acids were extracted from the urine and measured by gas-liquid chromatography of their methyl esters as described previously (10). Excretion of α-ketoisocaproic acid (KIC) and α-keto-β-methylvaleric acid (KMV), which averaged 200 mg/24 hr, fell progressively as thiamine administration increased.

In addition to this fall in urinary keto acid excretion, white blood cells isolated from the boys' blood displayed an increase in branched-chain amino acid decarboxylating activity, as shown in Table 3. White blood cells were isolated midway through the period of thiamine administration from 10 to 20 ml of heparinized blood as described previously (10). The cells were

Table 3. Increase in Branched-Chain Amino Acid Decarboxylating Activity (BCAA) in Older Brother after Thiamine Administration

Oral Thiamine, mg	White Blood Cell BCAA Decarboxylase Activity, % of normal control		
	Isoleucine	Leucine	Valine
Base line	5.5	2.3	4.7
50	9.3	25.0	12.2
100	7.6	14.4	19.6
150	23.0	16.6	25.7

washed and resuspended in Krebs phosphate buffer. The $^{14}CO_2$ produced from radiolabeled branched-chain amino acids was compared with that of an adult control who was not taking thiamine. The data are expressed as percentages of this normal control activity. The base-line decarboxylating activity in these uncultured peripheral cells for both affected children was approximately the same as is found in cultured skin fibroblasts, i.e., between 2 and 5% of normal activity. After administration of thiamine in large doses, activity rose to 23, 16.6, and 25.7% of control in the older brother's cells for isoleucine, leucine, and valine, respectively.

This *in vivo* effect of thiamine was also tested in three controls who were matched with respect to age, size, and general physical condition. Their nutritional status at home had included vitamin supplements (One-A-Day) before this study. They were given 150 mg thiamine/day for 3 weeks. Two of the control children had cerebral palsy from other causes. The results are shown in Fig. 1, where the patients' initials (R. G. M., J. W., and J. B.) are listed below bar graphs representing their white blood cell branched-chain amino acid decarboxylation activities as percentages of the activity of the same adult control, who did not receive additional thiamine. Open bars represent prethiamine activity; stippled bars show the activity after administration of thiamine for 3 weeks. Despite individual variations the white blood cells of the three children showed increased decarboxylating activity for all three branched-chain amino acids after 3 weeks of treatment with these pharmacologic levels of thiamine. This thiamine program also increased their tolerance to isoleucine loading.

The results of isoleucine tolerance tests in these three control patients are demonstrated in Fig. 2. This graph represents the results of two different isoleucine tolerance tests in each patient, in which 150 mg isoleucine/kg

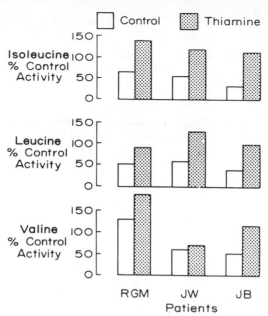

Figure 1. Branched-chain amino acid decarboxylating activity by white blood cells isolated from controls before and after 3 weeks of thiamine administration.

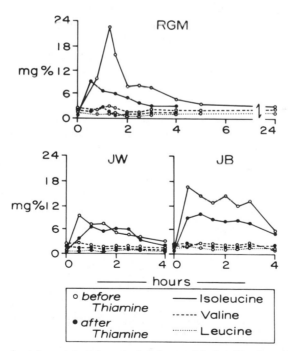

Figure 2. Isoleucine tolerance tests in controls before and during thiamine administration.

body weight was given *per ora*. Plasma levels of isoleucine, leucine, and valine, measured by ion-exchange chromatography, are plotted at the time points indicated on the abscissa. Note that maximal levels of blood isoleucine reached were higher before thiamine (indicated by open circles) than after thiamine (closed circles). If one calculates and compares the areas under the two curves, there are 87, 15, and 68% decreases in the level and duration of plasma isoleucine reached after prolonged thiamine administration in R. G. M., J. W., and J. B., respectively. These data in controls suggest that thiamine in some way enhances the utilization of isoleucine.

We then turned to the rat to see whether chronic pharmacologic amounts of thiamine would directly enhance the conversion of isoleucine's branched-chain keto acid, α-keto-β-methylvaleric acid, to CO_2. We measured the effects of parenteral thiamine administration *in vivo* on the rat's ability to produce $^{14}CO_2$ from [1-^{14}C]α-keto-β-methylvaleric. As shown in Table 4, seven littermate, male, Sprague-Dawley rats were kept on a constant Purina Chow diet. One group (ThPD-treated) was given 5 mg of thiamine propyl disulfide intraperitoneally for 8 days. This lipid-soluble thiamine derivative, whose therapeutic efficacy has been studied by Nose et al., was kindly provided by Takeda Industries of Japan (13). An age- and weight-matched control was given normal saline. Each animal was placed in a closed metabolic chamber. Expired $^{14}CO_2$ was trapped in hyamine after the injection into his tail vein of 1 mM [1-^{14}C]α-keto-β-methylvaleric, which we synthesized by previously described techniques (14). Two points should be made. First, thiamine did not alter the growth characteristics of these

Table 4. α-Keto-β-Methylvaleric Acid Decarboxylation *in Vivo* by Rats: Effect of Thiamine PropylDisulfide (ThPD)

Animal Pair	ThPD-Treated,[a] %/g	Weight, grams	Controls,[a] %/g	Weight, grams
1	0.281	135.1	0.218	157.7
2	0.225	195.1	0.194	206.2
3	0.253	233.2	0.208	226.5
4	0.288	181.1	—	—
	$\bar{X} = 0.262 \pm 0.029$		$\bar{Y} = 0.207 \pm 0.012$	

[a] The unit "%/gm" indicates the percentage of [1-^{14}C] α-keto-β-methylvaleric acid injected which was recovered in 1 hour as $^{14}CO_2$ per gram of animal weight.

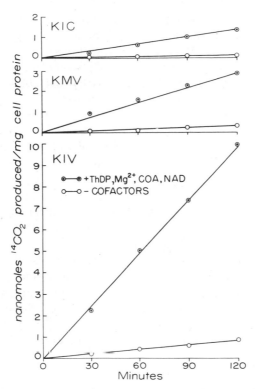

Figure 3. Reconstitution of branched-chain α-ketoacid dehydrogenase in a broken cell suspension of normal cultured skin fibroblasts.

animals, as is indicated by similar weight gains in both groups. Second, for each pair the percentage of $^{14}CO_2$ recovered was higher in the thiamine-treated animal than in his control; the treated animals averaged approximately 26% more $^{14}CO_2$ production. This was significant at the 95% probability level using paired t tests. These data for both man and rat suggest that chronic high doses of thiamine *in vivo* enhance the conversion of branched-chain amino acids and their keto acid derivatives to CO_2.

We then turned to cultured human skin fibroblasts, which reflect the genetic defects in branched-chain α-ketoacid dehydrogenase, to determine coenzyme requirements. We first studied a broken cell suspension of normal cultured skin fibroblasts in which decarboxylating activity required the presence of coenzymes for reconstitution, as shown in Fig. 3. Cells were grown to confluence in 690-cm² Belco disposable roller bottles, harvested, frozen in dry ice and acetone, and then thawed in 50 mM Tris-HCl 0.2 mM EDTA at pH 7.5. Reactions were initiated by the addition of 1 mM

[1-^{14}C]α-ketoisocaproate (KIC), [1-^{14}C]α-keto-β-methylvalerate (KMV), or [1-^{14}C]α-ketoisovalerate (KIV). The nanomoles of $^{14}CO_2$ released are plotted on the ordinate. Very low to absent base-line activity was seen without added cofactors (open circles). Optimum cofactor requirements were then established. When 0.2 mM CoASH and NAD$^+$ and 0.15 mM ThDP and Mg^{2+} were added (dotted circles), activity was markedly increased and was linear over a 2-hour incubation period. Reconstituted activity was linear over cell protein concentrations of 60 to 600 μg per reaction. Control systems for each buffer and with ceric sulfate and H_2O_2 were run in each experiment to establish base-line activity and to quantitate recovery of $^{14}CO_2$ from our synthesized substrates. Quantitative differences in activity for these substrates were seen, with lessening activity for KIV, KMV, and KIC, respectively. All membranes, including mitochondrial, were disrupted by freeze-thawing in hypotonic Tris, thus making possible the reconstitution experiments described here.

Cofactor requirements as well as relative activity also differed among the three substrates when CoASH and NAD$^+$ or ThDP and Mg^{2+} were added separately, as shown in Table 5. Added cofactors are indicated in the column heads, with the fully reconstituted system in the last column. Addition of Mg^{2+}, ThDP, CoASH, or NAD$^+$ singly failed to return activity. Activity above the base line in nanomoles $^{14}CO_2$/(mg cell protein)

Table 5. Coenzyme Requirements for Branched-Chain α-Ketoacid Dehydrogenase in Freeze-Thawed Skin Fibroblasts[a]

	ThDP/Mg^{2+},	CoASH/NAD,	ThDP/Mg^{2+} and CoASH/NAD,
	nM $^{14}CO_2$/(60 min)(mg protein)		
[1-^{14}C] α-KIV			
Mutants (13)	0	0	0
Controls (34)	0	1.76	3.92
[1-^{14}C] α-KIC			
Mutants (5)	0	0	0
Controls (13)	0	2.15	2.86
[1-^{14}C] α-KMV			
Mutants (8)	0.74	0	1.09
Controls (19)	0.53	0.39	1.71

[a] Numbers in parentheses indicate numbers of observations in two mutant cell lines and four control cell lines.

(60 min) is depicted for both control lines and cells, designated "mutant," derived from the two brothers with maple syrup urine disease. Notice first the qualitative difference in cofactor requirements among the substrates. In control cells ThDP and Mg^{2+} alone failed to reconstitute KIV and KIC activity, whereas CoASH and NAD alone reconstituted 45% of KIV and 75% of KIC activity. In control cells ThDP and Mg^{2+} alone reconstituted 30% of KMV activity, whereas CoASH and NAD reconstituted 23%. More importantly, note that in the mutant cell lines cofactors either singly or in concert failed to return decarboxylating function for either KIV or KIC. By contrast, KMV decarboxylating activity in mutant cells was similar to that in controls in the presence of ThDP and Mg^{2+} alone, but was absent in the presence of CoASH and NAD alone. This $ThDP/Mg^{2+}$ stimulable KMV decarboxylase function was saturable and was present in mutant cells over a wide substrate range. When 1.0 mM [1-^{14}C]pyruvate was used as substrate, similar cofactor requirements for reconstitution were found. Activity was 6 times that observed when KIV was used as substrate. More importantly, control and mutant cell lines had identical activity, clearly delineating separate genetic control for pyruvate and branched-chain α-ketoacid dehydrogenase function.

Several hypothetical models regarding the mutation in this family can be made from these data. Since the mutation affects the decarboxylation of all three substrates, at least one polypeptide must be common to the branched-chain α-ketoacid dehydrogenase complex for all three substrates. There are, however, qualitative differences in cofactor requirement and absolute activity among the three substrates. One hypothetical model assumes that surface decarboxylases have different affinities for their substrates and are oriented around a core of transacylases which could influence their affinities for the three substrates through protein-protein and enzyme-coenzyme interaction. With this model, the presence of normal ThDP and Mg^{2+} reconstituted KMV decarboxylase in the mutant cells suggests that the mutation affects a core transacylase rather than the surface decarboxylase. It is relevant that freeze-thawed preparations of heterozygous cells in this family were successfully discriminated from control cells when reconstituted by CoASH and NAD^+ alone at low (0.01 mM) substrate concentrations.

To solve these hypothetical models, better resolution of this enzyme complex is needed. Initial attempts at solubilization of activity from fibroblasts were unsuccessful. As an alternative method, subcellular fractionation was undertaken, as shown in Table 6. In these experiments cells were mass-produced in roller bottles, harvested with trypsin, and pelleted to between 1 and 2 grams of wet weight. Whole cells were suspended in a 0.27 M mannitol, 1.0 mM Tris-HCl, 0.1 mM EDTA buffer at pH 7.3 to a volume of 10 ml per 0.4 gram of wet weight. The cell

Table 6. Subcellular Distribution of KMV Dehydrogenase in Cultured Human Skin Fibroblasts

Cell Fraction	Specific Activity, nM CO_2/(30 min)(mg)
Whole homogenate	1.05
Mitochondrial	2.24
Inner membrane	8.50
Outer membrane	0.00
Microsomal + cytosol	0.00

suspension was then treated with 0.1 mg protease/ml buffer for 7 minutes at 0° according to the method of Millis, and the homogenate was doubled in volume with mannitol-Tris-EDTA buffer (15). Nuclear material and undisrupted cells were removed by centrifugation at 700 × g. The supernatant was then subjected to 12 minutes of centrifugation at 10,000 × g, which produced the mitochondrial pellet and microsomal + cytosol fraction. No activity was found in the microsomal + cytosol fraction. Inner membrane matrix particles were prepared by a modification of the method of Schnaitmann and Greenawalt, using 1 mg recrystallized digitonin/mg mitochondrial protein (16). The solution was centrifuged at 10,000 × g for 15 minutes. The pellet contained inner membrane matrix and was resuspended in mannitol-Tris-EDTA at 60 to 200 μg protein/250 μl reaction. The supernatant contained outer membrane fragments. Although Johnson and Connelly had reported 3 to 8% of activity in a soluble fraction, we found all branched-chain α-ketoacid decarboxylase activity in the mitochondrial inner membrane (17). These procedures produced an 8.5-fold increase in specific activity based on whole homogenate. The mitochondrial inner membrane preparation was used in subsequent experiments.

Unfortunately these inner mitochondrial membrane particles from fibroblasts were quite unstable in our Tris-EDTA buffer system, as shown in Fig. 4. On the ordinate are the results of enzyme activity in nanomoles CO_2 per milligram per 15 minutes for the three substrates KIV, KMV, and KIC, as expressed by mitochondrial inner membrane derived from the normal (white bars) or from the mutant (black bars) cell lines. On the abscissa are the minutes of incubation in buffer at 37°C that preceded the enzyme assay. To the left are the results obtained without added cofactors; to the right (stippling), those obtained when ThDP and magnesium were added to the buffer. The ThDP and Mg^{2+} had little effect on the loss of either KIV or KIC decarboxylating activity in normal or mutant cells but did stabilize KMV decarboxylating function. Here, rather than a fall to the base line as expressed for KIV and KIC, approximately 50% of control activity was preserved after 100 minutes of prior incubation in thiamine and magnesium. The mutant cell line which had 25% of normal activity at 5 minutes of preincubation had the same activity as did normal cells after 100 minutes of incubation when ThDP and Mg^{2+} were added to the buffer. These data demonstrate a stabilizing effect of ThDP and Mg^{2+} on both normal and mutant KMV decarboxylating activity, which is apparently selective for that substrate in mitochondrial inner membrane from cultured skin fibroblasts.

The mutant ThDP/Mg^{2+}-stabilized KMV decarboxylating activity shared several characteristics with the normal enzyme. Both pH optima were between 7.2 and 7.6. Heats of inactivation were similar in normal and mutant cells. Thirty percent inactivation was found at 40° for 10 minutes, and complete inactivation at 50°. This KMV decarboxylating activity in

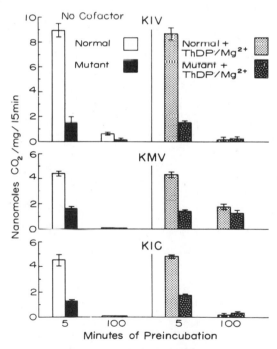

Figure 4. Instability of branched-chain α-ketoacid dehydrogenase in mitochondrial inner membrane from normal and mutant cultured skin fibroblasts. Stabilization by ThDP/Mg^{2+} of KMV dehydrogenase.

mutant mitochondrial membrane was not due to a pyruvate dehydrogenase, since addition of 1 mM ATP selectively deactivated pyruvate dehydrogenase without affecting KMV decarboxylation by either normal or mutant mitochondrial membranes.

There was a difference in the kinetic characteristics of the normal and mutant KMV decarboxylase. The mutant cells had a reduced apparent V_{max} of 2 nmoles/(mg) (15 min), as compared to 10 in the normal cells. An apparent K_m of 1 mM for KMV decarboxylation was similar in mitochondrial inner membrane from both normal and mutant fibroblasts.

At this point we could not demonstrate a direct *in vitro* effect of ThDP/Mg^{2+} on normal or mutant branched-chain α-ketoacid dehydrogenase in mitochondrial inner membrane from cultured skin fibroblasts. We then turned to mitochondria isolated from human liver biopsy material. As shown in Fig. 5, the mitochondrial inner membrane

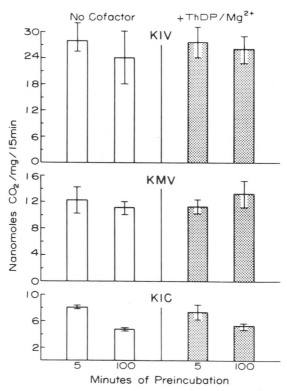

Figure 5. Stability of branched-chain α-ketoacid dehydrogenase in mitochondrial inner membrane from normal human liver.

Table 7. Thiamine Stabilization of Branched-Chain α-Ketoacid Dehydrogenase in Human Hepatic Mitochondrial Inner Membranes[a]

Oral Thiamine	KIV,	KMV, nM $^{14}CO_2/(mg)$ (15 min)	KIC,
Base line (6)	18.92 ± 5.34	9.53 ± 2.15	8.25 ± 2.73
5–7 days (9)	19.84 ± 3.90	8.38 ± 2.24	6.88 ± 1.24
18–28 days (3)	35.29 ± 6.96	12.79 ± 2.65	14.89 ± 2.61

[a] Numbers in parentheses indicate number of patients in each category. (See reference number 18).

from normal human liver obtained at surgery for diagnostic purposes was more stable and had 2 to 3 times more activity than did membranes from fibroblasts. With this preparation we were able to show stoichiometry between CO_2 production and NAD^+ reduction (18). The bars to the left represent mitochondrial inner membrane activity for decarboxylation of KIV, KMV, and KIC from three control biopsies, each measured in triplicate at 5 and 100 minutes of preincubation. To the right are the same specimens assayed when ThDP and Mg^{2+} were added to the medium. No significant *in vitro* effects of added ThDP and Mg^{2+} were observed in these liver membranes. We had demonstrated, therefore, an *in vitro* requirement for ThDP, Mg^{2+}, CoASH, and NAD^+ only in the reconstitution of freeze-thawed whole-cell preparations. Except for stabilization of KMV decarboxylation in the unstable fibroblast inner mitochondrial membrane, ThDP and Mg^{2+} caused no direct augmentation of enzyme activity.

How, then, did thiamine produce its observed *in vivo* effects in both control patients and patients affected by maple syrup urine disease? An answer to this question was sought by comparing the specific activities of branched-chain α-ketoacid dehydrogenase from hepatic inner mitochondrial membrane obtained from patients homozygous normal for branched-chain α-ketoacid dehydrogenase before and during prolonged ingestion of pharmacologic doses of thiamine. The results are shown in Table 7. In this table, CO_2 produced from KIV, KMV and KIC in nanomoles per milligram per 15 minutes is expressed as the mean and standard deviation for each of three experimental conditions: six patients receiving no added thiamine; nine patients receiving 100 mg/day of thiamine for 5 to 7 days; and three patients receiving this amount of thiamine for 18 to 28 days. The specific activity was similar for both base-line conditions and for patients receiving thiamine for less than 7 days. However, 89%, 34%, and 80% increases in the specific activity of KIV, KMV, and KIC decarboxylation, respectively, were seen in hepatic mitochondrial inner membrane from patients treated for more than 18 days. This difference is significant at confidence limits of 99.9% or better (18).

We conclude that pharmacologic amounts of thiamine given over a 3-week period will increase *in vivo* utilization of branched-chain amino acids by both control patients and patients homozygous for maple syrup urine disease, that this effect is directly related to increased activity of a proposed branched-chain α-ketoacid dehydrogenase complex, and that ThDP and Mg^{2+} do not directly augment dehydrogenase of either fibroblast or hepatic mitochondrial inner membrane. Therefore the increased hepatic enzyme specific activity seen after prolonged administration of thiamine results from an increase in either the biological half-life or the rate of synthesis of the enzyme complex.

Acknowledgments

These studies were supported by U.S. Public Health Service research grants: NICHD grant HD-06416, Research Career Development Award HD-35,615 (Dr. Elsas), and Clinical Research Center grant RR-00039, and by gifts from the local United Airlines Stewardess Clipped Wings Association and the National Foundation-March of Dimes.

References

1. L. J. Reed, *Adv. Enzymol.*, **18**, 319 (1957).
2. H. Fernandez-Moran, L. J. Reed, M. Koike, and C. R. Willms, *Science*, **145**, 930 (1964).
3. M. Koike, L. J. Reed, and W. R. Carroll, *J. Biol. Chem.*, **235**, 1924 (1960).
4. J. H. Menkes, P. L. Hurst, and J. M. Craig, *Pediatrics*, **14**, 462 (1954).
5. J. Dancis, J. Hutzler, and T. Rokkones, *New Engl. J. Med.*, **276**, 84 (1967).
6. J. D. Schulman, T. J. Lustberg, U. L. Kennedy, M. Museles, and J. E. Seegmiller, *Am. J. Med.*, **49**, 118 (1970).
7. H. W. Ruediger, U. Langenbeck, D. Brackertz, and H. W. Goedde, *Biochim. Biophys. Acta*, **264**, 220 (1972).
8. Y. Namba, K. Yoshizawa, A. Ejima, T. Hayashi, and T. Kaneda, *J. Biol. Chem.*, **244**, 4437 (1969).
9. J. L. Connelly, D. J. Danner, and J. A. Bowden, *J. Biol. Chem.*, **243**, 1198 (1968).
10. L. J. Elsas, B. A. Pask, F. B. Wheeler, D. P. Perl, and S. Trusler, *Metabolism*, **21**, 929 (1972).
11. S. E. Snyderman, *Am. J. Dis. Child.*, **113**, 68 (1967).
12. C. R. Scriver, S. Mackenzie, C. L. Clow, and E. Delvin, *Lancet*, **i**, 310 (1971).

13. Y. Nose and A. Iwashima, *J. Vitam.* (Kyoto), **11**, 165 (1965).

14. L. J. Elsas, J. H. Priest, F. B. Wheeler, D. J. Danner, and B. A. Pask, *Metabolism,* **23**, 569 (1974).

15. A. J. T. Millis and D. A. Pious, *Biochim. Biophys. Acta,* **292**, 73 (1973).

16. C. Schnaitman and J. W. Greenawalt, *J. Cell. Biol.,* **38**, 158 (1968).

17. W. A. Johnson and J. L. Connelly, *Biochemistry,* **11**, 1967 (1972).

18. D. J. Danner, E. D. Davidson, and L. J. Elsas, *Nature,* **254**, 529 (1975).

DISCUSSION

Chapter 23

Dr. Kark. If you treat patients with high doses of thiamine and then return them to a normal diet, how long does it take the enzyme levels in the white blood cells to return to pretreatment values? Or has the analogous experiment been done with fibroblasts?

Dr. Elsas. We have only preliminary data on one control and the two affected brothers. We discontinued thiamine and retested 3 weeks later. White blood cell enzyme activity was still greater than before treatment in all three. The question of the biological half-life of this enzyme complex is extremely difficult to answer at this point. We would have to label a protein of the multienzyme complex and follow its biological half-life.

24. Subacute Necrotizing Encephalomyelopathy

J. R. COOPER, Ph.D.
J. H. PINCUS, M.D.

Departments of Pharmacology and Neurology
Yale University School of Medicine
New Haven, Connecticut

Subacute necrotizing encephalomyelopathy (SNE), or Leigh's disease, is a fatal, genetic (autosomal recessive), neurological disease first described in 1951. In the majority of cases, the symptomatology of the disease starts before the age of 2 years and is characterized by a large variability in the clinical picture. Feeding problems, weakness, visual disturbances, ataxia, convulsions, swallowing difficulties, and peripheral neuropathy—all have been reported in different combinations. Until recently, the diagnosis of SNE has rested entirely on autopsy findings of necrotizing lesions, mainly in the midbrain and lower brain-stem regions, the spinal cord, and the basal ganglia. These lesions are almost identical to those seen in Wernicke's encephalopathy, the classical thiamine deficiency disease. The major differences are that in SNE the mammillary bodies are almost never involved, while the substantia nigra and basal ganglia are usually lesioned, whereas the reverse is true in Wernicke's encephalopathy. However, because of the similarities of the lesions in the two diseases, some clinicians have suspected that SNE represents aberrant thiamine metabolism, despite the findings that patients with SNE have normal thiamine levels in their blood and normal thiamine diphosphate (ThDP)-dependent enzyme activities in the brain. Furthermore, the administration of moderate amounts of thiamine to patients with SNE has no ameliorating effect on their clinical status.

Our interest in SNE came about in a somewhat indirect fashion. For the past several years we have been pursuing the hypothesis that thiamine has a role in nervous tissue that is distinct from its function as a coenzyme in intermediary metabolism. At the same time that we were examining this hypothesis, we were also engaged in the isolation and characterization of the enzymes involved in thiamine metabolism. We partially purified thiamine diphosphatase and thiamine triphosphatase from brain, but, more importantly, as will be shown, we found the enzyme system in brain that catalyzes the synthesis of thiamine triphosphate (ThTP) from ThDP. This enzyme, found also in liver, kidney, and heart, is referred to as a ThDP-ATP phosphoryltransferase and plays a major part in our understanding of SNE.

Shortly after our identification of the phosphoryltransferase, a patient was admitted to the Yale-New Haven Hospital who apparently had SNE, since she showed symptomatology identical to that of her sister, who had died about a year previously and in whom SNE had been diagnosed on histological grounds. In an attempt to see whether we could uncover any relationship between thiamine and SNE, we tested the blood, urine, and cerebrospinal fluid (CSF) of this patient against the enzyme systems involved in thiamine phosphate metabolism. We found that minute amounts (0.1 ml) of these body fluids markedly inhibited the phosphoryltransferase activity of rat brain, whereas normal blood, urine, or CSF had absolutely no effect. The "inhibitor" that is present in the fluids is nondialyzable, unstable, and extractable into chloroform-methanol. Our current impression is that it may be either a lipid or a proteolipid. Since the inhibitor prevents the synthesis of ThDP, it could be inferred that the patient had a deficiency of ThTP in her brain. When the child died, we examined her brain, liver, and kidney for thiamine phosphate content. In all tissues the total thiamine content was normal, as was the percentage of ThDP, thiamine monophosphate (ThMP), and free thiamine. However, although her liver and kidney had the usual content of ThTP, this compound was absent from her brain. Thus, although all these tissues contain phosphoryltransferase, the inhibitor affected only the brain enzyme. Since this finding we have had the opportunity to examine the brains of five other patients who died of SNE, and in each case a deficiency of ThTP was noted as compared to control brains. A rough correlation was also observed between the severity of the lesion in specific areas of the brain and the ThTP content.

With the observation of the inhibition of ThTP synthesis from the urine of patients with SNE, we now had a possibly useful diagnostic test for the disease. Since 1968 we have tested over 500 urine samples from medical centers in North America, Europe, and Asia and now have a fairly clear picture of the specificity of this diagnostic assay.

The overall rate of false positives is about 6%; to date we have encountered one false negative, although the histological data on which the diagnosis of SNE was made are not yet available to us. We have found that the inhibitor is not detectable in amniotic fluid, so that amniocentesis cannot be used to predict the development of SNE. In addition, the presence of the inhibitor in parents of afflicted children is variable so that the urine test is of limited value is identifying carriers.

When patients with SNE are treated with large daily doses of either thiamine or a derivative of the vitamin, thiamine tetrahydrofurfural disulfide, a marked improvement in their clinical status is observed after about 5 weeks on the regimen. This improvement can be maintained for variable periods, ranging from 3 months to 2 years, and is correlated with the CSF level of thiamine. Most patients, however, become refractory after a time, so that, regardless of the dose of the vitamin administered, the CSF level of thiamine cannot be maintained at the level obtained when treatment was initiated. This finding suggests either that large doses of the vitamin may induce an enzyme that destroys thiamine or that transport of thiamine into the brain has been affected. A curious finding has been that, once patients are on thiamine therapy, we can no longer detect this inhibitor in their urine.

In determining the thiamine content in different brain areas, we uncovered a possible explanation for the histological lesions in the mammillary bodies in Wernicke's encephalopathy. Whereas in children affected by SNE the thiamine content in various regions of the brain ranges from 0.4 to 1.8 μg/g, in the mammillary bodies the range is from 6 to 8 μg/g. Furthermore, on thiamine therapy the level in the mammillary bodies rises to 30 μg/g, whereas the content in other areas of the brain (e.g., cerebellum, cortex, and pons) increases only to 1 to 3 μg/g. The mammillary bodies therefore seem to be outside the blood-brain barrier in that they have a high thiamine content under normal circumstances which can be raised even higher on thiamine therapy. Since they can be easily repleted with the vitamin, it follows that they can just as readily be depleted on a thiamine-deficient diet. Thus in Wernicke's encephalopathy, a thiamine-deficiency disease, it is easy to understand why the mammillary bodies are heavily involved.

Our current studies on SNE involve the isolation and identification of the inhibitor and a determination of its interaction with the phosphoryltransferase that catalyzes the synthesis of ThTP.

References

1. J. R. Cooper, Y. Itokawa, and J. H. Pincus, *Science,* **164,** 72 (1969).

2. J. H. Pincus, Y. Itokawa, and J. R. Cooper, *Neurology,* **19,** 841 (1969).

3. J. R. Cooper, J. H. Pincus, Y. Itokawa, Y. Hashitani, and K. Piros, *N. Engl. J. Med.,* **283,** 793 (1970).

4. J. H. Pincus, G. B. Solitaire, Y. Itokawa, Y. Hashitani, and J. R. Cooper, *Neurology,* **21,** 444 (1971).

5. J. H. Pincus, *Develop. Med. Child Neurol.,* **14,** 87 (1972).

6. J. H. Pincus, J. R. Cooper, J. V. Murphy, E. F. Rabe, D. Lonsdale, and H. G. Dunn, *Pediatrics,* **51,** 716 (1973).

7. J. H. Pincus, J. R. Cooper, K. Piros, and V. Turner, *Neurology,* **24,** 885 (1974).

DISCUSSION

Chapter 24

Dr. Dreyfus. I have been following a family afflicted with Leigh's encephalopathy. The diagnosis was established at postmortem examination in an older sibling who died before the diagnosis was established clinically. This child's younger brother, age 4 years, has been followed by us since early infancy, and the hallmarks of the disease (i.e., ophthalmoplegia, ataxia, and peripheral neuropathy) were detected at about 2 years of age. Urine samples sent to Dr. Pincus' laboratories before the patient was given large doses of thiamine failed to reveal the inhibitory factor. Possibly the inhibitory factor was destroyed by the transport of the urine from California to Connecticut. There is, of course, a distinct possibility that the second child is suffering from a variant of Leigh's encephalopathy. As you know, a variety of biochemical lesions have been demonstrated in this disease. A year or two ago, Dr. Lardy, from the University of Wisconsin, published the findings in a child afflicted with Leigh's disease. He demonstrated elevated levels of lactic acid and pyruvate and low levels of cholesterol in the blood in the absence of pyruvate carboxylase in the liver. When he placed the child on large doses of glutamate and vitamin B$_6$, improvement ensued, suggesting that oxaloacetate had been formed by an alternative metabolic route. It is entirely possible that patients afflicted with pyruvate carboxylase deficiency do not show the inhibitor and that their thiamine triphosphate levels in the brain are normal.

Recently, Dr. O'Brien's laboratories in La Jolla indicated that they had observed decreased levels of pyruvic decarboxylase activity in the fibroblasts of children presumably afflicted with Leigh's encephalopathy. A skin biopsy from our child and one from his mother have been sent to Dr. O'Brien's laboratories for determinations of pyruvic decarboxylase activity in cultured fibroblasts. As yet the results of these tests are not available. Perhaps Dr. O'Brien's patients represent yet another variety of the same syndrome. Perhaps Dr. Cooper would like to comment on this particular point.

Dr. Cooper. One possibility is something rather curious that we have run into: on at least three occasions we have had a urine sample from a sibling of a patient who had died of SNE, and the sibling seemed to have the same symptoms, according to the pediatrician, but we could not find the inhibitor. It turned out that when these patients died they had some other disease but not SNE. The second point is, in terms of the syndrome, that one of the instances where we have found the inhibitor is in the genetic form of "Ondine's curse," primary alveolar hypoventilation, and for those of you who are a little weak on mythology I should explain what this is. Ondine was a nymph who fell in love with a mortal; the mortal unfortunately fell in love with another mortal, so Ondine put a curse on him, saying that he would be perfectly normal except when he went to sleep, in which case he would not be able to breathe. This is the situation with Ondine's curse. These patients are perfectly normal except when they go to bed at night. They either have to be put on a tilt bed to keep their diaphragm going or to be implanted with a phrenic nerve pacemaker. We have had a total of five patients with Ondine's curse. Ondine's curse, by the way, is a syndrome, not a disease, and there are other ways in which one can get primary alveolar hypoventilation besides a genetic defect. In three of our five patients, we have found the inhibitor. One patient died, and in her brain we found no ThTP. This may be a variant of SNE of the sort you were mentioning. There may be a number of variants of SNE with the pyruvic carboxylase situation. This is something I find difficult to accept as a primary problem. I think that it may be a secondary problem in SNE.

Dr. Patel. I would like to support your statement. We studied a documented case of SNE about 2 years ago (Grover et al., *J. Pediatr.,* **81**, 39, 1972). Contrary to earlier findings of Dr. Tada in Japan (Tohoku, *J. Exp. Med.,* **97**, 99, 1969) and Dr. Hommes in Europe (*Arch. Dis. Child.,* **43**, 423, 1968), in which the activity of pyruvate carboxylase was shown to be low or almost absent in liver, we found normal amount of pyruvate carboxylase in liver biopsy at the age of about 10 months. However, at the time of autopsy, which was at age 38 months, pyruvate carboxylase was found in negligible amounts not only in liver but also in kidney and brain. It appears that the reduction in pyruvate carboxylase activity was secondary to the disease process. It also suggests that there are variants of this disease.

Dr. Barchi. First of all, I want to congratulate you and your laboratory on your work on this disease. I think it is one of the most compelling pieces of evidence that we have that ThTP has something to do with the nervous system, and it encourages all of us. There is something that we probably should try to resolve while we are here and to see if we can draw on each other's experience in the same area, i.e., the nature of the enzyme that we are dealing with. We have looked fairly hard, as I know you have also, for an enzyme which synthesizes ThTP, using methods that attempt to identify the synthesized compound. In other words, we started with ThDP and ATP and looked for the production of ThTP, and we have been unable to document the production of ThTP. We have also worked a little bit with the enzyme system which you use, a coupled set of enzyme reactions which looks at the disappearance of ATP while using an ATP-regenerating system while does not actually identify the ThTP, and have had considerable difficulty with the system. There is large background activity, which you mentioned before, and sometimes one gets activity that is not really reproducible and sometimes one gets no activity at all.

There is no question from your work that there is an inhibitory factor in the urine of these patients. I think there is also no question that there is little or no ThTP in the brain and the regions which you have indicated. The question arises as to what the inhibitory factor inhibited and what enzyme we are talking about—whether we actually have thiamine triphosphate synthetase that we can put our fingers on. If not, what kind of problems are we dealing with? And if so, where do the difficulties in trying to identify ThTP lie?

Dr. Cooper.   I think maybe it would be well to postpone discussion of the enzyme until after Dr. Itokawa's paper, and then we can bring out some of these points.

Dr. Blass.   Some of these problems may be semantic. There is a group of children who are basically defined by the fact that if one looks at their brains at autopsy one sees changes similar to those that Dennis Leigh described in 1953. The picture is very reminiscent of that for patients who died with Wernicke-Korsakoff syndrome. There is also a group of children who have a neurological disease, and in whose urine Drs. Cooper and Pincus, notably, demonstrated an inhibitor. There is a large overlap between these two categories. Furthermore, there are some children in whom a number of laboratories have found defects in hepatic pyruvate carboxylase. And there are also children in whom it is possible to demonstrate a defect of pyruvate decarboxylase. Finally, there are children who fall into more than one of these categories. Beyond this, we are disputing not what happens—on which we can all agree—but what to call it. The same situation existed with the lipidoses. I am sure that you all know the literature, including symposia on the relationship between Tay-Sachs and Nieman-Pick diseases. I would argue that, as the chemistry is done, such questions resolve themselves. I do not know whether we can resolve them now with logic. Do we have the data to come to firmer conclusions?

Dr. Elsas.   A genetic factor is of importance, and you mentioned that it might have been a carrier. It would be of great value to have the ability to predict and to identify the carriers for the recessive trait.

Dr. Cooper.   No, the presence of inhibitor is variable. Sometimes one finds it in parents, and sometimes on retesting one does not find it.

Dr. Elsas.   Has the amniotic fluid been tested for inhibitor?

Dr. Cooper.   Yes, we tested it on three occasions. The first two times the result was negative for the amniotic fluid of mothers who had previously had a child with SNE, and both younger children grew normally. The third time we tested, we again could not find the inhibitor, but this child ultimately developed SNE. Thus we cannot use amniocentesis to detect the disease.

25. Assay Method and Some Properties of Thiamine Diphosphate-Adenosine Triphosphate Phosphoryltransferase in Rat Brain

YOSHINORI ITOKAWA, M.D.

Department of Hygiene
Faculty of Medicine
Kyoto University
Kyoto, Japan

Thiamine diphosphate-adenosine triphosphate phosphoryltransferase is of particular interest since it has been found that patients with subacute necrotizing encephalomyelopathy contain a factor in their blood, urine, and spinal fluid which inhibits the enzyme (1–4). This enzyme was first discovered in yeast (5) and then in brain (6); however, little is known about its properties. In this report, we introduce a revised procedure for assay and describe some properties of this enzyme.

1. Principle

The principle of the assay method is based on the original procedure of Itokawa and Cooper (7), as follows:

$$\text{Thiamine diphosphate (ThDP)} + \text{ATP} \xrightarrow{\text{PT}} \text{thiamine triphosphate (ThTP)} + \text{ADP}$$

$$\text{ADP} + \text{phosphoenolpyruvate} \xrightarrow{\text{PK}} \text{ATP} + \text{pyruvic acid}$$

$$\text{Pyruvic acid} + \text{NADH} \xrightarrow{\text{LDH}} \text{lactic acid and NAD}^+$$

where PT = ThDP-ATP phosphoryltransferase,   PK = pyruvate kinase,
    LDH = lactate dehydrogenase.

2. Procedure

The complete system usually used in our laboratory was composed of acetate buffer, pH 5.0 (200 μmoles), $MgCl_2$ (10 μmoles), ThDP (20 μmoles), ATP (2 μmoles), NaF (3 μmoles), rat brain mitochondria (2 mg protein), and Krebs-Ringer solution to a final volume of 3.0 ml. The ThDP was omitted from a control tube, and we also took zero time control. Incubation was carried out for 15 minutes at 37°C and terminated by the addition of 3 ml of 1 N $HClO_4$. After centrifugation, 5 ml of supernatant was pipetted into another test tube, and 1 ml of solution containing 500 μM of triethanolamine HCl plus 2 μM of K_2CO_3 was added. This was chilled for 10 minutes and filtered. Phosphoenol pyruvate (2 μmoles), KCl (260 μmoles), $MgSO_4$ (80 μmoles), NADH (0.5 μmoles), and LDH (0.02 mg) were added to 2 ml

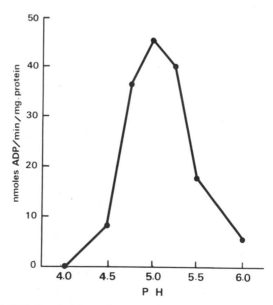

Figure 1. ThPP-ATP phosphoryltransferase as a function of pH.

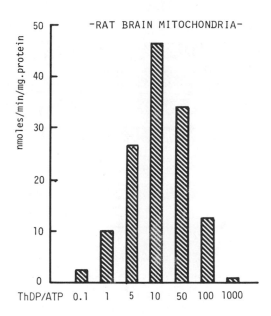

Figure 2. Effect of ThDP/ATP ratio in reaction mixture on ThDP-ATP phosphoryl-transferase activity.

filtrate, followed by water to a final volume of 2.5 ml. The solution was then mixed. After 5 minutes the optical density was measured at 340 nm (E_1); 0.02 ml of pyruvate kinase (1 mg/ml) was then added, and the optical density read again at 340 nm (E_2). $E_1 - E_2 \times 435.4$ μmoles/l is the amount of ThDP formed in the reaction.

3. Critical Studies

Figure 1 shows the optimal pH for this enzyme; it is between 4.75 and 5.25. Under pH 4.0 and over pH 6.0 the activity is very little. The optimal ratio of ATP and ThDP with rat brain mitochondria was 1:10, as shown in Fig. 2. When a 1:1 ratio was used, only 20% of the maximum activity could be obtained.

The effect of calcium, magnesium, or Krebs-Ringer solution on the activity is shown in Fig. 3. When 10 μmoles of $MgCl_2$ was omitted from the reaction mixture, the activity decreased to about 80%, although some magnesium was present in the Krebs-Ringer solution. Calcium could not be

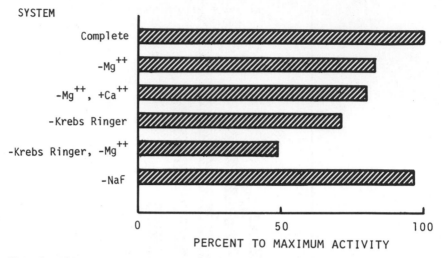

SYSTEM

Figure 3. ThDP-ATP phosphoryltransferase activity in various systems.

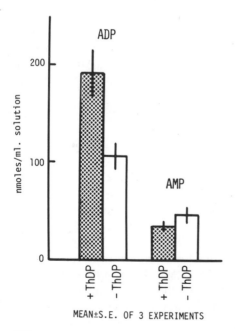

Figure 4. ADP and AMP in reaction mixture (ThDP-ATP phosphoryltransferase).

substituted for magnesium. When water was used instead of Krebs-Ringer solution, the activity decreased to 75%. When both magnesium and Krebs-Ringer solution were omitted, the activity was reduced to 50%. This fact suggests that this enzyme requires magnesium and some other minerals present in Krebs-Ringer solution. Fluoride has no effect on this enzyme, whereas ThDPase was inhibited more than 90% at the same concentration of fluoride.

There was a possibility that our spectrophotometric assay might have measured an effect of ThDP on adenylate kinase. Therefore we assayed adenylate kinase with and without the addition of ThDP, and it became clear that ThDP has no effect on adenylate kinase in this medium.

If the enzyme catalyzing the reaction below exists in our mitochondrial preparation, the data will be influenced:

$$\text{Thiamine diphosphate} + \text{ADP} \rightarrow \text{thiamine triphosphate} + \text{AMP}$$

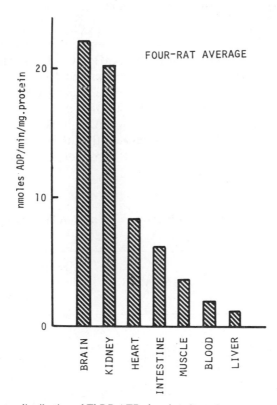

Figure 5.   Organ distribution of ThDP-ATP phosphoryltransferase.

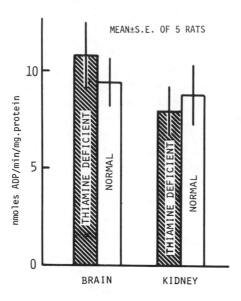

Figure 6. ThDP-ATP phosphoryl-transferase in normal and thiamine-deficient rats.

To eliminate this possibility, we compared AMP levels in the same reaction mixture with a brain mitochondrial preparation and found that changes in AMP levels in tubes with ThDP added were negligible as compared to changes in AMP levels in tubes in which ThDP was omitted. In contrast, the ADP level was significantly higher with ThDP in the mixture than with ThDP omitted (Fig. 4). These facts suggest that the greater part of the activity we were measuring was ThDP-ATP phosphoryltransferase.

Table 1. Subcellular Localization of ThDP-ATP Phosphoryl-transferase[a]

Cell Fraction	Total Activity, %	Specific Activity, nmoles/(mg protein) (min)
Nuclei	11.2	6.3
Mitochondria (crude)	70.5	39.4
Microsome	9.4	5.2
Supernatant	8.7	4.8

[a] Values represent averages of four experiments.

Table 2. Localization of ThDP-ATP Phosphoryltransferase Activity in Crude Mitochondrial Subfractions in Rat Brain[a]

Subfraction	Total Activity, %	Specific Activity, nmoles ADP liberated/(mg protein) (min)
Myelin membranes	1.6	1.1
Synaptosomes	23.4	15.3
Mitochondria	74.9	49.1

[a] Three-rat average.

4. Properties of the Enzyme

Figure 5 shows the organ distribution of ThDP-ATP phosphoryltransferase. The activity is highest in brain, followed by kidneys, heart, intestine, and muscles. It is lowest in blood and liver. In brain subcellular fractions, about 70% of this enzyme is localized in the crude mitochondrial fraction, as described by Itokawa and Cooper (6) (Table 1) When the crude mitochondrial fraction is further purified, the activity is localized in the pure mitochondrial fraction (Table 2). The enzyme activity in brain and kidney was not altered even when rats were placed on a thiamine-deficient diet for 1 month, as shown in Fig. 6.

Acknowledgment

The author wishes to express his gratitude to Professor Motonori Fujiwara, Kyoto University, and Professor Jack R. Cooper, Yale University, for their valuable support and advice. Thanks are due also to Miss Liang Fang Tseng for technical assistance.

References

1. J. R. Cooper, Y. Itokawa, and J. H. Pincus, *Science,* **164,** 72 (1969).

2. J. H. Pincus, Y. Itokawa, and J. R. Cooper, *Neurology,* **19,** 841 (1969).

3. J. R. Cooper, J. H. Pincus, Y. Itokawa, and K. Piros, *New Engl. J. Med.,* **283,** 793 (1970).

4. J. H. Pincus, J. R. Cooper, Y. Itokawa, and M. Gumbinas, *Arch. Neurol.*, **24**, 511 (1971).

5. T. Yusa, *Plant Cell Physiol.*, **3**, 95 (1962).

6. Y. Itokawa and J. R. Cooper, *Biochim. Biophys. Acta*, **158**, 180 (1968).

7. Y. Itokawa and J. R. Cooper, in S. P. Colwick and N. D. Kaplan, Eds., *Methods Enzymol.*, **18A**, 226 (1970).

26. Initial Process Formation on Neuroblastoma Cells with Glia Cells in Thiamine-Deficient Medium

T. NAKAZAWA, M.D.
T. YAMAUCHI, M.D.

Department of Neuropsychiatry
Fujita-Gakuen University School of Medicine
Toyoakeshi, Aichi-Ken, Japan

In the study of cytodifferentiation in heterogeneous cell populations, such as nervous tissue, it is clear that culture techniques provide an indispensable tool for precise analysis. Neurons under suitable conditions *in vivo* and *in vitro* tend to adhere to glial cells, giving rise to a histoformation. This communication between neuron and glia extends by a cell-line which can be induced to differentiate from a cell that has some properties of a mature neuron. The initial process formation by neuroblastoma cells in tissue culture has been termed morphological differentiation, and its importance as a model for neural differentiation has been reported by many researchers (1, 2). The purpose of the present report is to extend observations on the effect of thiamine in tissue culture on the differentiation of mammalian neurons with special reference to glia.

1. Materials and Methods

Experiments were carried out with neuroblastoma C-1300, clone N-18 (kindly supplied by Dr. T. Amano), and glial cells, clone C-6 [kindly supplied by Dr. P. Benda (3)], grown in Falcon 60-mm tissue culture dishes

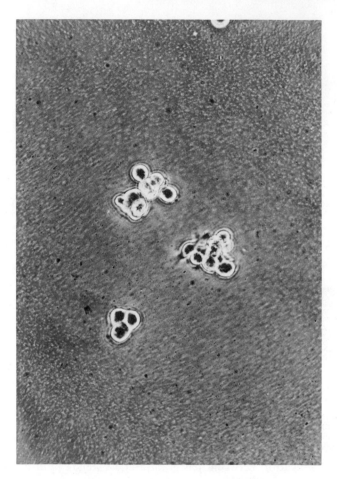

Figures 1 and 2. Morphological differentiation of neuroblastoma cells. Fig. 1. Three aggregate neurons surrounded by a clear halo of light in 48-hour culture. Fig. 2. The neurons send out long processes induced by 0% serum in culture medium.

in Eagle's medium, supplemented with 10% calf serum in a humidified atmosphere of 5% CO_2–95% air at 37°C. Considering the morphological differentiation of neurons, we tried the conditioning medium from glial cell culture. For comparison, several cell types—normal fetal glia, normal rat glia, neuroblastoma cells (N-18), HeLa cells, mouse fibroblast cells, and hamster kidney cells—were used. To determine the percentage of cells undergoing morphological differentiation, 40,000 trypsinized neuroblastoma cells were plated per 60-mm dish. After 16 hours of incubation, the medium was replaced by the medium to be tested, and 48 hours later all cells, with

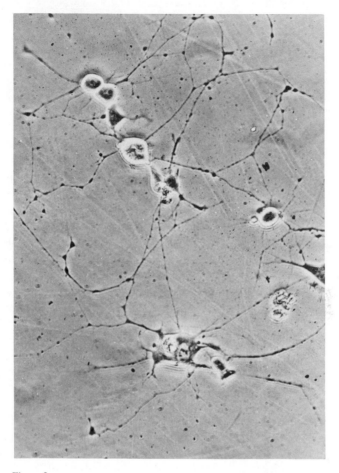

Figure 2

and without processes, were counted in at least five randomly selected areas of each culture plate. Cells having processes longer than the diameter of the cell body were considered morphologically differentiated. A total of 300 cells was counted per dish. The reported values represent the percentages of differentiated cells determined in three parallel cultures. The average doubling time of neuroblastoma cells and glia cells was 24 hours. Thiamine-deficient medium was made from Eagle components except thiamine, and the G-100 fraction of crude protein extracted from mouse submaxillary gland and glial cells was purified by the method of Varon, Nomura, and Shooter (4).

2. Results and Discussion

Neuroblastoma cells usually consist of two types of cells, quite different in morphology. One type has a round cell body without processes, and the other sends out processes up to 3 mm in length and thus assumes the morphology of mature neurons. The proportion of neurons with processes was found to vary greatly, depending on the condition of the cell culture (see Figs. 1 and 2).

A model of neural differentiation is shown in Fig. 3. Removal of serum and the addition of dibutyryl adenosine 3´,5´-cyclic monophosphate (BcAMP) can induce a similar process formation. All these treatments are unphysiological, even at a low degree of morphological differentiation, and the rate of cell proliferation is inversely related to the serum concentration and the treatment with BcAMP.

The induction of morphological differentiation of neuroblastoma cells occurs via glia-conditioning medium, filtered through a sterile 0.22-μm Millipore membrane. The rate of morphological differentiation obtained with this medium, after 48 hours, is much higher than that obtained with the removal of serum or with BcAMP treatment (Table 1). Under these circumstances, conditioning medium does not affect the growth rate of the neuroblastoma cells (see Fig. 4).

When comparing media from the several cells tested, the morphological differentiation is found to induce less or no effect. However, media from mouse submaxillary gland cells induce a high rate of morphological differentiation.

In general, the thiamine requirement of cultured neurons is relatively higher than that of glia cells, as shown in Fig. 5. The morphological differentiation of neuroblastoma cells is induced by the conditioning medium of glia cultivated in thiamine-deficient medium of the third culture generation, but not over the fifth culture generation (Table 2). After glial cells had been cultivated in thiamine-deficient medium for the fifth generation, and then returned to normal medium within 72 hours, this medium again induced a high degree of morphological differentiation in neuroblastoma cells under normal growth conditions. These results support the assertion that thiamine in glia cells performs a significant role in regulating the transfer of a factor between neuron and glia.

Nerve growth factor (NGF), described by Levi-Montalcini (5) and Cohen (6), and purified from mouse submaxillary gland, also shows activity for the induction of process formation and hypertrophy of ganglion cells. Sensory and sympathetic ganglion cells respond maximally to NGF during the period in which the outgrowth of axons normally occurs. This period also corresponds with the period of glial proliferation. Furthermore, it is well known that Schwann cells and glial cells act as guides for regenerating axons (7).

Glial cells were scraped with a "rubber policeman" from Raux culture bottles under an atmosphere of 5% CO_2 and were homogenized with 20 volumes of H_2O. The supernatant fluid was removed by centrifugation, and dissolved in Tris-buffer (pH 7.4, 50 mM) after freezing and drying. This

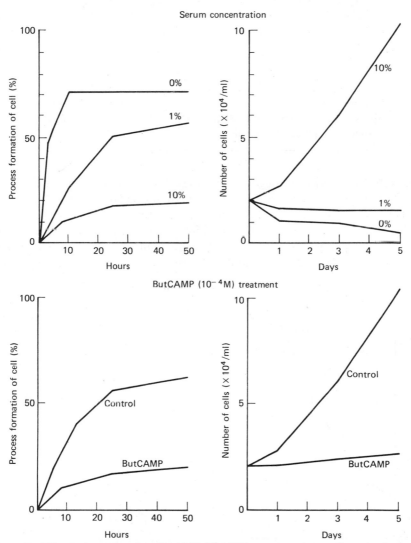

Figure 3.   Effects of serum and cyclic AMP (BcAMP) concentration on the rate of process formation and cell proliferation.

Table 1. Effect of Medium Conditioned by Different Cell Cultures on Process Formation of Neuroblastoma Cells

Cell Type	Cells with Processes, %
Control fresh medium	14.4 ± 1.6
C-6 glia cells[a]	82.3 ± 7.1
Human fetal normal glia	27.5 ± 3.2
Rat normal glia	29.8 ± 1.9
n-18 neuroblastoma cells	18.7 ± 1.4
HeLa cells	14.9 ± 2.3
Mouse fibroblast cells	9.7 ± 0.6
Hamster kidney cells	42.6 ± 3.6
Mouse submaxillary gland cells[a]	80.3 ± 7.7
Human spongioblastoma cells[a]	67.9 ± 6.2

solution was passed through a Sephadex G-100 column. Its mobility in acrylamide gel showed that it corresponds to mouse NGF.

This glial protein and crude NGF, extracted by the same technique, induced the morphological differentiation of neuroblastoma cells as shown in Table 3. Morphologically, the cells were similar to those incubated with the conditioning medium of glial cells. By contrast, the protein extracted

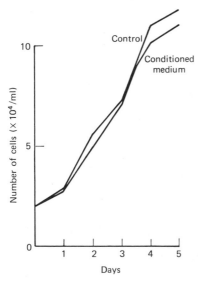

Figure 4. Growth of neuroblastoma cells in conditioned or normal medium.

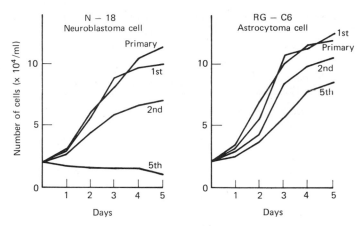

Figure 5. Thiamine requirements on neuroblastoma (N-18) and glioma (astrocytoma C-6) cells in culture. Primary: continuous culture maintained in normal medium; 1st, 2nd, and 5th: number of culture generations in thiamine-deficient medium.

from glial cells in thiamine-deficient medium was mostly inhibited, and also the rate of differentiation was lower than that of glial cells within a concentration of 1 μmolc/ml of pyrithiamine, treated simultaneously. The results of neural differentiation under thiamine-deficient conditions indicate that there are some inevitable disruptions, other than of thiamine metabolism, in glia cells over a long term.

In 1974, Longo and Ponhoet reported that rat glioma tumor contains a protein which cross-reacts with antibody against mouse 2.5S NGF prepared

Table 2. Effect of Medium Conditioned by Different Culture Generations of Glia Cells in Thiamine-Deficient Medium

Number of Generation	Cells with Processes, %
Control	82.3 ± 7.1
1st	84.1 ± 9.3
2nd	79.7 ± 10.5
3rd	46.8 ± 3.1
5th	14.3 ± 2.2
After 5th generation, retreated control conditioned medium within 72 hours	72.4 ± 11.6

Table 3. Effect on Process Formation of Neuroblastoma
Cells Treated with Different Proteins

Cell Type	Cells with Processes, %
Control fresh medium	15.2
C-6 glia cells	79.6
Basic protein of C-6 glia cells (25 μg/ml)	84.1
Crude NGF of mouse submaxillary gland (5 μg/ml)	80.7
Basic protein of C-6 glia cells in thiamine-deficient medium	7.9
Basic protein of C-6 glia cells (25 μg/ml) with pyrithiamine (1 μM/ml)	18.4

from rabbit by microcomplement fixation assays and has isoelectric points analogous to those of all the hybrids of 2.5S NGF (8). These findings, based on glioma *in vivo,* were confirmed by our *in vitro* experiments.

Glioma induced by transplantation of C-6 glial cells into rat brain resulted mainly in astrocytoma. Astrocytes in general are divided into two kinds of cell types, protoplasmic and fibrous. The protoplasmic astrocytes have a tendency to fibrillate in the aging process and are high in vital potentiality, and cell proliferation of astrocytes occurs only in the protoplasmic stage. The transformation of astrocytes between protoplasmic and fibrous type is also reversible under physiological conditions (9, 10).

It is well known that NGF is present at high levels in submaxillary glands of mice only after puberty, and removal of these glands from newborn animals has no effect on sympathetic development. This suggests that an alternative site of synthesis exists during development. The glia-visible protein, whose isoelectric point was indistinguishable from the NGF band on acrylamide gel, was precisely released from astrocytes at one stage of cell proliferation. However, since the glia protein is crude and contains substances other than NGF, definitive proof of biological identity must await purification of the glial NGF to homogeneity. The finding that thiamine-deficient conditions effects decrease or stoppage of neural differentiation of glial cells supports the assumption that the thiamine requirement of glial cells was elevated in the limiting stage, such as glia protein synthesis, used for morphological differentiation.

In conclusion, glial cells release into their culture medium a factor that induces a high degree of morphological differentiation in neuroblastoma cells under normal growth conditions. This factor contains a protein with an isoelectric point indistinguishable from that of the nerve growth factor band on acrylamide gel. The protein extracted from glial cells in thiamine-deficient medium for a limited number of culture generations inhibits the morphological differentiation of neuroblastoma cells.

References

1. D. Schubert, S. Humphreys, C. Baroni, and M. Cohn, *Proc. Natl. Acad. Sci. U.S.*, **64**, 316 (1969).
2. N. W. Seeds, A. G. Gilman, T. Amano, and M. W. Nierenberg, *Proc. Natl. Acad. Sci. U.S.*, **66**, 160 (1970).
3. P. Benda, J. Lightbody, G. Sato, L. Levine, and W. Sweet, *Science,* **161**, 370 (1968).
4. S. Varon, J. Nomura, and E. M. Shooter, *Biochemistry,* **6**, 2202 (1967).
5. R. Levi-Montalcini and V. Hamburger, *J. Exp. Zool.,* **116**, 321 (1951).
6. S. Cohen, *Proc. Natl. Acad. Sci. U.S.,* **46**, 302 (1960).
7. S. Kuffler and J. Nicholls, *Ergeb. Physiol. Biol. Chem. Exp. Pharmakol.,* **57** (1960).
8. A. M. Longo and E. E. Penhoet, *Proc. Natl. Acad. Sci. U.S.,* **71**, 2347 (1974).
9. T. Nakazawa, "Biological response on oligodendrocyte and astrocyte in tissue culture," in J. Nakai, Ed., *Morphology of Neuroglia.* Igaku Shoin, Tokyo, 1961, p. 103.
10. J. Tominaga, *Psychiat. Neurol. Jap ,* **69**, 770 (1967).

CLOSING REMARKS

Motonori Fujiwara, M.D.
Department of Hygiene
Kyoto University
Kyoto, Japan
Japan Coordinator
Second United States-Japan Seminar on Thiamine

I am very pleased to have the opportunity to make a few remarks at the end of this conference. The 3 days since it began have flown so swiftly!

During the seminar, I was deeply impressed by the following points: how greatly the field of thiamine research has broadened, how directly investigations on thiamine benefit mankind, and how many difficult problems remain to be solved in this field of study. I believe that we all share similar impressions.

I think that we have succeeded in making this conference a very profitable one, not only for the study of thiamine, but also for the promotion of mutual understanding among researchers. Furthermore, much of the knowledge shared at this conference will be helpful in future studies.

On this occasion, on behalf of all of our participants and the Vitamin B Research Committee of Japan, I wish to express once more our deepest thanks to Professor Gubler for his untiring efforts, which made this conference possible, and to Professor Dreyfus, who devoted so much of his time to the organization of the seminar. My heartfelt thanks go also to all of you for the kindness you have shown during this conference.

My one hope for all of us is that the next 5 years will be as happy and fruitful as the past 5 years have been, and that we shall have the opportunity to meet again at a third seminar in Japan.

Please be assured that I shall pray for your happiness and good luck in the future.

Pierre M. Dreyfus, M.D.

**Department of Neurology
School of Medicine
University of California
Davis, California
Assistant United States Coordinator
Second United States-Japan Seminar on Thiamine**

Many have contributed to making this conference both successful and stimulating. Professors Gubler and Fujiwara made an excellent selection of topics and speakers. The National Science Foundation, the Japan Society for the Promotion of Science, Hoffmann-La Roche, Inc., Brigham Young University, the School of Medicine of the University of California at Davis, and Mr. Jerry Hawthorne of Beckman Instruments provided the essential financial assistance. And, finally, all of the participants at this conference have been instrumental in fostering continued cooperation between Japan and the United States in the field of thiamine research.

During the past 3 days we have been made aware of the fact that thiamine research continues to expand in many directions. The results of this expansion are bound to provide the stimulus necessary for further investigation and the solutions to many problems and the answers to many questions. It is obvious that we need to know a great deal more about the noncoenzymatic role of thiamine and its phosphate esters, particularly triphosphothiamine, in the function of the normal mammalian nervous system before we can assess their importance in the pathophysiology of the thiamine-deficient state. The fact that thiamine diphosphate has been found to be a cofactor for the branched-chain ketoacid dehydrogenases suggests that the vitamin may also be necessary for other enzyme systems which have not as yet been defined.

Abnormal thiamine triphosphate metabolism has been implicated in a genetically determined disease of the nervous system—Leigh's disease, or subacute necrotizing encephalomyelopathy. A deficiency of the thiamine-dependent enzyme pyruvate decarboxylase has been held responsible for a neurological disorder characterized by intermittent episodes of ataxia. It would not be surprising, therefore, to discover genetic disorders affecting the nervous system in which some other aspect of thiamine metabolism or a deficiency of a different thiamine-dependent enzyme could be implicated. Vitamins have figured heavily in the ever-burgeoning field of molecular neurology.

As knowledge concerning the biochemical pathology of genetically determined metabolic disorders accumulates, important interrelationships between various vitamins, cofactors, and essential substances seem to emerge, further complicating an already obfuscated field.

Meetings such as this provide us with a unique opportunity to communicate in a free and informal manner with other investigators in the field who belong to a variety of different scientific disciplines. They keep us informed of the latest findings; above all, they stimulate thought for future investigations. I sincerely hope that it will be possible for us to meet again within the next 5 years in order to learn from each other by reviewing and criticizing the fruits of our labors. To all of you, and to those who have helped us with this conference, once again many thanks and *sayonara*!

ACKNOWLEDGMENTS

Thanks are gratefully extended to the National Science Foundation, Office of International Programs; the United States-Japan Cooperative Science Program; and the Japan Society for the Promotion of Science for making this seminar possible. We are grateful also to Hoffmann-LaRoche, Inc., Nutley, N.J.; University of California School of Medicine, Davis, California; Brigham Young University, Provo, Utah; and Mr. Jerry Hawthorne of Beckman Instruments for financial assistance in regard to physical arrangements, publications, and other matters related to the seminar.

Dr. Motonori Fujiwara, Japan Coordinator
Dr. Clark J. Gubler, United States Coordinator
Dr. P. M. Dreyfus, Assistant United States Coordinator

INDEX